Antimicrobial Prescribing, Population Use and Resistance, Impact in Global Health

Antimicrobial Prescribing, Population Use and Resistance, Impact in Global Health

Juan Manuel Vázquez-Lago
Ana Estany-Gestal
Angel Salgado-Barreira

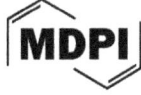

Basel • Beijing • Wuhan • Barcelona • Belgrade • Novi Sad • Cluj • Manchester

Editors

Juan Manuel Vázquez-Lago
Preventive Medicine and
Public Health
University of Santiago
de Compostela
Santiago de Compostela
Spain

Ana Estany-Gestal
Health Research Institute of
Santiago de Compostela
University of Santiago
de Compostela
Santiago de Compostela
Spain

Angel Salgado-Barreira
Medicine Preventive and
Public Heatlh
University of Santiago
de Compostela
Santiago de Compostela
Spain

Editorial Office
MDPI AG
Grosspeteranlage 5
4052 Basel, Switzerland

This is a reprint of articles from the Special Issue published online in the open access journal *Antibiotics* (ISSN 2079-6382) (available at: www.mdpi.com/journal/antibiotics/special_issues/K4C102TZIY).

For citation purposes, cite each article independently as indicated on the article page online and as indicated below:

Lastname, A.A.; Lastname, B.B. Article Title. *Journal Name* **Year**, *Volume Number*, Page Range.

ISBN 978-3-7258-2286-7 (Hbk)
ISBN 978-3-7258-2285-0 (PDF)
doi.org/10.3390/books978-3-7258-2285-0

© 2024 by the authors. Articles in this book are Open Access and distributed under the Creative Commons Attribution (CC BY) license. The book as a whole is distributed by MDPI under the terms and conditions of the Creative Commons Attribution-NonCommercial-NoDerivs (CC BY-NC-ND) license.

Contents

About the Editors vii

Preface ix

Ana Estany-Gestal, Angel Salgado-Barreira and Juan Manuel Vazquez-Lago
Antibiotic Use and Antimicrobial Resistance: A Global Public Health Crisis
Reprinted from: *Antibiotics* 2024, *13*, 900, doi:10.3390/antibiotics13090900 1

Juan M. Vázquez-Lago, Rodrigo A. Montes-Villalba, Olalla Vázquez-Cancela, María Otero-Santiago, Ana López-Durán and Adolfo Figueiras
Knowledge, Perceptions, and Perspectives of Medical Students Regarding the Use of Antibiotics and Antibiotic Resistance: A Qualitative Research in Galicia, Spain
Reprinted from: *Antibiotics* 2023, *12*, 558, doi:10.3390/antibiotics12030558 3

Maryam Farooqui, Zaffar Iqbal, Abdul Sadiq, Abdul Raziq, Mohammed Salem Alshammari and Qaiser Iqbal et al.
Hospital Pharmacists' Viewpoint on Quality Use of Antibiotics and Resistance: A Qualitative Exploration from a Tertiary Care Hospital of Quetta City, Pakistan
Reprinted from: *Antibiotics* 2023, *12*, 1343, doi:10.3390/antibiotics12081343 15

Rajeev P. Nagassar, Amanda Carrington, Darren K. Dookeeram, Keston Daniel and Roma J. Bridgelal-Nagassar
Knowledge, Attitudes, and Practices in Antibiotic Dispensing amongst Pharmacists in Trinidad and Tobago: Exploring a Novel Dichotomy of Antibiotic Laws
Reprinted from: *Antibiotics* 2023, *12*, 1094, doi:10.3390/antibiotics12071094 30

Nazym Iskakova, Zaituna Khismetova, Dana Suleymenova, Zhanat Kozhekenova, Zaituna Khamidullina and Umutzhan Samarova et al.
Factors Influencing Antibiotic Consumption in Adult Population of Kazakhstan
Reprinted from: *Antibiotics* 2023, *12*, 560, doi:10.3390/antibiotics12030560 46

Brady Page and Simeon Adiunegiya
Antimicrobial Resistance in Papua New Guinea: A Narrative Scoping Review
Reprinted from: *Antibiotics* 2023, *12*, 1679, doi:10.3390/antibiotics12121679 58

Mohamed A. Hussain, Ahmed O. Mohamed, Omalhassan A. Abdelkarim, Bashir A. Yousef, Asma A. Babikir and Maysoon M. Mirghani et al.
Prevalence and Predictors of Antibiotic Self-Medication in Sudan: A Descriptive Cross-Sectional Study
Reprinted from: *Antibiotics* 2023, *12*, 612, doi:10.3390/antibiotics12030612 77

Alfredo Jover-Sáenz, María Ramirez-Hidalgo, Alba Bellés Bellés, Esther Ribes Murillo, Meritxell Batlle Bosch and Anna Ribé Miró et al.
Effects of a Primary Care Antimicrobial Stewardship Program on Meticillin-Resistant *Staphylococcus aureus* Strains across a Region of Catalunya (Spain) over 5 Years
Reprinted from: *Antibiotics* 2024, *13*, 92, doi:10.3390/antibiotics13010092 90

Lindsey A. Laytner, Kiara Olmeda, Juanita Salinas, Osvaldo Alquicira, Susan Nash and Roger Zoorob et al.
Acculturation and Subjective Norms Impact Non-Prescription Antibiotic Use among Hispanic Patients in the United States
Reprinted from: *Antibiotics* 2023, *12*, 1419, doi:10.3390/antibiotics12091419 107

Carlotta Gamberini, Sabine Donders, Salwan Al-Nasiry, Alena Kamenshchikova and Elena Ambrosino
Antibiotic Use in Pregnancy: A Global Survey on Antibiotic Prescription Practices in Antenatal Care
Reprinted from: *Antibiotics* **2023**, *12*, 831, doi:10.3390/antibiotics12050831 . . . . **126**

Nirmin F. Juber, Abdishakur Abdulle, Amar Ahmad, Fatme AlAnouti, Tom Loney and Youssef Idaghdour et al.
Associations between Polycystic Ovary Syndrome (PCOS) and Antibiotic Use: Results from the UAEHFS
Reprinted from: *Antibiotics* **2024**, *13*, 397, doi:10.3390/antibiotics13050397 . . . . **145**

About the Editors

Juan Manuel Vázquez-Lago

I graduated with Honors in Medicine and Surgery from the University of Santiago de Compostela in 2004. I trained as a Specialist in Preventive Medicine and Public Health at the Clinical Hospital of Santiago and achieved the official title in 2009. During this period, I combined this training with a Master's degree in Public Health (Official Sanitary) at the National School of Health, the Carlos III Health Institute (ISCIII), in 2006. I also completed doctoral courses in Public Health at the University of Santiago de Compostela, obtaining a Diploma of Advanced Studies-Research Proficiency (DEA) in 2008 and a Diploma in Statistics in Health Sciences from the Autonomous University of Barcelona in 2014. Additionally, I completed a Master's in Clinical Trials at the University of Seville in 2014. I earned a Ph.D. in Epidemiology and Public Health from the University of Santiago de Compostela in 2021. Currently, I hold the position of Specialist in Preventive Medicine and Public Health at the University Clinical Hospital of Santiago in the Santiago and Barbanza Health Area. I am involved in healthcare activities, teaching, and training specialists in health sciences, serving as a teaching tutor in the specialty of Preventive Medicine and Public Health and as a collaborating tutor in the specialties of Family and Community Medicine and Family and Community Nursing. I have been the coordinator and leader of the research group of the Santiago Health Research Institute Foundation (FIDIS), named AC10-Healthy Aging, Frailty, and Chronicity, Primary Care Research, since October 3, 2016. My teaching activities are focused on postgraduate continuing education in the National Health System, as well as various collaborations in several Master's degree programs at the University of Santiago de Compostela. My research work is centered on quantitative and qualitative perspectives of public health problems, health risk behaviors, and health education programs.

Ana Estany-Gestal

I graduated with a Bachelor's degree in Pharmacy (2006) and earned my PhD in Epidemiology in 2012 from the University of Santiago (USC). I also completed my training with a Master's in Public Health from USC in 2008, Design and Analysis of Research in Health Science from the Autonomous University of Barcelona (UAB) in 2011, and Clinical Trials from the University of Sevilla (US) in 2016.

I am currently responsible for the Research Methodology Platform and am also a postdoc researcher in the Research Methodology group at the Health Research Institute of Santiago (IDIS). Additionally, I have been a member of the Research Ethics Committee of two areas of health since its creation (2014), and I have served as technical secretary since 2019. In addition to my scientific and technical professional work as an epidemiologist and expert in bioethics, I am involved in education by coordinating and participating as a teacher in accredited courses mainly on research methodology and bioethics. I am a tutor for the Master's program in Public Health at USC, and I have co-supervised two doctoral theses in the field of clinical epidemiology and dental public health. I am also a member of the Training Commission of my workplace, IDIS. I participate as an evaluator in different agencies both national (Carlos III Health Institute) and autonomic (Canarian Health Research Foundation, Basque Research Foundation).

In the field of clinical research, I am a researcher of competitive projects financed by public and private organizations as well as a member of the organizational structure of national research (SCReN) and innovation (ITEMAS) units. I have published around 50 scientific articles, many of them in the first decile. My research work consists of proposing innovative design and analysis methodologies to solve research questions in the field of clinical care.

Angel Salgado-Barreira

Angel Salgado-Barreira graduated with a Bachelor's degree in Pharmacy and a PhD in Public Health from the University of Santiago de Compostela. He is currently a professor in the Department of Preventive Medicine and Public Health at the University of Santiago de Compostela. Most of his studies and professional career have been focused on research, particularly in the fields of biostatistics and epidemiology, as well as in the evaluation of healthcare technologies. He has worked at the Galician Agency for Health Technology Assessment (avalia-t) and as a methodologist and statistician at the Methodology and Statistics Unit of the Galicia Sur Health Research Institute. Before joining the University of Santiago de Compostela, he was an associate professor at the University School of Nursing in Vigo (from 2011 to 2021) and the University School of Nursing in Ourense (from 2015 to 2021), both of which are a part of the University of Vigo. In recent years, he has collaborated and participated in numerous national projects, including two European projects, and has been a member of the working group in four industry-sponsored clinical trials. He is the author or co-author of several articles in national and international journals, three books published by the Ministry of Health and Consumer Affairs, and a clinical practice guideline. Additionally, he has been a member of the Research Committee of the Vigo Healthcare Area and the training and quality commissions of the Galicia Sur Health Research Institute.

Preface

This Special Issue collects research articles focused on antimicrobial prescribing, population use, resistance, and their impact on global health. Antimicrobial resistance (AMR) has emerged as one of the most urgent public health threats worldwide, driven largely by the misuse and overuse of antibiotics. The articles in this issue examine the factors contributing to the rise of AMR and explore innovative approaches aimed at improving antibiotic use and reducing resistance.

The objective of this Special Issue is to provide valuable insights into the current state of antimicrobial prescribing and the interventions being developed to address misuse. The selected studies cover a wide range of topics, from clinical prescribing patterns to public health initiatives and monitoring systems that track resistance trends. Through these diverse perspectives, this issue highlights key challenges and potential solutions to mitigate AMR on a global scale.

AMR is a complex issue influenced by medical practices, societal factors, and policy regulations. This issue reflects this complexity by incorporating research from different regions and healthcare settings, offering a comprehensive overview of the problem. The articles address the variations in antibiotic use across different populations and healthcare systems, emphasizing the need for tailored strategies to combat resistance. By sharing these diverse experiences, this Special Issue seeks to promote global collaboration and improve stewardship practices worldwide.

This publication is aimed at researchers, healthcare professionals, and policymakers who are actively involved in the fight against AMR. The findings and recommendations presented here are intended to guide future interventions, improve antibiotic use, and inform public health policies. The studies included provide evidence-based insights that will help strengthen antimicrobial stewardship programs and support more rational antibiotic prescribing.

We would like to express our heartfelt thanks to the Section Managing Editor of *Antibiotics* for their invaluable support throughout the development of this Special Issue. I am also deeply grateful to the authors for their hard work and dedication, as well as the reviewers whose insightful feedback has ensured the high quality of the research included here. Lastly, we extend our appreciation to the institutions and organizations that provided the necessary support for this project.

We hope that this Special Issue will contribute to the ongoing efforts to reduce antimicrobial resistance and inspire further research in this critical area of public health.

Juan Manuel Vázquez-Lago, Ana Estany-Gestal, and Angel Salgado-Barreira
Editors

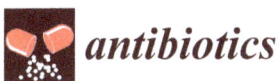

Editorial

Antibiotic Use and Antimicrobial Resistance: A Global Public Health Crisis

Ana Estany-Gestal [1], Angel Salgado-Barreira [2] and Juan Manuel Vazquez-Lago [1,3,*]

1. Health Research Institute of Santiago de Compostela (IDIS), 15706 Santiago de Compostela, Spain
2. Department of Preventive Medicine and Public Health Service, Faculty of Pharmacy, University of Santiago de Compostela, Campus Vida s/n, 15705 Santiago de Compostela, Spain
3. Department of Preventive Medicine and Public Health Service, University Hospital of Santiago de Compostela, Rua da Choupana s/n, 15705 Santiago de Compostela, Spain
* Correspondence: juan.manuel.vazquez.lago@sergas.es

The discovery of antibiotics revolutionized modern medicine, effectively treating bacterial infections that were once fatal. However, the widespread misuse and overuse of these drugs have led to the emergence and spread of resistant microorganisms, compromising the efficacy of current treatments [1]. The World Health Organization (WHO) has identified antimicrobial resistance as one of the top ten global health threats [2].

The indiscriminate use of antibiotics in human medicine, veterinary practices, and agriculture is a key driver of antimicrobial resistance (AMR) [3]. Antibiotics are dispensed without a prescription in many countries, facilitating unnecessary use [4]. Additionally, in the agricultural sector, the prophylactic and growth-promoting use of antibiotics in animals is widespread, significantly contributing to the spread of resistance [5]. The impact of inappropriate antibiotic use is further exacerbated by the lack of education and awareness among healthcare professionals and the general public [6,7]. A recent study found that many patients still mistakenly believe that antibiotics are effective against viral infections, such as the common cold [8]. This misunderstanding drives unnecessary demand for these drugs, pressuring healthcare providers to prescribe them even when they are not needed.

Consequently, AMR has a devastating global impact on developed and developing countries. It is estimated that antimicrobial-resistant infections cause approximately 1.27 million deaths annually [9]. Moreover, AMR prolongs the duration of illnesses, increases mortality, and imposes a significant economic burden due to the additional costs associated with prolonged treatment and hospitalization [10]. In developing countries, the impact of AMR is particularly severe due to limited access to second-line drugs, accurate diagnostics, and robust healthcare systems. Based on this premise, the Bellagio Group for Accelerating AMR Action met in April 2024 to develop the ambitious but achievable 1-10-100 unifying goals to galvanize global policy change and investments for antimicrobial resistance mitigation [11].

Addressing AMR requires a multifaceted approach that includes regulating antibiotic use, investing in R&D for new drugs, and implementing global educational programs [12]. Policies promoting the rational use of antibiotics are essential to limit inappropriate prescriptions and reduce unnecessary demand [13]. At the global level, initiatives such as the WHO Global Action Plan on Antimicrobial Resistance aim to strengthen surveillance and research, reduce infection incidence, and optimize antimicrobials in human, animal, and environmental health [14]. However, effectively implementing these strategies requires international collaboration and a firm commitment from all sectors involved.

This Special Issue presents a compendium of multidisciplinary research on the use of antibiotics, the resistance they generate, and the impact this has on a global level. The collected works serve as a comprehensive resource for scholars engaged in this field, and the Guests Editors are grateful for the interest and contributions received.

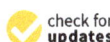

Citation: Estany-Gestal, A.; Salgado-Barreira, A.; Vazquez-Lago, J.M. Antibiotic Use and Antimicrobial Resistance: A Global Public Health Crisis. *Antibiotics* 2024, 13, 900. https://doi.org/10.3390/antibiotics13090900

Received: 3 September 2024
Accepted: 19 September 2024
Published: 21 September 2024

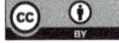

Copyright: © 2024 by the authors. Licensee MDPI, Basel, Switzerland. This article is an open access article distributed under the terms and conditions of the Creative Commons Attribution (CC BY) license (https://creativecommons.org/licenses/by/4.0/).

Funding: This research received no external funding.

Conflicts of Interest: The authors declare no conflicts of interest.

References

1. Morehead, M.S.; Scarbrough, C. Emergence of Global Antibiotic Resistance. *Prim. Care.* **2018**, *45*, 467–484. [CrossRef] [PubMed]
2. World Health Organization. Ten Threats to Global Health in 2019. 2019. Available online: https://www.who.int/news-room/spotlight/ten-threats-to-global-health-in-2019 (accessed on 2 September 2024).
3. Machowska, A.; Stålsby Lundborg, C. Drivers of Irrational Use of Antibiotics in Europe. *Int. J. Environ. Res. Public Health* **2019**, *16*, 27. [CrossRef] [PubMed]
4. Li, J.; Zhou, P.; Wang, J.; Li, H.; Xu, H.; Meng, Y.; Ye, F.; Tan, Y.; Gong, Y.; Yin, X. Worldwide dispensing of non-prescription antibiotics in community pharmacies and associated factors: A mixed-methods systematic review. *Lancet Infect. Dis.* **2023**, *23*, e361–e370. [CrossRef] [PubMed]
5. Landers, T.F.; Cohen, B.; Wittum, T.E.; Larson, E.L. A review of antibiotic use in food animals: Perspective, policy, and potential. *Public Health Rep.* **2012**, *127*, 4–22. [CrossRef] [PubMed]
6. Gonzalez-Gonzalez, C.; López-Vázquez, P.; Vázquez-Lago, J.M.; Piñeiro-Lamas, M.; Herdeiro, M.T.; Arzamendi, P.C.; Figueiras, A.; GREPHEPI Group. Effect of Physicians' Attitudes and Knowledge on the Quality of Antibiotic Prescription: A Cohort Study. *PLoS ONE* **2015**, *10*, e0141820. [CrossRef] [PubMed]
7. Vazquez-Cancela, O.; Souto-Lopez, L.; Vazquez-Lago, J.M.; Lopez, A.; Figueiras, A. Factors determining antibiotic use in the general population: A qualitative study in Spain. *PLoS ONE* **2021**, *16*, e0246506. [CrossRef] [PubMed]
8. McCullough, A.R.; Pollack, A.J.; Plejdrup Hansen, M.; Glasziou, P.P.; Looke, D.F.; Britt, H.C.; Del Mar, C.B. Antibiotics for acute respiratory infections in general practice: Comparison of prescribing rates with guideline recommendations. *Med. J. Aust.* **2017**, *207*, 65–69. [CrossRef] [PubMed]
9. Antimicrobial Resistance Collaborators. Global burden of bacterial antimicrobial resistance in 2019: A systematic analysis. *Lancet* **2022**, *399*, 629–655. [CrossRef] [PubMed]
10. Pulingam, T.; Parumasivam, T.; Gazzali, A.M.; Sulaiman, A.M.; Chee, J.Y.; Lakshmanan, M.; Chin, C.F.; Sudesh, K. Antimicrobial resistance: Prevalence, economic burden, mechanisms of resistance and strategies to overcome. *Eur. J. Pharm. Sci.* **2022**, *170*, 106103. [CrossRef] [PubMed]
11. Rogers Van Katwyk, S.; Poirier, M.J.P.; Chandy, S.J.; Faure, K.; Fisher, C.; Lhermie, G.; Moodley, A.; Sarkar, S.; Sophie, M.; Strong, K.; et al. 1-10-100: Unifying goals to mobilize global action on antimicrobial resistance. *Glob. Health* **2024**, *20*, 66. [CrossRef] [PubMed]
12. Holmes, A.H.; Moore, L.S.; Sundsfjord, A.; Steinbakk, M.; Regmi, S.; Karkey, A.; Guerin, P.J.; Piddock, L.J. Understanding the mechanisms and drivers of antimicrobial resistance. *Lancet* **2016**, *387*, 176–187. [CrossRef] [PubMed]
13. World Health Organization. Fact Sheets: Antimicrobial Resistance. 2021. Available online: https://www.who.int/news-room/fact-sheets/detail/antimicrobial-resistance (accessed on 1 September 2024).
14. World Health Organization. World Antimicrobial Awareness Week 2023. 2023. Available online: https://www.who.int/campaigns/world-amr-awareness-week/2023 (accessed on 1 September 2024).

Disclaimer/Publisher's Note: The statements, opinions and data contained in all publications are solely those of the individual author(s) and contributor(s) and not of MDPI and/or the editor(s). MDPI and/or the editor(s) disclaim responsibility for any injury to people or property resulting from any ideas, methods, instructions or products referred to in the content.

Knowledge, Perceptions, and Perspectives of Medical Students Regarding the Use of Antibiotics and Antibiotic Resistance: A Qualitative Research in Galicia, Spain

Juan M. Vázquez-Lago [1,2,*], Rodrigo A. Montes-Villalba [3], Olalla Vázquez-Cancela [1], María Otero-Santiago [1], Ana López-Durán [4] and Adolfo Figueiras [2,5,6]

[1] Service of Preventive Medicine and Public Health, Clinic Hospital of Santiago de Compostela, 15706 Santiago de Compostela, Spain
[2] Health Research Institute of Santiago de Compostela (IDIS), 15706 Santiago de Compostela, Spain
[3] Service of Admission and Clinical Documentation, Clinic Hospital of Santiago de Compostela, 15706 Santiago de Compostela, Spain
[4] Department of Clinical Psychology and Psychobiology, University of Santiago de Compostela, 15782 Santiago de Compostela, Spain
[5] Department of Preventive Medicine and Public Health, University of Santiago de Compostela, 15782 Santiago de Compostela, Spain
[6] Consortium for Biomedical Research in Epidemiology & Public Health (CIBER en Epidemiología y Salud Pública—CIBERESP), 28029 Madrid, Spain
* Correspondence: juan.manuel.vazquez.lago@sergas.es; Tel.: +34-9-8195-0037

Abstract: Antibiotic resistance is a significant public health concern, with numerous studies linking antibiotic consumption to the development of resistance. As medical students will play a pivotal role in prescribing antibiotics, this research aimed to identify their perceptions of current use and factors that could influence future inappropriate use of antibiotics. The study employed a qualitative research approach using Focus Group discussions (FGs) consisting of students from the final theoretical course of the Medicine degree. The FGs were conducted based on a pre-script developed from factors contributing to antibiotic misuse identified in previous studies. All sessions were recorded and transcribed for analysis by two independent researchers, with all participants signing informed consent. Seven focus groups were conducted, with a total of 35 participants. The study identified factors that could influence the future prescription of antibiotics, including the low applicability of knowledge, insecurity, clinical inertia, difficulties in the doctor-patient relationship, unawareness of available updates on the topic, and inability to assess their validity. The students did not perceive antibiotic resistance as a current problem. However, the study found several modifiable factors in medical students that could explain the misuse of antibiotics, and developing specific strategies could help improve their use.

Keywords: antibiotic resistance; antibiotics; knowledge; perceptions; attitudes; medical students; qualitative

1. Introduction

Antibiotic resistance is an increasingly significant public health issue worldwide [1,2], with substantial implications for morbidity, mortality, and costs [3,4]. There is now little doubt that the consumption of antibiotics is strongly linked to the development of resistance [3,5].

Spain's antibiotic consumption is higher than the European Community average, despite no difference in infection prevalence [6,7]. This abuse and misuse of antibiotics is a complex issue that pertains to different groups, including doctors, healthcare users, pharmacists, veterinarians, and health authorities, and is related to knowledge, attitudes, and practices [3,8–11]. Medical students are an ideal population to implement educational strategies during their university studies to improve antibiotic prescription and use in the future. They are trained in the functionality of antibiotics, and their appropriate prescription [12,13] and are aware of the issue of antibiotic resistance. However, they may still lack confidence in selecting the right antibiotic for each case, providing instructions, and communicating with patients [12–14]. A systematic review of medical students' knowledge, beliefs, and attitudes regarding antibiotics and resistance showed a need for more training to raise awareness of this public health problem [15].

Accordingly, our research aimed to explore the factors that influence the students of the last theoretical course of degree in Medicine on the future prescription of antibiotics and resistances in order to identify knowledge gaps on which to design future strategies.

2. Results

A total of 35 final-year medical students participated in seven focus groups, with each group consisting of 4 to 6 participants (see Table 1). 62.86% were women. None of the students invited to participate declined to take part in the study.

Table 1. Focal Groups characteristics.

	n	M-F
FG1	5	2-3
FG2	5	0-5
FG3	5	2-3
FG4	4	2-2
FG5	6	4-2
FG6	5	2-3
FG7	5	1-4

FG. Focal Groups; M: Male; F: Female.

The initial group served as a pilot study, during which we introduced certain modifications to the script. Due to the qualitative methodology's flexibility [16], we were able to incorporate new topics that emerged in this group into the subsequent sessions.

Through analysis of the transcripts, we identified students' perceptions of current antibiotic use and the main factors that could lead medical professionals to abuse or misuse antibiotics in the future. Drawing on participants' insights from the focus group, we compiled Table 2 to summarize the reasons behind this trend.

2.1. Knowledge about the Use of Antibiotics

All seven groups indicated that they were familiar with the general mechanism of action of antibiotics, the concept of "antibiotic resistance," and the biological mechanisms of its development. However, a few students shared common misconceptions found among the general population concerning the symptoms that indicate the necessity for antibiotic treatment: "[...] *sputum if it is dense, green, then, antibiotic*" (F2, FG1); "*green mucus in children, earache, sore throat*" (M2, FG3), such claims were not refuted, nor discussed by their peers, who were sympathetic to them. They expressed their opinions about the mechanisms regarding the development of antibiotic resistance: "*if you always give fosfomycin, maybe that patient tends to generate a resistance to fosfomycin; if he has been taking it all his life, you also have to be careful with that.*" (F2, FG1).

Table 2. Factors identified with respect to knowledge and attitudes regarding antibiotic use among medical students.

Knowledge		They claim to know the concept of antibiotic resistance and the mechanisms by which they are developed.
Perception	Use	They perceive abuse of antibiotics. They perceive pressure for the prescription to which it is yielded. They perceive inertia on the part of professionals.
	Responsibility	Multifactorial: ○ Doctors. ○ Patients: adherence, leftover kits. ○ Food sector.
	Magnitude	Aware of the seriousness of the advance of the resistance. Unaware of the degree of presence of resistance in their healthcare environment.
Training	Theoretical	They claim to have received good theoretical training. They believe that their knowledge has no practical applicability.
	Skills and tools	They report poor practical training: they lack skills and assertiveness. Insecurity before the diagnosis.
	Updating	They perceive little updating among doctors. Through congresses, clinical sessions, and clinical guidelines. Lack of information search tools and critical reading.
Perspectives	Doctor-patient relationship	They consider it essential. They report lacking the necessary skills and time.
	Training Industry	Awareness of the existence of biases. Perceived as necessary.

2.2. Perception of Current Antibiotic Use

All seven groups concurred on the prevalence of antibiotic misuse, which they attributed to various factors, including both healthcare professionals and patients. The students linked the inappropriate use of antibiotics with certain behaviors they observed during medical consultations. For instance, they noted that inadequate patient histories and physical examinations often resulted in uncertain diagnoses, making it challenging to determine the appropriate treatment: *"[...] in the end what decides what is done is the time of anamnesis and exploration. It makes you more certain whether to give an antibiotic or not. If you have little time, you give things without evidence or don't look for it so much."* (M1, FG1).

They also pinpointed the insufficient explanations from doctors regarding the diagnosis, prognosis, treatment, and the significance of adhering to the prescribed dosage as another issue of antibiotic use. This inadequacy obstructs the doctor-patient relationship and results in noncompliance with the treatment plan *"[...] there are patients who, when they leave, have that desire of a better explanation of what they have and with a simple explanation they would better understand what they have, or they would be calmer"* (M2, FG6).

Two additional interconnected topics were identified: complacency in prescription and patient demand for antibiotics. Four groups referred to the issue of complacency in prescription *"[...] it is very tempting to give the antibiotic, and also the patient leaves with a smile. I know it shouldn't be done, but I see people do it because of that: you watch your back and leave the patient happy."* (M1, FG7). They said that doctors often succumb to this type of pressure on numerous occasions. Furthermore, it was noted that there is anticipation or expectation of patient demand *"if you think it will be driving you nuts for half an hour and you will end up giving it, then already ... you give it to him directly, don't you?"* (M2, FG1).

In four groups, doctors' lack of confidence in establishing the diagnosis and selecting treatment was identified as a contributing factor to prescription abuse. This lack of confidence was linked to the perceived specificity of symptoms, inadequate patient histories and physical examinations, and the absence of access to rapid tests, *"and I wonder: Doctor's insecurity? The <I'm not sure, I'm not going to go out on a limb>, will that imply a lot? In theory, everything seems very easy, but a guy who is complaining there and you don't know what he has ..."*. Closely linked to the issue of insecurity, another concept emerged and was repeated in five groups: "defensive medicine." This term refers to the practice of taking precautions to minimize the consequences for the doctor if their diagnostic hypothesis proves to be incorrect. The challenges of dealing with dissatisfied patients and providing additional assistance were also noted: *"in addition, you do not want to find him again in consultation if he returns and you did not give him an antibiotic ..."* (M1, FG5). This is also related to the reduction of risk for the patient. They reported that by prescribing antibiotics, they were providing coverage against potential complications of the patient's condition: *"[...] many times, a pathology that has a very viral characteristic or seems very viral, to take care of health, they prescribe antibiotics. And that I think is one of the problems we have in the face of resistance: doctors are afraid of failing, or that a banal pathology gets complicated"* (F2, FG4), *"on the one hand, it is defensive of doctors, to save themselves in case this does not worsen, well."* (F2, FG2).

The students mentioned that medical professionals might lack knowledge or experience circumstances that create doubt, ultimately leading to a prescription of antibiotics. This decision may be made in an effort to protect both themselves and the patient: *"what I saw in Primary Care was that many times they commented that there was a clear difference between the guidelines and clinical practice, and that was also manifested ... there are some dogmas, and you block yourself to the theory."* (M2, FG4).

Three groups identified inertia as a factor contributing to antibiotic misuse. However, it was noted that this was mentioned unconsciously in all three cases, as it was not subsequently linked to poor practices: *"[...] you give the best known by custom. So, you give this one out of habit because it goes well, it doesn't have to be caused by the same bacteria, but you know it, it goes well, so I continue to use it."* (F1, FG1).

Five groups commented on the perception that the Pediatrics department is a service in which the use of antibiotics is commonly abused, primarily due to pressure or complacency from parents: *"Especially in Paediatrics, more than anything to calm parents, it's like if you don't give them antibiotics, you're not doing your job properly."* (F1, FG3).

2.3. Attribution of Responsibility for the Evolution of Antibiotic Resistance

Six groups assured that the current situation and the trajectory of antibiotic resistance development has a shared responsibility and a multifactorial cause *"is a bit everyone's responsibility: what he says, patients taking them wrong, and doctors prescribing inappropriately, or because they ask for them... it's something that affects everybody"* (F2, FG6).

The other group mentioned that once the healthcare sector became aware of the severity of the problem and began to regulate the use of antibiotics more strictly, the primary responsibility shifted to the general population. The public was perceived to be abusing antibiotics, not following treatment guidelines, and demanding them unnecessarily.

In three groups, the livestock sector was identified as a significant contributor to antibiotic resistance. Additionally, three students from different groups specifically highlighted the livestock sector as the primary source of antibiotic resistance *"partly the doctor, but also treatments to animals and the meat industry, which gives medicine and antibiotics to grow better, and I think it is also a fundamental part of the resistance."* (F2, FG2).

2.4. Perception of the Magnitude of the Problem of Antibiotic Resistance

Although most participants acknowledged the severity of antibiotic resistance, their statements were not consistently aligned. Specifically, undergraduate Medicine students acknowledged the seriousness of the problem, recognizing that the advancement of resistance is outpacing the development of new antibiotics, which could result in a post-antibiotic era reminiscent of pre-antibiotic times: *"yes, we will return almost to the pre-antibiotic era."* (F1, FG4).

Regarding the prevalence of antibiotic resistance in our environment, participants stated that it is a medium to long-term problem. While they were aware of outbreaks of multidrug-resistant bacteria in the environment, they believed that these situations were specific and self-limited, part of a gradual progression, and that, in general, they had not observed them during their clinical practices. *"I, for example, think it is something rather global because I have never found a case in my training where I had to say <now this one does not work anymore>."* (F1, FG4).

2.5. Training

2.5.1. Theoretical Training

The students acknowledged that their theoretical training was extensive and detailed. *"I think that they harped upon us a lot and informed us quite well."* (M2, FG3). However, they also expressed that the knowledge they gained lacked practical application. *"adapting an antibiotic to a pathology is something I think that we were not taught at any time."* (F4, FG2). As a result, we assessed their theoretical education as insufficient in terms of preparing them for professional practice: *"I believe that the training period is bad. I think that the training regarding antibiotics the form is not good, (...); I do not see the practical purpose of that way, and it is a problem during the whole degree, not only in the case of antibiotics."* (M1, FG1).

Several students have expressed their perception of a significant disparity between the theoretical knowledge they have acquired and the practical skills exhibited by the doctors they have worked with. Additionally, these students have shared their concerns (fear) about feeling compelled to act in a manner that may contradict their own beliefs or values to adhere to hierarchical structures: *"we were in the health center in clinical sessions, and doctors always made a distinction between what is practice and theory in the prescription of antibiotics. I find it curious because they end up determining misuse because many of the theoretical criteria are not met in practice"* (M2, FG4).

2.5.2. Tools and Skills

The students unanimously reflected that they lacked the essential skills required to translate their theoretical knowledge into practical applications and establish effective doctor-patient relationships. They also noted that they lacked social and communicative skills that are essential for dealing with the pressures that arise in clinical settings. The students expressed their belief that their practical training had been inadequate in these areas, leaving them ill-prepared for the challenges of real-world practice: *"in the end, it's a job where you deal with public face to face, and these skills are facing the public. They don't put a lot of emphasis on this in training."* (M1, GF6), *"during the degree we are not taught any communicative skill. They teach you to study; you learn that, and... you would have to know and understand it very well to be able to change it and explain it with your words well. And we don't do that during the degree."* (F2, FG6).

2.5.3. Update

According to the observations made during their practices, the most frequently utilized sources of information by the students for updates were conferences, clinical sessions, and clinical practice guidelines. These sources were considered to be both accessible and reliable, and the students expressed a willingness to continue using them in the future.

However, the students also reported being uninformed about other available resources and lacking the necessary training to effectively utilize them for ongoing learning and professional development. They further noted that their reliance on note-taking as a primary study method had led them to overlook alternative sources of information beyond textbooks: *"That is, it would be good to know those websites or databases that are more reliable, other than searching on Medline or Wikipedia"* (M1, FG6).

2.6. About the Doctor-Patient Relationship

Without exception, the students acknowledged the critical importance of establishing and maintaining a positive doctor-patient relationship as a means of managing stress and effectively communicating to patients that antibiotic treatment may not be necessary for their particular condition during consultations: *"if you have confidence in your doctor, you trust him blindly and if he says no, that means no"* (M2, FG3).

2.7. Solutions

When asked about potential solutions to reduce antibiotic abuse, students identified education of the population and packaging tailored to the treatment duration as the most effective measures.

Table 3 demonstrates the saturation of information gathered on factors contributing to inappropriate future prescriptions by medical students. This section may be subdivided into headings to provide a clear and concise description of the experimental results, their interpretation, and the conclusions that can be drawn from the experiment.

Table 3. Saturation of information on identified factors contributing to inadequate future prescribing.

Contributing Factors to Future Bad Prescribing	FG1	FG2	FG3	FG4	FG5	FG6	FG7
Low practical applicability of knowledge	X	X	-	X	X	X	X
Lack of social and communication skills	X	X	X	X	X	X	X
Lack of knowledge of updating tools and continuous training	-	X	X	X	X	X	X
Need for the industry as a trainer	-	X	X	X	X	X	X
Insecurity	X	X	X	X	X	X	X
Clinical inertia as a valid tool	X	X	-	X	-	X	X
Patient demands	X	X	X	X	X	X	X
Lack of awareness of the current presence of antibiotic resistance in the direct environment	X	-	X	X	-	X	X

3. Discussion

This is the first qualitative study in Spain to examine the factors that influence medical students in their attitudes toward antibiotic use and resistance. The findings indicate that students recognize their role in combating antibiotic resistance but are hindered by a lack of understanding of basic concepts, limited practical experience, insecurity, inertia, and challenges in the doctor-patient relationship. Identifying these factors can inform the development of targeted strategies to improve antibiotic use and enhance the impact of interventions aimed at addressing these deficiencies.

Some beliefs have been identified in a similar study on the general population [10]. This study conducted on the general population has identified certain beliefs that are incorrect because they are based on outdated knowledge and not supported by current scientific evidence. For instance, some people believe that the color of mucus in upper respiratory tract infections is correlated with its etiology. Given that medical students are a group that falls midway between the general population and medical professionals, it is logical that they may share some of these opinions. This finding is consistent with other studies that evaluated the knowledge of medical students regarding the effectiveness of antibiotics in treating colds, influenza, and coughs. Surprisingly, only 47–60% of students knew that antibiotics were not the preferred treatment option [17–19].

Furthermore, despite claiming to know about the appropriate use of antibiotics and antibiotic resistance, some students' statements indicate clear ignorance of these topics. For instance, confusion between the terms antibiotic resistance and tolerance, as well as resistance, pan-resistance, and therapeutic failure, has been identified among certain students. Confusion between some of these terms has been perceived equally among the general population [10,11]. This lack of understanding is consistent with findings from a systematic review by Nogueira–Uzal et al. [15], published in 2020, which reported a general lack of knowledge regarding the diagnosis and treatment of infectious diseases, particularly upper respiratory tract infections, among medical students, regardless of their level of study.

Students are aware of the abuse and misuse of antibiotics and how it leads to increased antibiotic resistance, which they associate with both doctors and patients. Although they agree that prescribers bear direct responsibility, they only partially attribute it to clinicians and attribute bad practices to external causes, primarily the lack of time during consultations. Previous studies have also identified a lack of time as a crucial factor in antibiotic prescription [20]. This not only limits the doctor-patient relationship but also hinders proper anamnesis and exploration and instruction of patients. In general, students relate the shortage of personnel to these issues.

According to the students, insecurity among doctors is one of the main causes of antibiotic prescription abuse. Although they have received extensive theoretical training and possess the necessary knowledge to manage infectious diseases and antibiotics, they express insecurity when faced with the actual clinical environment. Previous studies on medical students have also identified similar insecurities regarding the selection and dosage of antibiotic drugs, attributed to a low transferability of knowledge to practical environments [12,13,21,22]. However, some studies suggest that overconfidence may also contribute to poor prescribing practices [13,22].

The students also expressed their opinion that antibiotic abuse is more prevalent in pediatric services due to the demands made by parents for prescriptions. However, a similar study on parents of primary school children in the same community observed that this group is more aware of the function of antibiotics and is more likely to conform to the explanations provided by the clinician, especially if it comes from their usual Pediatrician. Nonetheless, pediatricians acknowledge that parents often request antibiotics out of fear [11].

The lack of communication and social skills necessary to establish a good doctor-patient relationship and convince demanding patients of the unnecessary use of antibiotics is another contributing factor to prescription abuse. The students claim that they have not been trained in this area. Both the students and other studies have emphasized that the doctor-patient relationship is crucial for proper antibiotic prescription by professionals and their appropriate use by patients [9,20,23]. This lack of communication skills often leads to giving in to patient pressure and promotes complacency in prescribing, which has also been observed in pharmacists and primary care physicians [9,24,25].

Although the students are aware of the severity and consequences of the increase in antibiotic resistance, they view it as a medium-to-long-term problem. They are uncertain about the extent to which it currently affects their healthcare environment, a belief shared by medical professionals across different fields [25–27]. Similar findings were reported in a systematic review, which revealed that students acknowledge antibiotic resistance as a global public health concern but do not express concern about its impact in their immediate workplace or learning environment, such as their teaching hospital [15].

Strengths and Limitations

The students who participated in the focus groups were recruited from a single university and may not necessarily represent all students from public universities in the country. Therefore, caution should be taken when generalizing the results to other regions or countries. Nevertheless, qualitative methods aim to capture a range of perspectives, and generalizability is not typically an expected attribute of this type of research.

The methodology and design used in this study met all the points of the Consolidated Criteria for Reporting Qualitative Research (COREQ) scale [28], indicating that it adhered to the quality criteria required for qualitative studies (Table S1).

Qualitative methodology is of great interest as a tool for exploring and identifying attitudes related to the use of antibiotics that cannot be identified "a priori" by epidemiological studies with quantitative methodology included in the literature review since people's behavior is strongly influenced by the cultural characteristics of the population where they live and the interpersonal relationships that are generated. This methodology seeks to understand reality and phenomena from the perspective of the individuals who experience them [29–31].

Seven focus groups were conducted, which accounted for the number of enrolled students. This allowed for the collection of information from a diverse range of perspectives about students' perceptions and perspectives on antibiotic use at the end of their university academic stage. A total of 35 medical students participated. The sampling method used was simple random sampling and convenience sampling. In qualitative research, is a greater interest in analyzing and delving into the study cases without any loss of scientific rigor. As explained by Hernández, Fernández, and Baptista: *"In qualitative studies, the sample size is not important from a probabilistic perspective because the researcher's interest is not to generalize the results of their study to a wider population. What is sought in qualitative research is depth. We are concerned with cases (participants, people, organizations, events, animals, facts, etc.) that help us understand the phenomenon under study and answer research questions.* [32]"

In this context, the sample size is therefore determined by the ability of the different focus groups to generate the necessary information (data) for the study. Information collection through focus groups involves forming groups, each with between 4 and 10 participants until information saturation is reached. This means that all possible ideas that we explore have already emerged from group discourses or discussions and that no new ideas are emerging. Therefore, if we continue to form focus groups, they will no longer provide new data for the study. In our case, this occurred with seven groups, totaling 35 medical students. Sample size in this type of study is not fixed "a priori" based on statistical calculations but rather is determined "a posteriori" by reaching the sample size considered correct when no new information is generated [33,34].

4. Materials and Methods

4.1. Research Design

A qualitative study was conducted using FG discussions to collect narrative data from students in the final theoretical course of their Medicine degree. This approach allowed for an exploration of the beliefs and perceptions of the student population regarding the use and misuse of antibiotics. The objective was to obtain a comprehensive and detailed description of the student's beliefs and perspectives and to develop a theory-based justification using systematically collected information. The use of FGs enabled an in-depth exploration of the topic and provided valuable insights into the participants' perspectives.

4.2. Target Population

FGs were conducted at the University of Santiago de Compostela (USC), which is the only university in Galicia, a region in northwest Spain, that offers a degree in Medicine. From 2010-2017, the university offered an average of 353.75 places per year, making it the public faculty with the highest number of places offered for this degree in the country.

4.3. Selection, Sample and Procedure

The Medicine degree program is a six-year curriculum that includes internships in health centers, clinical settings, and surgical services during the final year. For this study, participants were recruited from the School of Medicine at USC and were in their fifth year of study. This year of study is focused on theoretical training and is common to all participants, which created a relaxed atmosphere and facilitated the open expression of opinions and beliefs. Additionally, participants' similar age, levels of knowledge, and educational experiences allowed for the discussion of diverse perspectives without communication limitations [16].

To guide the focus group discussions, a script was developed by drawing on findings from previous studies involving family doctors [9,35], community pharmacists from Galicia and Portugal [9], the general population [10], and parents of primary school students [11].

The script aimed to explore the reasons that may lead students to misuse antibiotics toward the end of their medical training. Additionally, the script aimed to examine whether the improper use of antibiotics observed among primary care doctors could be attributed to inadequate training or the adoption of certain practices and misuse of resources once in practice.

The focus groups were conducted in A Coruña between February and May 2018 using a random selection procedure. The students were personally contacted during their face-to-face practicals on Preventive Medicine and Public Health subject and were invited to participate in the study by the researchers, who were independent of the teaching staff and faculty. The researchers explained the study's objectives and the nature of their participation. It is worth noting that the students did not have any previous relationship with the researchers.

FGs sessions took place in a classroom located in the University Clinical Hospital of Santiago, which allowed for the participation of students who attended their theoretical classes in a building attached to the hospital. The room was occupied solely by the participants and the researchers, and contact information, such as email addresses, was collected from each group member. The focus groups were conducted by 2 resident physicians of Preventive Medicine and Public Health, 1 female (OVC) and 1 male (RAMV), both of whom had prior experience leading focus groups. One researcher acted as the interviewer, while the other served as a moderator to ensure that all group members participated in a respectful and organized manner. This approach fostered an environment conducive to the free expression of opinions and facilitated accurate transcription of the recordings.

The FG sessions were recorded using a digital recorder and a mobile phone to ensure high-quality sound for transcription purposes. The average duration of the sessions was 39 min, and they continued until no new ideas were presented. No data management software was utilized in the study.

One of the researchers transcribed the sessions, and another researcher checked for accuracy. The FGs were identified as "StudentsGF 1-7", and each participant was assigned a code consisting of a letter "M" or "F" (to indicate male or female, respectively) and a number based on their speaking order in the audio files.

After each session, the two researchers discussed their initial impressions and noted down the group's characteristics. Additional focus groups were formed until "saturation" was achieved, meaning that no new information was provided by the participants. At this point, adding more units would have been redundant and would not have improved the quality of the study [36].

4.4. Ethical Considerations

The study underwent evaluation and received approval from the Santiago-Lugo Research Ethics Committee, registered under code 2014/386. Prior to participation, participants were informed of the study's objectives and the intention to record and transcribe sessions. They provided their consent to participate by signing an informed consent form. The study ensures the anonymity of all participants.

4.5. Analysis

The analysis of the transcripts was a repetitive process that involved two independent researchers. They were responsible for carefully reading the transcripts to ensure an appropriate structure of the data, which allowed for a deeper interpretation and reduced the risk of researcher bias.

Thematic and discursive content analysis was employed to examine the data, enabling the identification of different ideas and organization of the obtained data into relevant topics, supported by literal extracts serving as units of analysis [37]. The extracted ideas were then associated with the pre-established variables. In cases where there were disagreements between the researchers regarding the interpretation, they were debated and resolved by consensus. Given the limited number of focus groups, no software was used for data processing. The definition of the FGs was based on the participants' use of different concepts (Table 4).

Table 4. Concept coding.

Concept	Definition According to Its Use
Update	Methods they know or observe to keep knowledge up to date.
Complacency	Unnecessary prescription for meeting the expectations perceived in the patient.
Skills	Social and communicative skills available to establish a good doctor-patient relationship. Ability to set limits and not give in to patient demands.
Tools	Ability to bring their theoretical knowledge to the practical field. Means available to them to solve doubts individually.
Training Industry	Assessment and perception of the pharmaceutical industry as a method of updating and continuous training.
Inertia	Tendency to use the same treatments in similar situations without inquiring into the indication because: - had worked in the past in other cases. - a colleague would advise or order it. - is the usual treatment used in the service.
Magnitude	- Severity and extent perceived on antibiotic resistance.
Defensive Medicine	Proceeding perceived as: - less risky in possible repercussions for the professional. - of lower risk for the patient by covering possible complications.
Perception	What students claim to observe in clinical practice.
Pressure	User demand to be prescribed an antibiotic.
Responsibility	Attributed guilt to the development of antibiotic resistance.

5. Conclusions

This study highlights that Undergraduate medicine students lack adequate theoretical training in the prescription and use of antibiotics. Furthermore, they do not find the little training they receive clinically applicable. Additionally, they attribute their method of prescribing antibiotics to inertia, copying other professionals.

This study is a first step, which will allow the design of a validated questionnaire from which multifaceted interventions and strategies can be designed to improve the prescription of future medical professionals.

Supplementary Materials: The following supporting information can be downloaded at: https://www.mdpi.com/article/10.3390/antibiotics12030558/s1, Table S1: COREQ (COnsolidated criteria for REporting Qualitative research) Checklist.

Author Contributions: Conceptualization, J.M.V.-L., A.L.-D., and A.F.; methodology, J.M.V.-L. and A.L.-D.; formal analysis, O.V.-C. and R.A.M.-V.; investigation, O.V.-C. and R.A.M.-V.; resources, J.M.V.-L. and A.F.; data curation, O.V.-C. and R.A.M.-V.; writing—original draft preparation, O.V.-C. and R.A.M.-V and M.O.-S.; writing—review and editing, J.M.V.-L., M.O.-S., and A.F.; supervision, J.M.V.-L.; project administration, J.M.V.-L. and A.F.; funding acquisition, A.F. All authors have read and agreed to the published version of the manuscript.

Funding: This research was supported in part by the Instituto de Salud Carlos III (ISCIII) (PI081239, PI09/90609) Spanish State Plan for Scientific and Technical Research and Innovation and co-funded by The European Union (ERDF).

Institutional Review Board Statement: The study was conducted in accordance with the Declaration of Helsinki and approved by the Santiago-Lugo Research Ethics Committee under registry code 2014/386.

Informed Consent Statement: Informed consent was obtained from all subjects involved in the study.

Data Availability Statement: The transcriptions used and/or analyzed during the current study are available from the corresponding author upon reasonable request.

Conflicts of Interest: The authors declare no conflict of interest.

References

1. World Health Organization. Fact Sheets: Antimicrobial Resistance. 2021. Available online: https://www.who.int/news-room/fact-sheets/detail/antimicrobial-resistance (accessed on 10 February 2023).
2. Roca, I.; Akova, M.; Baquero, F.; Carlet, J.; Cavaleri, M.; Coenen, S.; Cohen, J.; Findlay, D.; Gyssens, I.; Heure, O.E.; et al. The global threat of antimicrobial resistance: Science for intervention. *New Microbes New Infect.* **2015**, *6*, 22–29. [CrossRef]
3. Ferri, M.; Ranucci, E.; Romagnoli, P.; Giaccone, V. Antimicrobial resistance: A global emerging threat to public health systems. *Crit. Rev. Food Sci. Nutr.* **2017**, *57*, 2857–2876, Erratum in *New Microbes New Infect.* **2015**, *8*, 175. [CrossRef]
4. European Center for Disease Prevention and Control. Rapid Risk Assessment: Carbapenem-Resistant Enterobacteriaceae—Second Update. 2019. Available online: https://www.ecdc.europa.eu/sites/default/files/documents/carbapenem-resistant-enterobacteriaceae-risk-assessment-rev-2.pdf (accessed on 28 February 2023).
5. Acharya, K.R.; Brankston, G.; Soucy, J.-P.R.; Cohen, A.; Hulth, A.; Löfmark, S.; Davidovitch, N.; Ellen, M.; Fisman, D.N.; Moran-Gilad, J.; et al. Evaluation of an OPEN Stewardship generated feedback intervention to improve antibiotic prescribing among primary care veterinarians in Ontario, Canada and Israel: Protocol for evaluating usability and an interrupted time-series analysis. *BMJ Open* **2021**, *15*, 11. [CrossRef]
6. Bruyndonckx, R.; Adriaenssens, N.; Versporten, A.; Hens, N.; Monnet, D.L.; Molenberghs, G.; Goossens, H.; Weist, K.; Coenen, S. ESAC-Net study group Consumption of Antibiotics in the Community, European Union/European Economic Area, 1997–2017. *J. Antimicrob. Chemother.* **2021**, *76* (Suppl. 2), ii7–ii13. [CrossRef]
7. European Centre for Disease Prevention and Control. *Antimicrobial Consumption in the EU/EEA (ESAC-Net)—Annual Epidemiological Report 2021*; ECDC: Stockholm, Sweden, 2022. Available online: https://www.ecdc.europa.eu/sites/default/files/documents/ESAC-Net_AER_2021_final-rev.pdf (accessed on 27 February 2023).
8. Servia-Dopazo, M.; Taracido-Trunk, M.; Figueiras, A. Non-Clinical Factors Determining the Prescription of Antibiotics by Veterinarians: A Systematic Review. *Antibiotics* **2021**, *10*, 133. [CrossRef]
9. Vazquez-Lago, J.M.; Lopez-Vazquez, P.; López-Durán, A.; Taracido-Trunk, M.; Figueiras, A. Attitudes of primary care physicians to the prescribing of antibiotics and antimicrobial resistance: A qualitative study from Spain. *Fam. Pract.* **2012**, *29*, 352–360. [CrossRef]
10. Vazquez-Cancela, O.; Souto-Lopez, L.; Vazquez-Lago, J.M.; Lopez, A.; Figueiras, A. Factors determining antibiotic use in the general population: A qualitative study in Spain. *PLoS ONE* **2021**, *16*, e0246506. [CrossRef]
11. Souto-López, L.; Vazquez-Cancela, O.; Vazquez-Lago, J.M.; López-Durán, A.; Figueiras, A. Parent-related factors influencing antibiotic use in a paediatric population: A qualitative study in Spain. *Acta Paediatr.* **2020**, *109*, 2719–2726. [CrossRef]
12. Abbo, L.M.; Cosgrove, S.E.; Pottinger, P.S.; Pereyra, M.; Sinkowitz-Cochran, R.; Srinivasan, A.; Webb, D.J.; Hooton, T.M. Medical students' perceptions and knowledge about antimicrobial stewardship: How are we educating our future prescribers? *Clin. Infect. Dis.* **2013**, *57*, 631–638. [CrossRef]
13. Dyar, O.J.; Pulcini, C.; Howard, P.; Nathwani, D.; Beovic, B.; Harbarth, S.; Hanberger, H.; Pagani, L.; Pardo, J.R.P.; Weschesler-Fördös, A.; et al. European medical students: A first multicentre study of knowledge, attitudes and perceptions of antibiotic prescribing and antibiotic resistance. *J. Antimicrob. Chemother.* **2014**, *69*, 842–846. [CrossRef]
14. Sánchez-Fabra, D.; Dyar, O.J.; del Pozo, J.L.; Amiguet, J.A.; Colmenero, J.D.D.; Fariñas, M.D.C.; López-Medrano, F.; Portilla, J.; Praena, J.; Torre-Cisneros, J.; et al. Perspective of Spanish medical students regarding undergraduate education in infectious diseases, bacterial resistance and antibiotic use. *Enferm. Infecc. Microbiol. Clín.* **2019**, *37*, 25–30. [CrossRef]
15. Nogueira-Uzal, N.; Zapata-Cachafeiro, M.; Vázquez-Cancela, O.; López-Durán, A.; Herdeiro, M.T.; Figueiras, A.; Nogueira-Uzal, N.; Zapata-Cachafeiro, M.; Vázquez-Cancela, O.; López-Durán, A.; et al. Does the problem begin at the beginning? Medical students' knowledge and beliefs regarding antibiotics and resistance: A systematic review. *Antimicrob. Resist. Infect. Control.* **2020**, *9*, 172. [CrossRef]
16. Cerdà, J.M.; Rodríguez, M.P.; García, M.H.; Gaspar, O.S. Técnicas cualitativas para la investigación en salud pública y gestión de servicios de salud: Algo más que otro tipo de técnicas. *Gac. Sanit.* **1999**, *13*, 312–319. [CrossRef]
17. Rusic, D.; Bozic, J.; Vilovic, M.; Bukic, J.; Zivkovic, P.M.; Leskur, D.; Perisin, A.S.; Tomic, S.; Modun, D. Attitudes and knowledge regarding antimicrobial use and resistance among pharmacy and medical students at the University of Split, Croatia. *Microb. Drug Resist.* **2018**, *24*, 1521–1528. [CrossRef]
18. Huang, Y.; Gu, J.; Zhang, M.; Ren, Z.; Yang, W.; Chen, Y.; Fu, Y.; Chen, X.; Cals, J.W.L.; Zhang, F. Knowledge, attitude and practice of antibiotics: A questionnaire study among 2500 Chinese students. *BMC Med Educ.* **2013**, *13*, 163. [CrossRef] [PubMed]
19. Chuenchom, N.; Thamlikitkul, V.; Chaiwarith, R.; Deoisares, R.; Rattanaumpawan, P. Perception, Attitude, and Knowledge Regarding Antimicrobial Resistance, Appropriate Antimicrobial Use, and Infection Control among Future Medical Practitioners: A Multicenter Study. *Infect. Control. Hosp. Epidemiol.* **2016**, *37*, 603–605. [CrossRef] [PubMed]

20. Bjorkman, I.; Berg, J.; Roing, M.; Erntell, M.; Lundborg, C.S. Perceptions among Swedish hospital physicians on prescribing of antibiotics and antibiotic resistance. *Qual. Saf. Health Care.* **2010**, *19*, e8. [CrossRef]
21. Afzal Khan, A.K.; Banu, G.; Reshma, K.K. Antibiotic Resistance and Usage-A Survey on the Knowledge, Attitude, Perceptions and Practices among the Medical Students of a Southern Indian Teaching Hospital. *J. Clin. Diagn. Res.* **2013**, *7*, 1613–1616. [CrossRef]
22. Wasserman, S.; Potgieter, S.; Shoul, E.; Constant, D.; Stewart, A.; Mendelson, M.; Boyles, T.H. South African medical students' perceptions and knowledge about antibiotic resistance and appropriate prescribing: Are we providing adequate training to future prescribers? *S. Afr. Med. J.* **2017**, *107*, 405–410. [CrossRef]
23. Shokouhi, E.; Zamani-Alavijeh, F.; Araban, M. Explaining family physicians' beliefs about antibiotic prescription. *Electron. Physician* **2017**, *9*, 5560–5567. [CrossRef]
24. Vazquez-Lago, J.; Gonzalez-Gonzalez, C.; Zapata-Cachafeiro, M.; López-Vázquez, P.M.; Taracido, M.; Lopez-Duran, A.; Figueiras, A. Knowledge, attitudes, perceptions and habits towards antibiotics dispensed without medical prescription: A qualitative study of Spanish pharmacists. *BMJ Open* **2017**, *7*, e015674. [CrossRef]
25. Gonzalez-Gonzalez, C.; Lopez-Vazquez, P.; Vazquez-Lago, J.M.; Piñeiro-Lamas, M.; Herdeiro, M.T.; Chavarri-Arzamendi, P.; Figueiras, A.; GREPHEPI Group. Effect of Physicians' Attitudes and Knowledge on the Quality of Antibiotic Prescription: A Cohort Study. *PLoS ONE* **2015**, e0141820. [CrossRef]
26. Menard, C.; Fégueux, S.; Heritage, Z.; Nion-Huang, M.; Berger-Carbonne, A.; Bonmarin, I. Perceptions and attitudes about antibiotic resistance in the general public and general practitioners in France. *Antimicrob. Resist. Infect. Control.* **2022**, *11*, 124. [CrossRef]
27. Simeoni, M.; Saragosa, M.; Laur, C.; Desveaux, L.; Schwartz, K.; Ivers, N. Coping with 'the grey area' of antibiotic prescribing: A theory-informed qualitative study exploring family physician perspectives on antibiotic prescribing. *BMC Prim. Care* **2022**, *23*, 188. [CrossRef]
28. Tong, A.; Sainsbury, P.; Craig, J. Consolidated criteria for reporting qualitative research (COREQ): A 32-item checklist for interviews and focus groups. *Int. J. Qual. Health Care* **2007**, *19*, 349–357. [CrossRef]
29. Chigbu, U.E. Visually hypothesising in scientific paper writing: Confirming and refuting qualitative research hypotheses using diagrams. *Publications* **2019**, *7*, 22. [CrossRef]
30. Prieto-Rodríguez, A.; March-Cerdá, J.C. Paso a paso en el diseño de un estudio mediante grupos focales. *Aten. Primaria* **2002**, *29*, 366–373. [CrossRef]
31. Carrillo-Pineda, M.; Leyva-Moral, J.M.; Medina-Moya, J.L. The analysis of qualitative data: A complex process. *Index Enferm.* **2011**, *20*, 96–100.
32. Hernández Sampieri, R.; Fernández, C.; Baptista, P. *Metodología de la Investigación*, 5th ed.; McGraw-Hill: Mexico City, Mexico, 2010.
33. Krueger, R.A. *Focus Groups: A Practical Guide for Applied Research*; Sage: London, UK, 1988.
34. Sim, J.; Saunders, B.; Waterfield, J.; Kingstone, T. Can sample size in qualitative research be determined a priori? *J. Soc. Sci. Res.* **2018**, *21*, 619–634. [CrossRef]
35. Rodrigues, A.T.; Roque, F.; Falcão, A.; Figueiras, A.; Herdeiro, M.T. Understanding physician antibiotic prescribing behaviour: A systematic review of qualitative studies. *Int. J. Antimicrob. Agents* **2013**, *4*, 203–212. [CrossRef]
36. Hennink, M.; Kaiser, B.N. Sample sizes for saturation in qualitative research: A systematic review of empirical tests. *Soc. Sci. Med.* **2022**, *292*, 114523. [CrossRef] [PubMed]
37. Corbin, J.M.; Strauss, A. Grounded theory research: Procedures, canons, and evaluative criteria. *Qual. Sociol.* **1990**, *13*, 3–21. [CrossRef]

Disclaimer/Publisher's Note: The statements, opinions and data contained in all publications are solely those of the individual author(s) and contributor(s) and not of MDPI and/or the editor(s). MDPI and/or the editor(s) disclaim responsibility for any injury to people or property resulting from any ideas, methods, instructions or products referred to in the content.

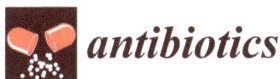

Article

Hospital Pharmacists' Viewpoint on Quality Use of Antibiotics and Resistance: A Qualitative Exploration from a Tertiary Care Hospital of Quetta City, Pakistan

Maryam Farooqui [1], Zaffar Iqbal [2], Abdul Sadiq [3], Abdul Raziq [4], Mohammed Salem Alshammari [1], Qaiser Iqbal [5], Sajjad Haider [5] and Fahad Saleem [5],*

[1] Department of Pharmacy Practice, Unaizah College of Pharmacy, Qassim University, Buraydah 52571, Saudi Arabia; m.farooqui@qu.edu.sa (M.F.); m.alshammari@qu.edu.sa (M.S.A.)
[2] Health Department, Government of Balochistan, Quetta 87100, Pakistan; zaffar_khosti@ymail.com
[3] Jhalawan Medical College Khuzdar, Khuzdar 89100, Pakistan; drabdulsadiq@gmail.com
[4] Department of Statistics, University of Balochistan, Quetta 87300, Pakistan; raziq@um.uob.edu.pk
[5] Faculty of Pharmacy & Health Sciences, University of Balochistan, Quetta 87300, Pakistan; qaiser.pharm@um.uob.edu.pk (Q.I.); sajjad.pharm@um.uob.edu.pk (S.H.)
* Correspondence: fahad.pharm@um.uob.edu.pk; Tel.: +92-3458326545

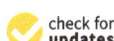

Citation: Farooqui, M.; Iqbal, Z.; Sadiq, A.; Raziq, A.; Alshammari, M.S.; Iqbal, Q.; Haider, S.; Saleem, F. Hospital Pharmacists' Viewpoint on Quality Use of Antibiotics and Resistance: A Qualitative Exploration from a Tertiary Care Hospital of Quetta City, Pakistan. *Antibiotics* **2023**, *12*, 1343. https://doi.org/10.3390/antibiotics12081343

Academic Editors: Juan Manuel Vázquez-Lago, Ana Estany-Gestal and Angel Salgado-Barreira

Received: 26 June 2023
Revised: 12 July 2023
Accepted: 13 July 2023
Published: 21 August 2023

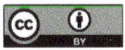

Copyright: © 2023 by the authors. Licensee MDPI, Basel, Switzerland. This article is an open access article distributed under the terms and conditions of the Creative Commons Attribution (CC BY) license (https://creativecommons.org/licenses/by/4.0/).

Abstract: Suboptimal antibiotics use and the development of antibiotic resistance is a universal calamity. The theoretical model of therapeutic efficacy correlates quality use of antibiotics with healthcare practitioners' understanding of antibiotic use and resistance. Keeping this phenomenon in mind, we aimed to evaluate hospital pharmacists' understanding of antibiotic use and resistance at a public healthcare institute in Quetta city, Pakistan. This was a qualitative study that employed a semi-structured interview guide for data extraction. The phenomenology-based approach commissioned in-depth, face-to-face interviews with hospital pharmacists stationed at the surgical unit of Sandeman Provincial Hospital, Quetta. The interviews were audio taped followed by transcribed verbatim and were then analyzed for thematic contents by the standard content analysis framework. Although the saturation was reached after the 10th interview, we conducted two additional interviews for definite validation. Content analysis revealed five major themes: (1) Defining antibiotics, quality use of antibiotics and resistance, (2) antibiotic use: awareness and concern, (3) antimicrobial resistance: awareness and concern, (4) responding to antibiotic use and resistance, and (5) barriers to quality use of antibiotics and prevention of antibiotic resistance. The knowledge of quality use of antibiotics and resistance was promising, and the respondents were eager to address the drastic situation. The respondents were aware of the critical situation and provided valuable insights that can offer valued input while promoting the quality use of antibiotics in a developing country. The current study managed to identify an adequate understanding of antibiotic use and resistance among hospital pharmacists. Additionally, prospective concerns and possible predictors of antibiotic resistance were also highlighted. The current findings must be disseminated to the policymakers and prescribers to take prompt restorative actions to address antibiotic use and the development of antibiotic resistance in a developing country like Pakistan.

Keywords: antibiotic use; antibiotics resistance; hospital pharmacists; qualitative; Quetta city; Pakistan

1. Introduction

The golden era of antibiotics regrettably did not last long as mankind was faced with the development of bacterial resistance against antibiotics [1]. Although Fleming, in his Nobel lecture, warned mankind by stating "it is not difficult to make microbes resistant to penicillin in the laboratory by exposing them to concentrations not sufficient to kill them" [2], minimum efforts were reported in the mid of 19th century to overcome antibiotic resistance [3]. Today, antibiotic resistance causes major risks to global safety and public health along with substantial societal impacts in the developing and developed world [4]. Kraker and associates in 2016 estimated that 10 million people will die due to antibiotic resistance by 2050 if restorative measures are not taken immediately [5]. Within this context, antibiotic resistance is driven by the inappropriate use of antibiotics in settings (hospitals and community) where antibiotics are not indicated, where guidelines for antibiotic use are not followed, or are considered clinically unnecessary for use among humans and animals [6]. Socioeconomic factors, self-medication, personal referrals, free availability of antibiotics, and unnecessary demands of the patients are also strong predictors of developing antibiotic resistance [7]. In a nutshell, antibiotic resistance is a multifactorial phenomenon that needs an imperative holistic approach and collaborative efforts of healthcare professionals, civil society, and community members to overcome the hazards presented to mankind and the generations to come.

Improving the quality use of antibiotics in hospitals and other healthcare settings in addition to limiting use in agriculture is a crucial area to safeguard antibiotics for future generations. In line with what is being discussed, the World Health Organization highlights the significant role of healthcare professionals in limiting the frequency of antibiotic resistance [8]. Healthcare professionals can reduce antibiotic resistance rates through evidence-based prescribing and adopting quality use of antibiotics. Moreover, being an educator, healthcare professionals are involved in reporting antibiotic-resistant infections to surveillance teams and educating patients and community members regarding antibiotic resistance and the hazards of misuse of antibiotics [8]. Today, the involvement of healthcare professionals in promoting the quality use of antibiotics is more inevitable than ever as the COVID-19 pandemic brought an alarming increase in antibiotic resistance. The Centers for Disease Control and Prevention reported a 15% increase in resistant infections from 2019 to 2020 among seven major pathogens because of a rush of antibiotic use while dealing with COVID-19 [9]. Therefore, controlling antibiotic resistance and promoting the quality use of antibiotics is a moral, ethical, and professional obligation of healthcare professionals.

Among healthcare professionals, hospital pharmacists occupy a conspicuous position in reducing the rates of antibiotic resistance [10]. Our claims are supported by the published literature where hospital pharmacists and their involvement during therapeutic plan development had a substantial positive effect on the healthcare system and disease management [11,12]. Shifting our concerns to the role of hospital pharmacists and antibiotic resistance, Sakeena and colleagues in their narrative review reported that aptly trained hospital pharmacists, when integrated into the health care system, can make a significant impact in minimizing inappropriate antibiotic use and resistance [13]. Hospital pharmacists promote the safe and cost-effective use of antibiotics, and this is acknowledged by the global healthcare systems [14–17]. However, such data are reported frequently from the developed world, and this is a major limitation faced by healthcare and social scientists around the globe. Developing countries have not yet implemented pharmacist-led initiatives whereby hospital pharmacists can play a key role in minimizing unnecessary prescribing of antibiotics and developing local prescribing guidelines according to diagnoses and local antibiotic susceptibility patterns [13]. Therefore, we strongly advocate using the expertise of hospital pharmacists as medicine counsellors to rationalize antibiotic use in the developing world.

Parallel to the published literature, the role of the hospital pharmacist in disease management and clinical decision-making is shadowed in a developing country like Pakistan. There is a paucity of data on hospital pharmacists' integration into the healthcare system. Moreover, the capability and proficiency of a hospital pharmacist are also questioned by other healthcare professionals. Based on this dearth of information, we aimed to evaluate how hospital pharmacists view the quality use of antibiotics and antibiotic resistance practicing at a local healthcare facility in Quetta city, Pakistan. Conducting this study had twofold reasons: to generate data that can be used as a potential reference for further studies, and to highlight what hospital pharmacists can offer while dealing with antibiotic resistance.

2. Results

2.1. Demographic Information

The demographics are given in Table 1. Fifteen participants were approached; however, three refused participations because of their busy schedule. Therefore, interviews were conducted with twelve participants. Although the saturation was reached at the 10th interview, two additional interviews were carried out for absolute validation.

Table 1. Demographic characteristics of the pharmacists.

Demographics	Frequency	Percentage
Gender		
Male	9	75%
Female	3	25%
Age		
25–35	10	80%
36–50	2	20%
Qualification		
Doctor of Pharmacy	7	58.3%
M.Phil	4	33.3%
Ph.D.	1	8.4%
Experience in years		
1–10 years	5	41.6%
11–20 years	7	58.4%
Designation		
Hospital pharmacist	11	91.6%
Chief pharmacist	1	8.4%

Most of the participants were male (75%), with age ranging from 25 to 35 years (80%). Half of the pharmacists had a Doctor of Pharmacy degree and had 11–20 years of experience.

The thematic content analysis revealed five themes and eight subthemes which are shown in Figure 1.

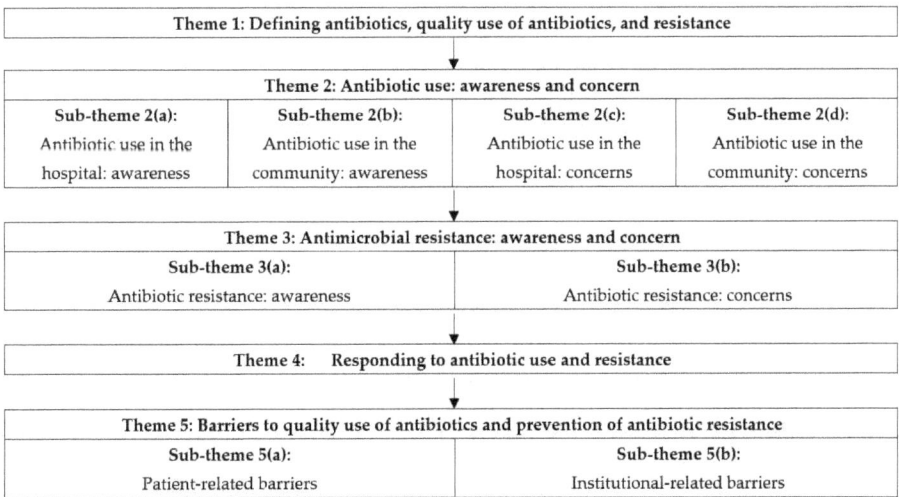

Figure 1. Schematic presentation of themes and sub-themes identified during data analysis.

2.2. Theme 1: Defining Antibiotics, Quality Use of Antibiotics, and Resistance

As expected, all pharmacists had a clear understanding of antibiotics, the quality use of antibiotics, and the development of antibiotic resistance. Additionally, the pharmacists mentioned routinely updating their knowledge about antibiotic use and resistance through updated information sources (journal articles, trusted websites, and books). This is encouraging because evidence-based information in pharmacy practice incorporates pharmacists' clinical expertise with the most accessible evidence. The availability of evidence-based information also helps in justifying the medication-related needs of the healthcare system, prescribing practices, and patients' predilections [18,19].

> "Antibiotics; Fleming' gift for mankind are static and cidal in nature. These are the drugs of choice against primary and secondary bacterial infections." (Pharmacist 1)

In parallel, pharmacists had decent knowledge about antibiotic resistance. It was obvious that pharmacists understood the phenomenon that can eventually help in the delivery of pharmaceutical care [20].

> "The over-use and misuse of antibiotics, bacterial mutations, and substantial use of antibiotics in agriculture and among animals (like poultry and livestock) result in developing antibiotic resistance." (Pharmacist 3)

2.3. Theme 2: Antibiotic Use: Awareness and Concern

2.3.1. Sub-Theme 2(a): Antibiotic Use in the Hospital: Awareness

Respondents of the current study acknowledged frequent use of antibiotics at the setting site. Furthermore, as the influx of inpatients is high compared to outpatients, the use of parenteral antibiotics was commonly reported. Among the commonly prescribed antibiotics were Ceftriaxone (3rd generation cephalosporin), Ciprofloxacin (fluoroquinolones), Vancomycin (glycopeptides), Meropenem (carbapenem), and Piperacillin-Tazobactam (β-lactam/beta-lactamase inhibitors).

> "The physicians prescribe oral antibiotics to the outpatients (based on the availability in the central pharmacy); however, Meropenem and Vancomycin are frequently used (inpatient) when compared to other antibiotics. It is estimated that every third or maybe fourth prescription contains these two drugs." (Pharmacist 6)

2.3.2. Sub-Theme 2(b): Antibiotic Use in the Community: Awareness

The absence of an effective surveillance system and poorly regulated legislature results in the free availability of antibiotics without prescription. Community pharmacies (medical stores) lack authorized personnel (community pharmacists) and are operated by laymen with no prior knowledge, qualification, or training in running a community pharmacy. Most of the pharmacists had information about antimicrobial dispensing rules according to Pakistan's Drug Act 1976 and the Drug Regulatory Authority of Pakistan Act 2012. However, few know the drug laws (schedule G and D) that elaborate the use and dispensing of antibiotics at the communal level.

> "From brands to generics, everything is freely available at the pharmacies. Everybody knows about it including policymakers and officials of the inspection teams. Till today, no one took serious action against the free availability and public sale of antibiotics." (Pharmacist 7)

2.3.3. Sub-Theme 2(c): Antibiotic Use in the Hospital: Concerns

The limited availability of antibiotics in the hospital and a high influx of patients requiring antibiotics was reported as a significant concern by all pharmacists. This is reasonable as the healthcare facilities are limited (in terms of human resources, utilities, and funding) and the prescribers have no or limited choice to prescribe antibiotics based on the availability in the central pharmacy.

"If I can recall, there are not more than 10 antibiotics available in the hospital. Therefore, antibiotic selection is based on availability and not on therapeutic needs. Rationally, yes this is malpractice, but what other choice do we have?" (Pharmacist 10)

2.3.4. Sub-Theme 2(d): Antibiotic Use in the Community: Concerns

The free availability of antibiotics, antibiotic sharing, and nonprofessional referrals of antibiotic use in the community was the primary concern of the pharmacists. These factors were linked to economic and therapeutic loss to society. Moreover, this free availability and frequent use of antibiotics were rated as important factors in developing antibiotic resistance. In comparison, antibiotic use in the community was ranked as a substantial problem when compared to antibiotic use in hospitals.

"Just name the antibiotic, the quantity and there you have it. There are zero concepts of the recommended dosage, treatment duration, and actual need for antibiotics. Community pharmacies are encouraging antibiotic resistance, and this is increasing day by day." (Pharmacist 8)

2.4. Theme 3: Antimicrobial Resistance: Awareness and Concern

2.4.1. Sub-Theme 3(a): Antibiotic Resistance: Awareness

The respondents agreed that antibiotic resistance is a significant issue and has increased after the pandemic. They were also of the opinion that the irrational use of antibiotics at the communal level is promoting antibiotic resistance and needs imperative attention.

"Irrational prescribing, self-medication, using leftovers, all results in antibiotic resistance. Other reasons are also reported in the literature, but we have to admit that the issue is serious and needs prompt actions." (Pharmacist 4)

2.4.2. Sub-Theme 3(b): Antibiotic Resistance: Concerns

"Last week a six-month child was subjected to cultural sensitivity. The kid was resistant to eleven tested antibiotics." (Pharmacist 5). The development of antibiotic resistance was taken seriously by all respondents that are resulting in suffering, deaths, and economic loss. Pharmacists also reported that antibiotic resistance at their practicing site is also emerging as treatment failure is often reported with the use of first or second-line antibiotics.

"I observed that compared to last year, antibiotics (specifically Ciprofloxacin and Ceftriaxone) are least effective. The physicians are now routinely prescribing Meropenem, Vancomycin, and Tazobactam. We must wake up because this is a serious concern and as I see it, there is no solution in near future too." (Pharmacist 1)

2.5. Theme 4: Responding to Antibiotic Use and Resistance

As evident from the above conversation, our respondents were versed in antibiotic use and resistance. Consequently, we wanted to extract pharmacists' viewpoints on how they respond to antibiotic use and the development of antibiotic resistance in their practice settings. Although all respondents agreed that they play a pivotal role in medicine management, mixed views were observed when the response to antibiotic use was investigated.

"Although I follow need and evidence-based medication (specifically when it comes to antibiotic), I must keep an eye on the generic availability in our stock." (Pharmacist 9)

Six pharmacists claimed that they often try to convince the patients about generic substitution to save costs as well as about the importance of completing the complete therapy. Most of the patients come from a meager income background; they have no idea about the quality use of antibiotics.

"I normally guide the patients about the importance of antibiotics, the hazards of antibiotic resistance, and the financial and social repercussions. I hope that a medically educated patient can help in halting the development of antibiotic resistance." (Pharmacist 11)

Three of the interviewees agreed that we could not control antibiotic resistance alone without implementing guidelines, laws, and legislation for antibiotic use. The interviewed hospital pharmacists also pointed out a few strategies to control the emergence of antibiotic resistance by involving all key stakeholders of the healthcare system.

"Alone, we cannot reduce antibiotic resistance. It is emerging at a high pace and a collective approach is needed to overcome this problem. The policymakers should target a mass population as well as an individualized strategy that must focus on community members and healthcare professionals to safeguard the use of antibiotics." (Pharmacist 9)

2.6. Theme 5: Barriers to Quality Use of Antibiotics and Prevention of Antibiotic Resistance

It is now acknowledged that antibiotic resistance can be reduced by prescribing antibiotics rationally based on established guidelines, antibiotic susceptibility testing, and clinical response. In parallel, the surveillance of antibiotic availability in healthcare settings, restrictive self-medication, and over-prescription is also needed. However, antibiotic resistance can only be controlled and minimized by the determined efforts of all healthcare professionals (physicians, pharmacists, nurses). Several barriers were identified by the study respondents while addressing the quality use of antibiotics and the development of antibiotic resistance and will be discussed consequently.

2.6.1. Subtheme 5(a): Patient-Related Barriers

Self-medication, using leftover antibiotics, referral of antibiotics (friends and families), expecting an antibiotic during the consultation, and demanding an antibiotic by themselves were identified as the key barriers to the quality use of antibiotics and antibiotic resistance. Patient education and counseling were last reported at the healthcare institutes and that was rated as a major factor in developing the false ideology about antibiotics as mentioned above.

"Our patients demand antibiotics and will go to different stores to get one. The physician is considered incompetent if an antibiotic is not prescribed. This mindset is shaping as a key barrier to quality use of antibiotics in our society." (Pharmacist 3)

Another barrier to rational use of antibiotics was related to the urgency of being cured. We must agree that when faced with a disease, expecting a quick recovery is obvious. However, this tendency does not allow misuse of antibiotics considering that it will pace up the recovery time. Nevertheless, patients are in the habit of using antibiotics for a fast pace of recovery, and this is shaping as a factor in developing antibiotic resistance.

"While being questioned (by physicians or nurses), using an antibiotic before coming to the hospital is usually reported by the patients. The reason is always the same (it cures everything). This is an issue that we are facing almost daily. Don't you think this is causing antibiotic resistance?" (Pharmacist 4)

2.6.2. Subtheme 5(a): Institutional-Related Barriers

Most of the respondents also emphasized certain institution-related deficiencies and limitations as barriers to the quality use of antibiotics and antibiotic resistance. The most reported barrier was the limited number of antibiotics available at the central pharmacy. Medicines are supplied annually based on hospital demand and because purchasing budgets are low, medicines are not adequately available. The availability is attained by reducing the quantity and types of medicines (when one class of antibiotic is available, the other class is inevitably rejected). However, this limits the choice of the prescribers, and they must prescribe what is available at the hospital.

"We work in a public hospital where 70–80% of medicine is provided by the hospital to the inpatients. However, we have financial limitations, and availability of antibiotics from all therapeutic classes is not possible." (Pharmacist 12)

Another barrier to the quality use of antibiotics was related to the limited capacity of cultural sensitivity. By practice, the developed guidelines advocate an initiation of empirical therapy followed by a culture sensitivity test. However, this was last performed at the study site, and without sensitivity reports being available, the practice promoted antibiotic resistance.

"We have limited the capacity of performing a culture sensitivity test. Because most of our patients belong to the below-average income group, ordering a sensitivity test is unaffordable for the patients. In such scenarios, we have no choice but to continue using the same antibiotics." (Pharmacist 10)

3. Discussion

For decades, healthcare and social scientists have been trying to minimize the burden of antibiotic resistance. Among those, numerous interventions and measures have been taken that too have reported their effectivity and effectuality [21–24]. However, with the development of new resistance mechanisms, antibiotic resistance is rising dangerously around the globe [8]. Additionally, the emergence of COVID-19 reported increased use of antibiotics that again resulted in augmenting antibiotic resistance [25,26]. Hence, the role of healthcare professionals in promoting the quality use of antibiotics remains crucial as they are the frontline specialists while tackling antibiotic resistance and its consequences. Among healthcare professionals, because of their duty for rationalizing antibiotic use, being medicine managers and patient educators, hospital pharmacists are critically placed and can play a key role in promoting the safe use of antibiotics. Within this context, we are aware that literature does mention hospital pharmacists' viewpoint on antibiotic use and resistance [27–30], but nothing is reported from the current study settings. We are also aware that several studies on the knowledge and practices of pharmacists are reported from Pakistan, but the target audience was different from what is reported in our study. Where Saleem et al. focused community pharmacists [31], Mubarak et al. targeted pharmacy students regarding their views of antibiotic use and resistance [32] and widely held information focused on antibiotic stewardship. Therefore, one distinct advantage of the current study is the pioneer study from Pakistan that evaluated the knowledge and attitudes of hospital pharmacists about antibiotic use and resistance along with the views and concerns on contributing factors.

Pharmacists' positive perception towards the quality use of antibiotics and antibiotic resistance was an encouraging finding of the current study. However, mixed observations were reported when the results of the current study were cross-compared with the published literature. Al-Tanni et al. in their study concluded that although pharmacists' knowledge of the quality use of antibiotics was satisfactory, the perception towards the spread of resistance was unsatisfactory [33]. Similarly, Tang et al. in their multi-centered study also identified significant knowledge gaps among pharmacists and the gap was prominent among work settings [34]. The European Centre for Disease Prevention and Control (ECDC) surveyed 1204 hospital pharmacists in 2019 and reported that although the respondents had good knowledge of antibiotics, ensuring the knowledge about resistance was highlighted as an area of improvement among the pharmacists [35]. Better knowledge of the current study respondents is a positive indication when correlating it with the goal of the Institute of Medicine (IMS) suggested in 2020. Accordingly, IMS proposed that by 2020, 90% of clinical decisions must be supported with accurate, timely, and up-to-date clinical information that should reflect the best available evidence to achieve the best patient outcomes [36]. Hospital pharmacists of the current study contained updated information (revealed during informal discussion) and that is an indication of providing an effective therapeutic plan when it comes to the quality use of antibiotics and containment of antibiotic resistance.

The results of this qualitative study revealed that the use of broad-spectrum antibiotics is widespread at the study site. Our respondents were aware and anxious about this imprudent use of antibiotics, and this is similar to the findings of Tarrant et al. [37]. The authors also reported frequent use of broad-spectrum antibiotics in three countries, which is supported by studies of the same nature [33,38]. Among the drivers, the use of broad-spectrum antibiotics was also mentioned by the current study respondents. A method of overcoming these issues is establishing medical education programs and providing credits to the prescribers that can act as a benchmark in annual assessment plans.

Another key finding of the current study was the limited availability of antibiotics in the hospital and hence a reduced choice for the prescribers while dealing with infectious diseases. In addition, poor culture sensitivity testing was highlighted. Unfortunately, the evidence-based data are lacking from Baluchistan, and we do not have an actual picture of such limitations. However, our personal observation goes parallel to what is reported by the respondents as there is a lack or limited number of antibiotics at the hospital. Within this context, the healthcare system of Pakistan is faced with severe financial limitations and is unable to cater to the needs of the patients [39]. Healthcare financing in Pakistan is mainly out-of-pocket, there are inequities at the healthcare levels, and at times care is not attained because of non-affordability [39]. The pandemic crisis and the current financial crunch are again posing a great threat to medicine availability at public healthcare facilities [40]. Although the reasons are genuine, limited availability, continuous use of the same antibiotics, and lack of sensitivity testing are posing an incessant threat to the development of antibiotic resistance. Frankly speaking, we do not see a solution to this threat soon, but it is true that there is going to be a continuous rise in antibiotic resistance. Healthcare professionals, policymakers, and financial stakeholders must realize the severity of this issue and propose concrete measures to ensure the appropriate availability of antibiotics at public healthcare institutions. Our suggestions are in line with the recommendations of the Pakistan Antimicrobial Resistance Surveillance System Surveillance Report of 2020 whereby the limitations were acknowledged and immediate actions to overcome the limitations were advocated.

Finally, patient-reported factors were rated as a predictor of antibiotic resistance by the study respondents. Among these, self-medications, personal referrals, and demanding an antibiotic were the major variables. These findings are not new, and the literature does support the claims of our study respondents. Nepal and Bhatta in their systematic review highlighted the high prevalence of self-medication of antibiotics in the WHO Southeast Asian Region and this hence was the leading cause of antibiotic resistance [41]. Similarly, Väänänen and Airaksinen also reported excessive and nonsensical self-medication of antibiotics in the European region [42]. Correspondingly, Nair and colleagues in their qualitative study confirmed that patients tend to demand antibiotics as they seek a fast cure [43]. Such comparable findings indicate a lack of communal knowledge of antibiotic use and resistance and the need for immediate attention from healthcare providers, especially pharmacists. Patients are to be provided ample medical education regarding antibiotic use and resistance and pharmacists must step up to engage their patients in education and counselling. In addition, the policymakers must ensure strict compliance with antibiotic sales at the community level and employ mass educational strategies to halt self-medication and referral of suggesting antibiotics to a friend, family, and societal members.

4. Materials and Methods

4.1. Study Design and Settings

Because of the scarcity of information, a qualitative study design (in-depth, face-to-face interviews) was the ultimate choice. Being amenable, qualitative methods can extract attitudes, experiences, and intentions that are often missed in a quantitative phase [44,45].

Because the research team was faced with limited published literature, using a qualitative design was appropriate as it can generate a wide range of ideas and opinions and divulging viewpoints [46,47]. As we were aiming for inductive approaches to generate ideologies and concepts, a qualitative design was also adopted because it has more potential for research than any other models [48]. Additionally, the COREQ checklist was used to describe the qualitative methodology and that is presented as Appendix A.

The research was conducted at the Surgical Department of Sandeman Provincial Hospital, Quetta (SPHQ). Centrally located, SPHQ is a tertiary care hospital and provides generalized healthcare facilities. Additionally, being a public institute, SPHQ is a choice for most of the population [49].

4.2. Study Participants, Criteria, and Sampling

Hospital pharmacists stationed and practicing at the surgical unit and consenting to participate in the study were approached for data collection. Based on our objective, it was apparent to adopt the purposive sampling method [50]. Pharmacists on rotations and not willing to participate were excluded.

4.3. The Interview Guide (Validation, Reliability, and Pilot Study)

We constructed a semi-structured interview guide after an extensive literature review [51–55], through expert panel discussion and experience sharing [56–58]. To extract maximum information, we intentionally constructed the guide with widely framed, open-ended questions. Additionally, pharmacists were allowed to provide their narratives and to share information relevant to antibiotic use and resistance.

The guide was constructed in the English language and was subjected to face and content validity through a panel of experts (senior pharmacists). Once the validity was ensured, the guide was piloted with four pharmacists to ensure that the topics to be discussed were at the level that respondents would comprehend with ease. The preliminary data and conclusion confirmed that the discussion topics were enough and appropriately phrased to answer research questions and minimize validity and reliability threats. As the validity and reliability of the discussion guide were ensured, it was made available for the main study. Data and participants of the pilot study were not included in the final analysis.

4.4. Interview Procedure, Data Collection, and Analysis

ZI (male, a certified medical practitioner, District Health Officer, certified in Qualitative methods) and FS (male, academic pharmacist with a PhD having experience of qualitative research with numerous published articles) conducted the interviews. FS was also involved in carrying out field notes during the interviews.

Interviews were conducted at the pharmacist's office in the surgical unit. All participants were briefed about the study objectives before the interviews. A debriefing session was again conducted at the end of the discussion. The interviews started with an ice-breaking session. Probing questions were asked in between conversations to clarify the meanings of responses and to gain insight into the topic being discussed.

The phenomenology-based approach commissioned in-depth, face-to-face interviews. All interviews were audio-taped followed by transcribed verbatim and were then analyzed for thematic contents by the standard content analysis framework. Each interview lasted for approximately half an hour. To draw in-depth views, the freedom to express additional reviews and comments was given. Interviews were conducted until thematic saturation was reached [59,60]. No repeat interviews were carried out.

The research team analyzed the recordings (verbatim) and later arranged an informal gathering where pharmacist were presented with the finalized interview scripts [61]. They were asked for confirmation of the precision and accuracy of words, ideas, and jargon used during the script analysis. Once confirmed, the transcripts were subjected to content analysis whereby four data coders were involved in the process [62,63]. NVivo® was used for coding and analysis through iterations [64] and inconsistencies were resolved through mutual consensus. Interviews were coded line-by-line, and an initial list of nodes was developed. Later, this augmented in developing the framework and transcripts were coded accordingly. New emerging nodes were added to the existing list and were categories as emerging themes. All emerging themes and subthemes were discussed among the research team for accuracy and were presented for data inference and interpretation.

5. Conclusions

The current study managed to identify an adequate understanding of antibiotic use and resistance among hospital pharmacists. Additionally, prospective concerns (limited availability of antibiotics) and possible predictors of antibiotic resistance (lack of sensitivity testing, self-medication, referrals, and demanding an antibiotic) were also highlighted factors contributing factors were also identified. As corrective measures, respondents of the current study focused on strict legislation to overcome the free availability and sales of antibiotics at the community level, ensuring the implementation of guidelines for the prescribers and copious availability of antibiotics and sensitivity testing facilities at the healthcare institutes. Therefore, we urge that these findings must be disseminated to policy-makers and prescribers to take restorative action as soon as possible. Antibiotic resistance is a global threat, and we need a holistic approach to tackle this issue for generations while combating infectious diseases with precision.

6. Limitations and Recommendations

Qualitative methods have their limitations. Although we ensured saturation, the convenience sampling approach does not offer views of the participants that are not interviewed. Likewise, generalizability is always an issue with qualitative methods. However, with rich data extraction, we are confident that the study has provided baseline information for prospective studies. Therefore, we are recommending an in-depth and detailed study (quantitative) focusing on a large cohort of hospital pharmacists to ensure the validity of the current findings.

Author Contributions: Conceptualization, M.F. and S.H.; methodology, M.S.A. and Q.I.; interviews, F.S. and Z.I., analyses, interpretation and transcription, A.S. and A.R., writing original draft, review of final manuscript, all authors. All authors have read and agreed to the published version of the manuscript.

Funding: This research received no external funding.

Institutional Review Board Statement: This study was conducted in accordance with the Declaration of Helsinki and was approved by the Institutional Review Board at the Faculty of Pharmacy & Health Sciences, University of Baluchistan, Quetta (FoP&HS/IRB/41/22).

Informed Consent Statement: Written consent was obtained from all subjects involved in the study. Furthermore, written informed consent has been obtained from the pharmacist(s) to publish this paper.

Data Availability Statement: The data are available from the corresponding author upon reasonable request.

Acknowledgments: The researchers would like to thank the Deanship of Scientific Research, Qassim University, Saudi Arabia for funding the publication of this project.

Conflicts of Interest: The authors declare no conflict of interest.

Appendix A

Table A1. The consolidated criteria for reporting qualitative studies (COREQ).

Topic	Guide Questions/Description	Remarks	Page No.
Domain 1: Research team and reflexivity			
(a) Personal Characteristics			
Interviewer/facilitator	Which author/s conducted the interview or focus group?	Two authors ZI and FS conducted the interviews.	9
Credentials	What were the researcher's credentials? e.g., Ph.D., MD	ZI: MBBS; MPH FS: Ph.D.	9
Occupation	What was their occupation at the time of the study?	ZI: Deputy District Health Officer, Government of Baluchistan FS: Academic/pharmacist	9
Gender	Was the researcher male or female?	ZI: Male FS: Male	9
Experience and training	What experience or training did the researcher have?	ZI: Certification in qualitative research methods (CQRM); attended workshop on NViVO for data analyses. FS: an experienced researcher in qualitative studies and has published numerous qualitative research articles.	9
(b) Relationship with participants			
Relationship established	Was a relationship established prior to study commencement?	The relationship was developed only for the current study.	N/A
Participant knowledge of the interviewer	What did the participants know about the researcher? e.g., personal goals, reasons for doing the research	None of the participants knew about the researchers.	N/A
Interviewer characteristics	What characteristics were reported about the interviewer/facilitator? E.g., Bias, assumptions, reasons, and interests in the research topic	The characteristics were presented as researchers and authors.	1
Domain 2: Study design			
(a) Theoretical framework			
Methodological orientation and Theory	What methodological orientation was stated to underpin the study? e.g., grounded theory, discourse analysis, ethnography, phenomenology, content analysis	Phenomenology and thematic content analysis.	9
(b) Participant selection			
Sampling	How were participants selected? e.g., purposive, convenience, consecutive, snowball	The participants were purposively selected.	9
Method of approach	How were participants approached? e.g., face-to-face, telephone, mail, email	The participants were approached face-to-face.	9
Sample size	How many participants were in the study?	12 participants were approached for the interviews.	3
Non-participation	How many people refused to participate or dropped out? Reasons?	We approached 15 participants. Three people refused as they were busy with their routine work.	3

Table A1. *Cont.*

Topic	Guide Questions/Description	Remarks	Page No.
(c) Setting			
Setting of data collection	Where was the data collected? e.g., home, clinic, workplace	Data were collected at the pharmacists' workplace.	9
Presence of non-participants	Was anyone else present besides the participants and researchers?	No-one else was present to ensure confidentiality of the responses.	N/A
Description of sample	What are the important characteristics of the sample? e.g., demographic data, date.	The important characteristics are presented in Table 1.	3
(d) Data collection			
Interview guide	Were questions, prompts, guides provided by the authors? Was it pilot tested?	A semi-structured interview guide was developed, and pilot tested with 4 pharmacists. Data of the pilot phase was not included in the final analysis.	9
Repeat interviews	Were repeat inter views carried out? If yes, how many?	No repeat interviews were carried.	9
Audio/visual recording	Did the research use audio or visual recording to collect the data?	All interviews were audio recorded.	9
Field notes	Were field notes made during and/or after the interview or focus group?	FS prepared then field notes during the interviews that assisted the transcription.	9
Duration	What was the duration of the inter views or focus group?	The duration of the in-depth interviews was approximately 30 min.	9
Data saturation	Was data saturation discussed?	Yes	3
Transcripts returned	Were transcripts returned to participants for comment and/or correction?	Yes, transcripts were return for confirmation of the precision and accuracy of words, ideas, and jargon used during the script analysis.	9
Domain 3: Analysis and findings			
(a) Data analysis			
Number of data coders	How many data coders coded the data?	Four data coders coded the data.	9
Description of the coding tree	Did authors provide a description of the coding tree?	Interviews were coded line-by-line, and an initial list of nodes was developed. Later, this augmented in developing the framework and transcripts were coded accordingly. New emerging nodes were added to the existing list and were categories as emerging themes.	9
Derivation of themes	Were themes identified in advance or derived from the data?	All themes were derived from the data.	4–7
Software	What software, if applicable, was used to manage the data?	NVivo® was used to manage the data.	9
Participant checking	Did participants provide feedback on the findings?	No	N/A

Table A1. *Cont.*

Topic	Guide Questions/Description	Remarks	Page No.
(b) Reporting			
Quotations presented	Were participant quotations presented to illustrate the themes/findings? Was each quotation identified? e.g., participant number	Yes, all quotations were cross matched with the respondent's demographics.	4–7
Data and findings consistent	Was there consistency between the data presented and the findings?	Yes	4–7
Clarity of major themes	Were major themes clearly presented in the findings?	Yes	4–7
Clarity of minor themes	Is there a description of diverse cases or discussion of minor themes?	Sub themes were identified and are presented and discussed in the manuscript.	4–7

References

1. Uddin, T.M.; Chakraborty, A.J.; Khusro, A.; Zidan, B.R.M.; Mitra, S.; Emran, T.B.; Dhama, K.; Ripon, M.K.H.; Gajdács, M.; Sahibzada, M.U.K. Antibiotic resistance in microbes: History, mechanisms, therapeutic strategies and future prospects. *J. Infect. Public Health* **2021**, *14*, 1750–1766. [CrossRef] [PubMed]
2. Action on Antibiotic Resistance. The Discovery of Antibiotics. Available online: https://www.reactgroup.org/antibiotic-resistance/course-antibiotic-resistance-the-silent-tsunami/part-1/the-discovery-of-antibiotics/#:~:text=In%20his%20Nobel%20lecture%20in,occasionally%20happened%20in%20the%20body (accessed on 17 December 2022).
3. Podolsky, S.H. The evolving response to antibiotic resistance (1945–2018). *Palgrave Commun.* **2018**, *4*, 1–8. [CrossRef]
4. Ben, Y.; Fu, C.; Hu, M.; Liu, L.; Wong, M.H.; Zheng, C. Human health risk assessment of antibiotic resistance associated with antibiotic residues in the environment: A review. *Environ. Res.* **2019**, *169*, 483–493. [CrossRef] [PubMed]
5. De Kraker, M.E.; Stewardson, A.J.; Harbarth, S. Will 10 million people die a year due to antimicrobial resistance by 2050? *PLoS Med.* **2016**, *13*, e1002184. [CrossRef] [PubMed]
6. Aslam, B.; Wang, W.; Arshad, M.I.; Khurshid, M.; Muzammil, S.; Rasool, M.H.; Nisar, M.A.; Alvi, R.F.; Aslam, M.A.; Qamar, M.U. Antibiotic resistance: A rundown of a global crisis. *Infect. Drug Resist.* **2018**, *11*, 1645. [CrossRef]
7. Ilić, K.; Jakovljević, E.; Škodrić-Trifunović, V. Social-economic factors and irrational antibiotic use as reasons for antibiotic resistance of bacteria causing common childhood infections in primary healthcare. *Eur. J. Pediatr.* **2012**, *171*, 767–777. [CrossRef]
8. World Health Organization. Antibiotic Resistance. Available online: https://www.who.int/news-room/fact-sheets/detail/antibiotic-resistance (accessed on 10 December 2022).
9. Centers for Disease Control and Prevention. COVID-19 Reverses Progress in Fight against Antimicrobial Resistance in U.S. Available online: https://www.cdc.gov/media/releases/2022/s0712-Antimicrobial-Resistance.html#:~:text=In%20the%20report%2C%20CDC%20analyzed,to%202020%20among%20seven%20pathogens (accessed on 5 December 2022).
10. Khan, N.; McGarry, K.; Naqvi, A.A.; Iqbal, M.S.; Haider, Z. Pharmacists' viewpoint towards their professional role in healthcare system: A survey of hospital settings of Pakistan. *BMC Health Serv. Res.* **2020**, *20*, 1–15. [CrossRef]
11. Clay, P.G. Turning the criticism into construction. *J. Am. Pharm. Assoc.* **2016**, *56*, 599–600. [CrossRef]
12. Greer, N.; Bolduc, J.; Geurkink, E.; Rector, T.; Olson, K.; Koeller, E.; MacDonald, R.; Wilt, T.J. Pharmacist-led chronic disease management: A systematic review of effectiveness and harms compared with usual care. *Ann. Intern. Med.* **2016**, *165*, 30–40. [CrossRef]
13. Sakeena, M.; Bennett, A.A.; McLachlan, A.J. Enhancing pharmacists' role in developing countries to overcome the challenge of antimicrobial resistance: A narrative review. *Antimicrob. Resist. Infect. Control* **2018**, *7*, 1–11. [CrossRef]
14. Ellis, K.; Rubal-Peace, G.; Chang, V.; Liang, E.; Wong, N.; Campbell, S. Antimicrobial stewardship for a geriatric behavioral health population. *Antibiotics* **2016**, *5*, 8. [CrossRef]
15. Okada, N.; Fushitani, S.; Azuma, M.; Nakamura, S.; Nakamura, T.; Teraoka, K.; Watanabe, H.; Abe, M.; Kawazoe, K.; Ishizawa, K. Clinical evaluation of pharmacist interventions in patients treated with anti-methicillin-resistant *Staphylococcus aureus* agents in a hematological ward. *Biol. Pharm. Bull.* **2016**, *39*, 295–300. [CrossRef]
16. Yen, Y.-H.; Chen, H.-Y.; Wuan-Jin, L.; Lin, Y.-M.; Shen, W.C.; Cheng, K.-J. Clinical and economic impact of a pharmacist-managed iv-to-po conversion service for levofloxacin in Taiwan. *Int. J. Clin. Pharmacol. Ther.* **2012**, *50*, 136. [CrossRef]
17. Zhou, Y.; Ma, L.Y.; Zhao, X.; Tian, S.H.; Sun, L.Y.; Cui, Y.M. Impact of pharmacist intervention on antibiotic use and prophylactic antibiotic use in urology clean operations. *J. Clin. Pharm. Ther.* **2015**, *40*, 404–408. [CrossRef]
18. Al-Quteimat, O.M.; Amer, A.M. Evidence-based pharmaceutical care: The next chapter in pharmacy practice. *Saudi Pharm. J.* **2016**, *24*, 447–451. [CrossRef]
19. Lewis, S.J.; Orland, B.I. The importance and impact of Evidence Based Medicine. *J. Manag. Care Pharm.* **2004**, *10*, S3–S5. [CrossRef]

20. Chan, A.H.Y.; Beyene, K.; Tuck, C.; Rutter, V.; Ashiru-Oredope, D. Pharmacist beliefs about antimicrobial resistance and impacts on antibiotic supply: A multinational survey. *JAC Antimicrob. Resist.* **2022**, *4*, dlac062. [CrossRef]
21. Borek, A.J.; Campbell, A.; Dent, E.; Butler, C.C.; Holmes, A.; Moore, M.; Walker, A.S.; McLeod, M.; Tonkin-Crine, S. Implementing interventions to reduce antibiotic use: A qualitative study in high-prescribing practices. *BMC Fam. Pract.* **2021**, *22*, 1–11. [CrossRef]
22. Raban, M.Z.; Gasparini, C.; Li, L.; Baysari, M.T.; Westbrook, J.I. Effectiveness of interventions targeting antibiotic use in long-term aged care facilities: A systematic review and meta-analysis. *BMJ Open* **2020**, *10*, e028494. [CrossRef]
23. Rogers Van Katwyk, S.; Grimshaw, J.M.; Nkangu, M.; Nagi, R.; Mendelson, M.; Taljaard, M.; Hoffman, S.J. Government policy interventions to reduce human antimicrobial use: A systematic review and evidence map. *PLoS Med.* **2019**, *16*, e1002819. [CrossRef]
24. Smith, R.D.; Coast, J.; Millar, M.R.; Wilton, P.; Karcher, A.-M. Interventions against Antimicrobial Resistance: A Review of the Literature and Exploration of Modelling Cost-Effectiveness. In *Global Forum for Health Research*; WHO: Geneve, Switzerland, 2001. Available online: https://apps.who.int/iris/handle/10665/66936 (accessed on 11 December 2022).
25. Getahun, H.; Smith, I.; Trivedi, K.; Paulin, S.; Balkhy, H.H. Tackling antimicrobial resistance in the COVID-19 pandemic. *Bull. World Health Organ.* **2020**, *98*, 442. [CrossRef] [PubMed]
26. Hashmi, F.K.; Atif, N.; Malik, U.R.; Saleem, F.; Riboua, Z.; Hassali, M.A.; Butt, M.H.; Mallhi, T.H.; Khan, Y.H. In pursuit of COVID-19 treatment strategies: Are we triggering antimicrobial resistance? *Disaster Med. Public Health Prep.* **2022**, *16*, 1285–1286. [CrossRef] [PubMed]
27. Broom, A.; Broom, J.; Kirby, E.; Plage, S.; Adams, J. What role do pharmacists play in mediating antibiotic use in hospitals? A qualitative study. *BMJ Open* **2015**, *5*, e008326. [CrossRef] [PubMed]
28. Broom, A.; Broom, J.; Kirby, E.; Scambler, G. The path of least resistance? Jurisdictions, responsibility and professional asymmetries in pharmacists' accounts of antibiotic decisions in hospitals. *Soc. Sci. Med.* **2015**, *146*, 95–103. [CrossRef]
29. Dooling, K.L.; Kandeel, A.; Hicks, L.A.; El-Shoubary, W.; Fawzi, K.; Kandeel, Y.; Etman, A.; Lohiniva, A.L.; Talaat, M. Understanding antibiotic use in Minya District, Egypt: Physician and pharmacist prescribing and the factors influencing their practices. *Antibiotics* **2014**, *3*, 233–243. [CrossRef]
30. Garau, J.; Bassetti, M. Role of pharmacists in antimicrobial stewardship programmes. *Int. J. Clin. Pharm.* **2018**, *40*, 948–952. [CrossRef]
31. Saleem, Z.; Hassali, M.A.; Hashmi, F.K.; Godman, B.; Saleem, F. Antimicrobial dispensing practices and determinants of antimicrobial resistance: A qualitative study among community pharmacists in Pakistan. *Fam. Med. Community Health* **2019**, *7*, e000138. [CrossRef]
32. Mubarak, N.; Arif, S.; Irshad, M.; Aqeel, R.M.; Khalid, A.; Ijaz, U.E.B.; Mahmood, K.; Jamshed, S.; Zin, C.S.; Saif-Ur-Rehman, N. How Are We Educating Future Physicians and Pharmacists in Pakistan? A Survey of the Medical and Pharmacy Student's Perception on Learning and Preparedness to Assume Future Roles in Antibiotic Use and Resistance. *Antibiotics* **2021**, *10*, 1204. [CrossRef]
33. Al-Taani, G.M.; Al-Azzam, S.; Karasneh, R.A.; Sadeq, A.S.; Mazrouei, N.A.; Bond, S.E.; Conway, B.R.; Aldeyab, M.A. Pharmacists' Knowledge, Attitudes, Behaviors and Information Sources on Antibiotic Use and Resistance in Jordan. *Antibiotics* **2022**, *11*, 175. [CrossRef]
34. Tang, K.L.; Teoh, T.F.; Ooi, T.T.; Khor, W.P.; Ong, S.Y.; Lim, P.P.; Abdul Karim, S.; Tan, S.S.A.; Ch'ng, P.P.; Choong, Y.C. Public hospital pharmacists' perceptions and knowledge of antibiotic use and resistance: A multicenter survey. *Antibiotics* **2020**, *9*, 311. [CrossRef]
35. Ashiru-Oredope, D.; Hopkins, S.; Vasandani, S.; Umoh, E.; Oloyede, O.; Nilsson, A.; Kinsman, J.; Elsert, L.; Monnet, D.L. Healthcare workers' knowledge, attitudes and behaviours with respect to antibiotics, antibiotic use and antibiotic resistance across 30 EU/EEA countries in 2019. *Eurosurveillance* **2021**, *26*, 1900633. [CrossRef]
36. McGinnis, J.M.; Goolsby, W.A.; Olsen, L. *Leadership Commitments to Improve Value in Health Care: Finding Common Ground: Workshop Summary*; National Academies Press: Washington, DC, USA, 2009.
37. Tarrant, C.; Colman, A.M.; Jenkins, D.R.; Chattoe-Brown, E.; Perera, N.; Mehtar, S.; Nakkawita, W.D.; Bolscher, M.; Krockow, E.M. Drivers of Broad-Spectrum Antibiotic Overuse across Diverse Hospital Contexts—A Qualitative Study of Prescribers in the UK, Sri Lanka and South Africa. *Antibiotics* **2021**, *10*, 94. [CrossRef]
38. Lubwama, M.; Onyuka, J.; Ayazika, K.T.; Ssetaba, L.J.; Siboko, J.; Daniel, O.; Mushi, M.F. Knowledge, attitudes, and perceptions about antibiotic use and antimicrobial resistance among final year undergraduate medical and pharmacy students at three universities in East Africa. *PLoS ONE* **2021**, *16*, e0251301. [CrossRef]
39. Malik, M.A.; Wasay, M. Economics of health and health care in Pakistan. *J. Pak. Med. Assoc.* **2013**, *63*, 814–815.
40. The Express Tribune. 'Pakistan in Financial Emergency'. Available online: https://tribune.com.pk/story/2389724/pakistan-in-financial-emergency (accessed on 2 January 2023).
41. Nepal, G.; Bhatta, S. Self-medication with antibiotics in WHO Southeast Asian Region: A systematic review. *Cureus* **2018**, *10*, e2428. [CrossRef]
42. Väänänen, M.H.; Pietilä, K.; Airaksinen, M. Self-medication with antibiotics—Does it really happen in Europe? *Health Policy* **2006**, *77*, 166–171. [CrossRef]

43. Nair, M.; Tripathi, S.; Mazumdar, S.; Mahajan, R.; Harshana, A.; Pereira, A.; Jimenez, C.; Halder, D.; Burza, S. Knowledge, attitudes, and practices related to antibiotic use in Paschim Bardhaman District: A survey of healthcare providers in West Bengal, India. *PLoS ONE* **2019**, *14*, e0217818. [CrossRef]
44. Berg, B.L.; Lune, H.; Lune, H. *Qualitative Research Methods for the Social Sciences*; Pearson: Boston, MA, USA, 2004; Volume 5.
45. Kitzinger, J. Qualitative research: Introducing focus groups. *Br. Med. J.* **1995**, *311*, 299–302. [CrossRef]
46. Krueger, R.A. *Focus Groups: A Practical Guide for Applied Research*; Sage Inc.: London, UK, 2009.
47. Stewart, D.W.; Shamdasani, P.N. *Focus Groups: Theory and Practice*; Sage Publications: Thousand Oaks, CA, USA, 2014; Volume 20.
48. Entwistle, V.A.; Renfrew, M.J.; Yearley, S.; Forrester, J.; Lamont, T. Lay perspectives: Advantages for health research. *Br. Med. J.* **1998**, *316*, 463–466. [CrossRef]
49. Shahzad, F.; Saleem, F.; Iqbal, Q.; Haque, N.; Haider, S.; Salman, M.; Masood, I.; Hassali, M.A.; Iftikhar, S.; Bashaar, M. A cross-sectional assessment of health literacy among hypertensive community of Quetta City, Pakistan. *Biomed. J.* **2018**, *11*, 8685–8693.
50. Brace-Govan, J. Issues in snowball sampling: The lawyer, the model and ethics. *Qual. Res. J.* **2004**, *4*, 52.
51. Asante, K.P.; Boamah, E.A.; Abdulai, M.A.; Buabeng, K.O.; Mahama, E.; Dzabeng, F.; Gavor, E.; Annan, E.A.; Owusu-Agyei, S.; Gyansa-Lutterodt, M. Knowledge of antibiotic resistance and antibiotic prescription practices among prescribers in the Brong Ahafo Region of Ghana; a cross-sectional study. *BMC Health Serv. Res.* **2017**, *17*, 422. [CrossRef] [PubMed]
52. Brooks, L.; Shaw, A.; Sharp, D.; Hay, A.D. Towards a better understanding of patients' perspectives of antibiotic resistance and MRSA: A qualitative study. *Fam. Pract.* **2008**, *25*, 341–348. [CrossRef] [PubMed]
53. Krockow, E.; Colman, A.; Chattoe-Brown, E.; Jenkins, D.; Perera, N.; Mehtar, S.; Tarrant, C. Balancing the risks to individual and society: A systematic review and synthesis of qualitative research on antibiotic prescribing behaviour in hospitals. *J. Hosp. Infect.* **2019**, *101*, 428–439. [CrossRef]
54. Moongtui, W.; Picheansathian, W.; Senaratana, W. Role of Nurses in Prevention of Antimicrobial Resistance. Available online: http://origin.searo.who.int/publications/journals/regional_health_forum/media/2011/V15n1/rhfv15n1p104.pdf (accessed on 15 July 2020).
55. Nair, M.; Tripathi, S.; Mazumdar, S.; Mahajan, R.; Harshana, A.; Pereira, A.; Jimenez, C.; Halder, D.; Burza, S. "Without antibiotics, I cannot treat": A qualitative study of antibiotic use in Paschim Bardhaman district of West Bengal, India. *PLoS ONE* **2019**, *14*, e0219002. [CrossRef]
56. Kallio, H.; Pietilä, A.M.; Johnson, M.; Kangasniemi, M. Systematic methodological review: Developing a framework for a qualitative semi-structured interview guide. *J. Adv. Nurs.* **2016**, *72*, 2954–2965. [CrossRef]
57. Morris, A. *A Practical Introduction to In-Depth Interviewing*; Sage: London, UK, 2015.
58. Voutsina, C. A practical introduction to in-depth interviewing. *Int. J. Res. Method Educ.* **2018**, *41*, 123–124. [CrossRef]
59. Nelson, J. Using conceptual depth criteria: Addressing the challenge of reaching saturation in qualitative research. *Qual. Res.* **2017**, *17*, 554–570. [CrossRef]
60. Saunders, B.; Sim, J.; Kingstone, T.; Baker, S.; Waterfield, J.; Bartlam, B.; Burroughs, H.; Jinks, C. Saturation in qualitative research: Exploring its conceptualization and operationalization. *Qual. Quant.* **2018**, *52*, 1893–1907. [CrossRef]
61. Guest, G.; MacQueen, K.M.; Namey, E.E. Introduction to applied thematic analysis. *Appl. Themat. Anal.* **2012**, *3*, 20.
62. Anderson, R. Thematic content analysis (TCA). *Descr. Present. Qual. Data* **2007**, *3*, 1–4.
63. Vaismoradi, M.; Turunen, H.; Bondas, T. Content analysis and thematic analysis: Implications for conducting a qualitative descriptive study. *Nurs. Health Sci.* **2013**, *15*, 398–405. [CrossRef]
64. Edhlund, B.; McDougall, A. *Nvivo 12 Essentials*; FORM & KUNSKAP AB: Stallarholmen, Sweden, 2019.

Disclaimer/Publisher's Note: The statements, opinions and data contained in all publications are solely those of the individual author(s) and contributor(s) and not of MDPI and/or the editor(s). MDPI and/or the editor(s) disclaim responsibility for any injury to people or property resulting from any ideas, methods, instructions or products referred to in the content.

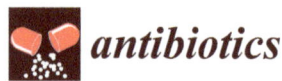

Article

Knowledge, Attitudes, and Practices in Antibiotic Dispensing amongst Pharmacists in Trinidad and Tobago: Exploring a Novel Dichotomy of Antibiotic Laws

Rajeev P. Nagassar [1,*], Amanda Carrington [2], Darren K. Dookeeram [3], Keston Daniel [4] and Roma J. Bridgelal-Nagassar [5]

1. Department of Microbiology, The Sangre Grande Hospital, The Eastern Regional Health Authority, Sangre Grande, Trinidad and Tobago
2. Department of Health Sciences, The University of Trinidad and Tobago, Trinidad and Tobago
3. Department of Emergency Medicine, The Sangre Grande Hospital, The Eastern Regional Health Authority, Sangre Grande, Trinidad and Tobago
4. The Public Health Observatory, The Eastern Regional Health Authority, Sangre Grande, Trinidad and Tobago
5. Manager, Medical Research and Audit, Directorate of Women's Health, The Ministry of Health, Trinidad and Tobago; bridgerom@yahoo.com
* Correspondence: rpnagassar@gmail.com

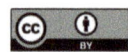

Citation: Nagassar, R.P.; Carrington, A.; Dookeeram, D.K.; Daniel, K.; Bridgelal-Nagassar, R.J. Knowledge, Attitudes, and Practices in Antibiotic Dispensing amongst Pharmacists in Trinidad and Tobago: Exploring a Novel Dichotomy of Antibiotic Laws. *Antibiotics* 2023, 12, 1094. https://doi.org/10.3390/antibiotics12071094

Academic Editors: Juan Manuel Vázquez-Lago, Ana Estany-Gestal and Angel Salgado-Barreira

Received: 17 May 2023
Revised: 20 June 2023
Accepted: 22 June 2023
Published: 23 June 2023

Copyright: © 2023 by the authors. Licensee MDPI, Basel, Switzerland. This article is an open access article distributed under the terms and conditions of the Creative Commons Attribution (CC BY) license (https://creativecommons.org/licenses/by/4.0/).

Abstract: The inappropriate consumption, use, and dispensing of antibiotics are problems faced globally, with a pattern of inappropriate consumption differing in higher-income countries due to the ease of accessibility of antibiotics. The main drivers of consumption and inappropriate use are the over-the-counter sales of antibiotics by pharmacies. Trinidad and Tobago (T&T), a twin island state in the Caribbean, has two Acts of Parliament that regulate antibiotics: the Antibiotics Act and the Food and Drug Act, yet the Over-the-Counter (OTC) sale of antibiotics still exists. This study sought to determine the knowledge, attitudes, and practices regarding the OTC dispensing of antibiotics in T&T. A cross-sectional study gathered data from pharmacists in both the private and public sectors of Trinidad over 7 months. The results showed that antibiotic resistance and antibiotic abuse were seen as significant problems. The level of experience, gender (female), and age (younger) were significantly associated with having good overall knowledge of good dispensing habits and antibiotic laws ($p = 0.036$, $p = 0.047$, and $p = 0.001$, respectively). Pharmacists generally agreed that antibiotics under the Food and Drug Act may have contributed to OTC dispensing in the private sector ($p = 0.013$) and that all antibiotics should be under the Antibiotic Act ($p = 0.002$). Additionally, it was found that the dispensing of antibiotics OTC in the private sector ($p = 0.006$) occurred: without doctors' advice and without requesting prescriptions; because it was perceived as lawful (especially by older pharmacists); and because of the perceived motivation of profit. Regulation enforcement was perceived as deficient. OTC dispensing for reasons, such as misunderstanding of laws, occurs in T&T.

Keywords: antibiotics; legislations; laws; dispensing; pharmacists

1. Introduction

The inappropriate use and dispensing of antibiotics are global problems, with antibiotics being one of the most commonly sold drugs worldwide [1,2]. Dache et al. found in their 2021 study that "pharmacies (57%) and family members or neighbors were common sources of antibiotics in low-income countries". Browne et al. (2021), however, found that higher levels of antibiotic consumption occurred in high-income countries, such as the United States of America, and lower consumption levels in lower-income countries, such as those in Sub-Saharan Africa, where they may be less accessible [3].

The inappropriate use of antibiotics has been seen as a complex problem involving various actors from the human, environmental, food, and veterinary sectors and fueled by the 'over-the-counter' sale of medication, dispensing by inappropriate pharmacy staff, and the use of leftover or borrowed antibiotics [2,4,5].

The most significant impact of dispensing, if not properly regulated, is the likelihood of people developing antibiotic resistance. In many cases, conflicting interests, such as profits for the prescriber and dispenser, are prioritized over preventing antimicrobial resistance and drive inappropriate dispensing behaviors [4–10]. These patterns will ultimately result in increased drug use and patient treatment costs in the future.

In Trinidad and Tobago, a high-income, developing country, the pharmacy is an important point of contact for patients, especially within the community. Legislative provisions in the country establish the powers and responsibilities of drug sales and distribution. This legal framework includes the "Food and Drugs Act (Act 8 of 1960), the Antibiotics Act (Act 18 of 1948), the Dangerous Drugs Act (Act 38 of 1991), the Narcotic Control (General Provisions) Regulations, the Narcotic Control (Licensing) Regulations, and the Pharmacy Board Act" (Act 7 of 1960) [6–14].

Antibiotics, however, are primarily regulated by the Drug Inspectorate Division (DID); this division plays a major role in private and public pharmacy inspections across the country. The Chemistry, Food, and Drug Division, another regulation agency with drug inspectors who have some operating power concerning the regulation of antibiotics, can be considered to operate within a "grey area" in the legislation. Both divisions operate under the Ministry of Health of Trinidad and Tobago but are considered to have separate roles and staff to conduct their monitoring and regulation activities. Even with the existence of two independent regulating bodies, the Trinidad and Tobago Pharmaceutical Country Profile states that antibiotics are often sold over the counter without the use of a prescription [6,7].

The WHO Policy Guidance on Integrated Antimicrobial Stewardship Activities lists the five (5) pillars of good antimicrobial stewardship as Commitment, Prevention, Detection, Optimization of Use, and Surveillance [8]. Pillars 2 and 3 (Prevention and Detection) will be mentioned in this study for the specific purpose of reviewing Antimicrobial Stewardship (AMS). These pillars are key to strengthening the Global Action Plan (GAP) to target the appropriate use of antimicrobials and thus strengthen antimicrobial stewardship (AMS) [8–10].

It is against this background that this Knowledge, Attitudes, and Practices (KAP) study aims to gather baseline data on the knowledge, attitudes, and practices of over-the-counter dispensing of antibiotics by pharmacists under a dichotomy of legislation in Trinidad and Tobago. It should be noted, however, that this study was conducted during the COVID-19 pandemic, with several restrictions preventing normal data collection. It also dealt with the sensitive issue of possible infringement of the law.

2. Results

A total of 104 responses were received from the public and private sectors. The response rate for the survey was (104/145) 71.7%, or approximately 72%. The majority (49%) of the respondents were between 21 and 40 years old, were female, had greater than 4 years of pharmacy dispensing experience, and worked in the private sector. Most respondents had four or more years of experience. Respondents were from the public, private, and both sectors.

2.1. Knowledge

Significant relationships were underlined. N/A means not applicable and is utilized as the response was 100% for a particular field, making this significant. The response to knowledge-related questions was yes or no and displayed as numbers and percentages, n (%). The responses are displayed in Table 1.

All respondents indicated that antibiotic resistance is a serious public health problem facing the world, regardless of age, gender, or the sector they were employed in.

Table 1. Significance tests showing the relationship between Knowledge of Antibiotic Resistance and the age, sex, experience, and sector of participants.

Knowledge	Yes n (%)	No n (%)	p-Values [+]			
			Age	Sex	Experience	Sector
Antibiotic Resistance is associated with inappropriate antibiotic use.	103 (99)	1 (1)	0.578	0.404	0.221	1.00
Repeated use of the same antibiotics results in resistance.	97 (93.3)	7 (6.7)	0.027 *	0.349	0.057	0.158
Antibiotics can speed up recovery from the flu or the common cold.	15 (14.4)	89 (85.65)	0.271	0.974	0.616	0.668
Antimicrobial Resistance results in Resistance to Antibiotics only.	32 (30.8)	72 (69.2)	0.360	0.206	0.255	0.017 **
Antibiotic resistance is a serious public health problem facing the world. ***	104 (100)	0 (0)	n/a	n/a	n/a	n/a
Antibiotics can speed up the recovery of people suffering from COVID-19.	23 (22.1)	81 (77.9)	0.446	0.349	0.870	0.684
Superbugs, such as MRSA and carbapenem-resistant Gram-negative bacilli, result in fewer antibiotic choices.	97 (93.3)	7 (6.7)	0.587	0.349	0.684	0.649
Superbugs, such as MRSA and carbapenem-resistant Gram-negative bacilli, result in increased costs.	94 (90.4)	10 (9.6)	0.125	0.515	0.173	0.760
Resistant Gram-negative bacilli result in an increased length of stay for patients on wards.	103 (99)	1 (1)	0.001 *	0.596	1.00	1.00
Vaccines can prevent unnecessary antibiotic use and, thus, antibiotic resistance.	70 (67.3)	34 (32.7)	0.130	0.112	0.440	0.001 **

[+] $p < 0.05$ is considered significant. The Chi^2 test was used to test the significance of relationships. Fisher's Exact t-test was used where cells have small values (less than or equal to 5). * Younger pharmacists were more knowledgeable than older pharmacists with regards to repeated use of antibiotics and increased length of stay on the wards. ** Pharmacists in both the private and public sectors significantly believed that antimicrobial resistance is not only to antibiotics, but more private sector pharmacists knew that vaccines could prevent unnecessary antibiotic use. *** All pharmacists agreed that antibiotic resistance is a serious worldwide problem.

2.1.1. Age

A Chi^2 test of independence was performed to examine the relationship between age and repeated use of the same antibiotic in terms of resistance ($p = 0.027$). Additionally, Fisher's Exact t-test showed that younger pharmacists displayed a significant difference in their knowledge of the fact that superbugs, such as MRSA and carbapenem-resistant Gram-negative bacilli, result in an increased length of stay for patients on wards ($p = 0.001$).

2.1.2. Sector

When pharmacists' responses to the statement "antimicrobial resistance results in resistance to antibiotics only" were compared with their sector of employment, a significant association was found for both the private and public sectors ($p = 0.017$). This was also true for the statement "vaccines can prevent unnecessary antibiotic use and thus antibiotic resistance" and their sector of work, where more private sector pharmacists responded affirmatively ($p = 0.001$). This is displayed in Table 1.

With regards to knowledge of the Antibiotic Act and Pharmacy Board Act, yes/no responses were gathered from the responding pharmacists and displayed as both numbers and percentages, n (%). No significant relationship was found between age, sex, experience, or sector and any question asked in this section. The Chi^2 value for the fields "The Pharmacy Board Act regulates the dispensing of antibiotics by pharmacists" and "Have you heard of the Antibiotic Inspectorate/Drug Inspectorate?" was used. Fisher's Exact t-test was used for the field "Have you heard of the Antibiotic Act?" The p values were insignificant, but over 80% of pharmacists in this study responded affirmatively to these fields, as displayed in Table 2.

Table 2. Knowledge of the Antibiotic Act and Pharmacy Board Act.

Knowledge about the Antibiotic and Pharmacy Board Acts	Yes n (%)	No n (%)	p-Values [+]			
			Age	Sex	Experience	Sector
The Pharmacy Board Act regulates the dispensing of antibiotics by pharmacists.	88 (84.6)	16 (15.4)	0.644	0.798	0.817	0.321
Have you heard of the Antibiotic Act?	101 (97.1)	3 (2.9)	0.146	1.00	0.827	1.00
Have you heard of the Antibiotic Inspectorate/Drug Inspectorate?	97 (93.3)	7 (6.7)	0.360	0.510	0.726	0.262

[+] $p < 0.05$ is considered significant. The Chi^2 test was used to test the significance of relationships. Fisher's exact t-test was used where cells had small values (less than or equal to 5).

With regards to knowledge of the Food and Drugs Act and Antibiotic Act (This is displayed in Table 3), questions were again answered yes or no, and the numbers and percentages displayed n (%).

Table 3. Knowledge of the Food and Drugs Act and Antibiotic Act.

Knowledge About Food and Drug Act	Yes n (%)	No n (%)	p-Values [+]			
			Age	Sex	Experience	Sector
Are All antibiotics registered under the Antibiotic Act?	31 (29.8)	73 (70.2)	0.461	0.507	0.374	0.398
Are any Antibiotics registered under the Food and Drug Act?	84 (80.8)	20 (19.2)	0.489	0.047 *	0.128	0.084
Are Antibiotics resisted under the Food and Drug Act under the purview of the Antibiotic Inspectorate/Drug Inspectorate?	59 (56.7)	45 (43.3)	0.051	0.254	0.036 **	0.509
Can you name an antibiotic registered under the Food and Drug Act?	73 (70.2)	31 (29.8)	0.292	0.128	0.222	0.141

[+] $p < 0.05$ is considered significant. This is denoted in red and underlined. The Chi^2 test was used to test the significance of relationships. Fisher's exact t-test was used where cells had small values (less than or equal to 5). * Female pharmacists significantly knew that antibiotics are also registered under the Food and Drugs Act. ** More experienced pharmacists significantly knew that antibiotics are resisted under the Food and Drug Act under the purview of the Antibiotic Inspectorate/Drug Inspectorate.

2.1.3. Age and Experience

Are Antibiotics registered under the Food and Drug Act under the purview of the Antibiotic Inspectorate/Drug Inspectorate? Notably, for this field with regards to age, there was no significant association for age ($p = 0.05$). With regards to the relationship between the responses to the question "Are antibiotics registered under the Food and Drug Act under the purview of the Antibiotic /Drug Inspectorate?" and years of experience, there was a significant relationship ($p = 0.036$). This is seen in Table 3.

2.1.4. Sex

When "Are any antibiotics registered under the Food and Drug Act?" was compared to the sex of the respondents, a significant relationship was noted ($p = 0.047$). Overall, 80.8% of pharmacists responded with the correct answer to this question (see Table 3).

The Chi^2 value and the p values were insignificant for most other values regarding knowledge of the various Acts of Parliament. The antibiotics named were ciprofloxacin, co-trimoxazole, o-amoxiclav, cefuroxime, azithromycin, and amoxicillin (Table 3). They were named incorrectly in most instances.

2.2. Attitudes

2.2.1. General

Pharmacists in this study unanimously agreed that there is currently abuse of antibiotics (104 (100%)). See Table 4.

Table 4. Attitudes to Antibiotic Dispensing.

Attitudes	Agree n (%)	Disagree n (%)	Do Not Know	p-Values +			
				Age	Sex	Experience	Sector
Antibiotics should be given to patients when they ask for them without a prescription.	3 (2.9)	101 (97.1)	0 (0)	0.216	0.356	1.00	0.320
When I have a cold or flu, antibiotics help me get better.	12 (11.5)	92 (88.5)	0 (0)	0.783	0.248	0.355	0.702
Antibiotics should be stopped as soon as a person feels better, not after the recommended course.	2 (1.9)	102 (98.1)	0 (0)	0.392	0.353	1.00	0.277
Skipping antibiotic doses does not contribute to resistance.	9 (8.7)	95 (91.3)	0 (0)	0.882	0.795	0.581	0.575
Antibiotic resistance is a problem in Trinidad and Tobago.	83 (79.8)	1 (1)	20 (19.2)	0.086	0.881	0.318	0.021 *
There is currently an abuse of antibiotics. **	104 (100)	0 (0)	0 (0)	n/a	n/a	n/a	n/a
The COVID-19 pandemic has worsened the problem of antibiotic abuse.	87 (83.7)	17 (16.3)	0 (0)	0.570	0.249	0.468	0.776
The public and I should vaccinate to avoid unnecessary antibiotic use.	71 (68.3)	33 (31.7)	0 (0)	0.518	0.63	0.692	0.102

+ $p < 0.05$ is considered significant. This is denoted in red and underlined. n/a means not applicable, as the response was 100%, and thus all pharmacists answered affirmatively. The Chi^2 test was used to test the significance of relationships. Fisher's exact t-test was used where cells had small values (less than or equal to 5). * Pharmacists, mainly in the private sector, believed that antibiotic resistance was a problem. ** Pharmacists, mainly in the private sector, agreed that there is abuse of antibiotics.

2.2.2. Experience and Sector

When the statement "Antibiotic resistance is a problem in Trinidad and Tobago" was compared with the sector of employment ($p = 0.021$). This was mainly in the private sector.

In reference to specific attitudes toward dual registration under the Food and Drug and Antibiotic Acts. The responses are displayed in Table 5.

Table 5. Percentages and Chi Square tests showing the relationships between Attitudes towards Dual Registration and age, sex, experience, and sector.

Attitudes to Dual Registration	Agree n (%)	Disagree n (%)	p-Values +			
			Age	Sex	Experience	Sector
Registration of Antibiotics under the Food and Drug Act and the Antibiotic Act is good.	76 (73.1)	28 (26.9)	0.681	0.755	0.804	0.416
Registration of Antibiotics Under the Food and Drug Act, pharmacists are allowed to give patients Antibiotics over the counter in a Public setting.	10 (9.6)	94 (90.4)	0.910	0.167	0.140	0.300
Registration of Antibiotics Under the Food and Drug Act, pharmacists are allowed to give patients Antibiotics over the counter in a private setting.	40 (38.5)	64 (61.5)	0.290	0.636	0.285	0.013 *
All antibiotics should be under the Antibiotic Act only.	67 (64.4)	37 (35.6)	0.090	0.981	0.241	0.002 *

+ $p < 0.05$ is considered significant. This is denoted in red and underlined. The Chi^2 test was used to test the significance of relationships. Fisher's exact t-test was used where cells had small values (less than or equal to 5). * Pharmacists (38.5%), mainly in the private sector, significantly believed that having antibiotics under the Food and Drug Act allowed pharmacists to give patients antibiotics over the counter in the private setting and that all antibiotics should be under one Act.

2.2.3. Sector

With regards to the field-tested finding that "registration of antibiotics under the Food and Drug Act allows pharmacists to give patients antibiotics over the counter in the private setting", there was a significant relationship between the private and public sectors ($p = 0.013$). This indicated that some pharmacists believed that registration of antibiotics under the Food and Drug Act allowed over-the-counter (OTC) dispensing. There was also a significant relationship seen between the responses to the statement "All antibiotics should be under the Antibiotic Act only" and the private sector ($p = 0.002$). A significant relationship existed between the attitude that registration under the Food and Drug Act did not allow over-the-counter dispensing and the attitude that all antibiotics should be registered under the Antibiotic Act only.

2.3. Practices

All responses in the area of practice showed no significant relationships concerning age. The results of these practices are displayed in Table 6.

Table 6. Practices of Pharmacists towards Antibiotic Dispensing and Chi Square tests comparing the relationships with age, sex, experience, and sector of work.

Practices	Never n (%)	Sometimes n (%)	Always n (%)	p-Values [+]			
				Age	Sex	Experience	Sector
Dispensing of antibiotics to patients over the counter in the private sector.	71 (68.3)	32 (30.8)	1 (1)	0.532	0.313	0.410	0.013 *
A presenting patient is always asked to get a doctor's advice before taking antibiotics.	1 (1)	26 (25)	77 (74)	0.344	0.454	0.693	0.007 *
A presenting patient is always asked to get a doctor's prescription before dispensing antibiotics.	1 (1)	28 (26.9)	75 (72.1)	0.105	0.543	0.858	0.008 *
Antibiotics are not dispensed over the counter without getting a doctor's advice.	13 (12.7)	31 (30.4)	58 (56.9)	0.504	0.305	0.055	0.029 *
Dispensing quinolones or sulfur drugs over the counter in the public sector.	94 (90.4)	9 (8.7)	1 (1)	0.620	0.690	0.674	1.00
Dispensing quinolones or sulfur drugs over the counter in the private sector. *	40 (38.5)	55 (52.9)	6 (5.8)	0.065	0.590	0.988	0.016 *
Dispensing quinolones or sulfur drugs over the counter as it is lawful.	45 (43.3)	52 (50)	7 (6.7)	0.475	0.783	0.981	0.008 *
Dispensing quinolones or sulfur drugs over the counter as it is profitable.	73 (70.2)	28 (26.9)	3 (2.9)	0.062	0.623	0.340	0.039 *

[+] $p < 0.05$ is considered significant. This is denoted in red and underlined. The Chi^2 test was used to test the significance of relationships. Fisher's exact t-test was used where cells had small values (less than or equal to 5).
* The private sector pharmacists were significantly associated with responses to over-the-counter dispensing and other possibly errant practices, such as dispensing without a prescription or doctors' advice.

Sector

The responses to the statement "Dispensing of antibiotics to patients over the counter in the private sector" showed a significant association with their sector of employment ($p = 0.013$). This association was important because it showed that pharmacists in this study significantly agreed that antibiotics were being dispensed OTC in the private sector. Most of the responding pharmacists were from the private sector. Their responses to the statements "A presenting patient is always asked to get a doctor's advice before taking antibiotics", "A presenting patient is always asked to get a doctor's prescription before dispensing antibiotics", and "Antibiotics are not dispensed over the counter without getting a doctor's advice" also showed a significant association with their sector of employment, with p-values ($p = 0.007$), ($p = 0.008$), and ($p = 0.029$) obtained, respectively.

The pharmacists' responses to the statements "Dispensing quinolones or sulfur drugs over the counter in the public sector" and "Dispensing quinolones or sulfur drugs over the counter as it is lawful" also showed significant relationships when compared to their sector of employment, with p-values ($p = 0.016$) and ($p = 0.008$) being obtained, respectively. Finally, when observing the responses to the statement "Dispensing of quinolones or sulfur drugs over the counter as it is profitable", there was a significant association seen with the pharmacists' sector of employment ($p = 0.039$). The results for the field practices showed a very significant relationship between the responses given and their sector of employment, particularly given that many of the responses supporting OTC dispensing were from those in the private sector.

2.4. Open-Ended Answers

Six main themes emerged from the questions that sought to group the answers to the second open-ended question in an ordered manner: 1. Dispensing with Prescription Only; 2. Allowance in Legislation for Legal OTC Dispensing; 3. Lack of Regulatory Enforcement; 4. Dispensing of Antibiotics OTC in Special Circumstances; 5. Doctors as Dispensers; 6. Suitcase Trade.

Some of these important themes will be discussed below, which are displayed in Figure 1. Notably, the theme "Lack of regulatory enforcement" was the most common, followed by "Dispensing with prescription only under one Act".

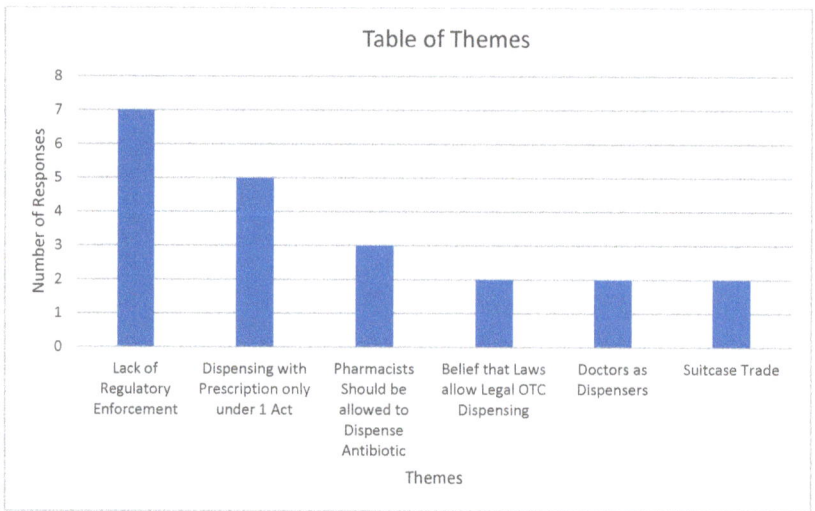

Figure 1. Graph of Themes for Open-Ended Questions. "Suitcase trade" refers to the illegal trade of pharmaceuticals.

Quinolones include ciprofloxacin, levofloxacin, and moxifloxacin. Aminoglycosides include gentamycin, while macrolides include clarithromycin and azithromycin.

Figure 2 shows the various antibiotic names, including quinolones, cefuroxime, and co-amoxiclav. One response stated: "There are no antibiotics under the Food and Drug Act".

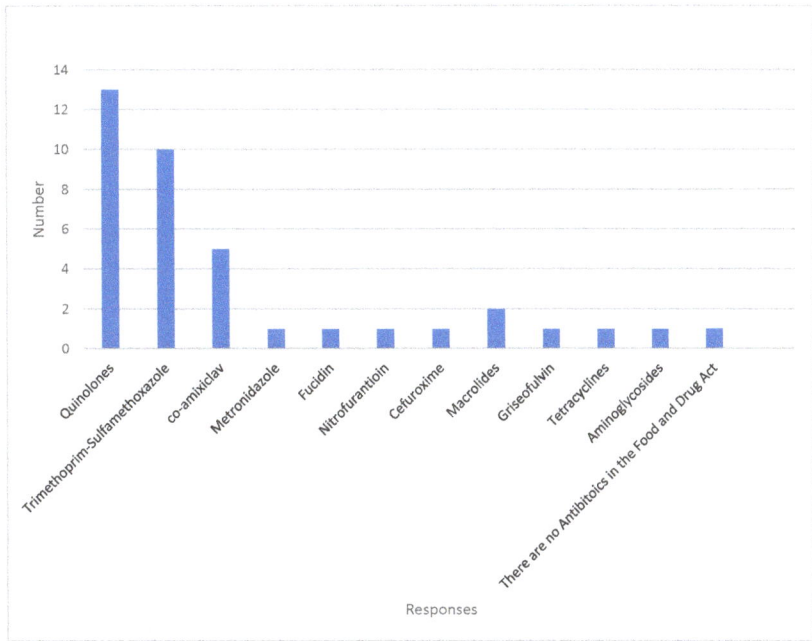

Figure 2. Responses to the Naming of Antibiotics under the Food and Drug Act.

3. Discussion

When the various demographic factors were analyzed with the knowledge, attitudes, and practices of pharmacists in the study, it was found that:

3.1. Knowledge

The results revealed good knowledge of general issues surrounding antimicrobial resistance (AMR) and antibiotic resistance (AR) among pharmacists. Ventola (2015) previously noted that antibiotic resistance and the misuse of antibiotics are serious problems facing the world [5]. The author further notes that there are increased burdens on individuals due to lost salaries and the increased cost of health services [5]. This good general knowledge is thus a good start for antibiotic stewardship efforts.

Knowledge was statistically tested against age, and 99% of respondents were significantly knowledgeable that the duration of hospitalization is affected if a resistant bug must be treated, with the majority being in the younger age group. Notably, at least one study from Trinidad and Tobago supports this knowledge that resistant bacteria lead to an increased duration of hospitalization [15]. The younger respondents were also significantly more knowledgeable about the fact that repeated use of the same antibiotics results in resistance.

Gajdács et al. (2020), similar to our study, indicated that older pharmacists were "less confident" in their knowledge of inappropriate antibiotic use [16]. Kosiyaporn et al. (2020) indicated that "awareness of antibiotic use" and the resulting impact of AMR have been useful in "designing interventions" to combat AMR and inappropriate antimicrobial use (AMU) [17]. Thus, the fact that the pharmacists were knowledgeable about inappropriate use is a good starting point for designing communication and health promotion strategies.

Voidăzan et al. (2019) showed that pharmacists were a major source of information on antibiotic resistance [18]. This information can be used strategically in Trinidad and Tobago to inform patients and combat inappropriate use [18]. Thus, the fact that younger pharmacists and, more importantly, pharmacists across all sectors are knowledgeable about these important issues is encouraging for future planning and intervention.

Knowledge about the Antibiotic and Food and Drug Acts

With regards to specific knowledge about the Antibiotic Act and the Food and Drug Act of Parliament, the responses showed variations in knowledge with experience and sex. Pharmacists with more experience had significantly more knowledge about antibiotics under the Food and Drug Act and Antibiotic Acts. With regards to knowledge of antibiotics registered under the Food and Drug Act, 84 (80.8%) respondents were aware that antibiotics are registered under this Act. Additionally, with regards to antibiotics registered under the Food and Drug Act and knowledge of the purview of the Antibiotic Inspectorate/Drug Inspectorate, 59 (56.7%) were knowledgeable. Thus, the majority of respondents were knowledgeable of the Food and Drug Act and the Antibiotic Act. Alternatively, 88 (84.6%) of respondents were knowledgeable about the Pharmacy Board Act and its role in antibiotic regulation.

Females were significantly more likely to be aware that some antibiotics are also registered under the Food and Drug Act, not just the Antibiotic Act. There is no specific comparison between sex and legislation in Trinidad and Tobago. Pham-Duc and Sriparamananthan (2021) and Zahreddine et al. (2018), however, have shown an association between greater knowledge and female sex [19,20].

Notably, the legal definition of antibiotics in the Food and Drug Act compared to the Antibiotics Act leads to the legal interpretation that there are no antibiotics registered in the Food and Drug Act [21]. This is supported by the open-ended statement from pharmacists that "there are no antibiotics under the Food and Drug Act".

In completing the first open-ended question, some pharmacists incorrectly named antibiotics registered under the Food and Drug Act. Interestingly, some pharmacists named antibiotics under the Antibiotic Act as being under the Food and Drug Act, such as co-amoxiclav and cefuroxime. This highlights an important area for the education of pharmacists.

3.2. Attitudes

Pharmacists with more experience and working in all sectors significantly displayed the attitude that antibiotic resistance is a problem in Trinidad and Tobago, with 79.8% of respondents agreeing. The pharmacists were also knowledgeable about the fact that this is a worldwide problem, including the abuse of antibiotics. Thus, knowledge and attitudes about antibiotic resistance are well established in this study.

The majority of pharmacists significantly disagreed that the registration of antibiotics under the Food and Drug Act allowed over-the-counter dispensing in the private sector (61.5%). However, 38.5% of pharmacists working in all sectors still agreed that registration of antibiotics under the Food and Drug Act does not lead to over-the-counter dispensing in the private sector. This question may have been sensitive, with possible legal repercussions perceived, and thus there may have been bias.

The majority of pharmacists in both the private and public sectors significantly agreed (64.4%) that all antibiotics should be under the Antibiotic Act only. This highlights the possibility of the dichotomous laws contributing to the perceived inappropriate dispensing and may make antibiotic regulation more complex and costly by having two separate divisions responsible for different antibiotics [6]. This is a complex and 'wicked' issue of dichotomy and legal regulations.

Mahmoud et al. (2018) have highlighted the regulatory issues that exist in Saudi Arabia even after the introduction of new legislation [22]. Mate et al. (2019) have highlighted the issue of poor enforcement and weak inspection of pharmacies in Mozambique, and Adhikari et al. (2021) have highlighted regulatory issues and over-the-counter dispensing in Nepal [23,24]. Similar regulatory issues exist internationally; however, none of these countries highlights a dichotomy of laws as in Trinidad and Tobago. The study from Saudi Arabia also highlights that changing a law may not be a short- or medium-term solution [22].

Open-Ended Response supporting Attitudes

Alkadhimi et al. (2021), in their study in Iraq, found that pharmacists believed that they "could dispense antibiotics OTC for diarrhea and tonsillitis; they believed that they could be given the leeway to dispense for emergencies also" [25]. This is similar to the findings in the open-ended questions where pharmacists believe that, as professionals, they should be given a certain amount of autonomy to dispense antibiotics OTC under special circumstances and is congruent with the theme "pharmacists should be allowed to dispense antibiotics OTC in special circumstances".

Notably, the issue of enforcement of current legislation was highlighted in the statement that "the relevant Acts need to be revaluated and enforced because presently there is no enforcement of any rules and regulations".

An issue in Trinidad and Tobago may be a lack of funding to adequately enforce prescriptions for appropriate antibiotic dispensing. The inspection role may also be inadequately staffed or funded [6,26].

3.3. Practices

3.3.1. Age

Within the private sector, the practice of dispensing quinolones or sulfur drugs over the counter was performed because it was considered profitable by most respondents. Additionally, younger respondents were less likely to dispense antibiotics for profit. Notably, the majority of respondents were younger than 40, indicating that there may have been a bias towards younger respondents. They were also more likely to be in a public practice where OTC dispensing is prohibited or were less likely to be owners of the pharmacy. In studies in Lebanon and Saudi Arabia, they stated, as mentioned previously, that pharmacists with greater years of experience were inclined to dispense over the counter, and additionally, those pharmacists between 30 and 35 years of age were less likely to dispense over the counter [20,27].

Torres et al. (2020) highlighted the "driver of profits" and its influence on owners of pharmacies in Mozambique. This may be similar in the private sector in Trinidad and Tobago [28].

3.3.2. Sector

Pharmacists dispense antibiotics over the counter in the private sector for profit and because of the perception that it is lawful, but not in the public sector. Notably, in the RHAs, the dispensing of antibiotics OTC is not allowed by policy. This allows accountability for the antibiotics in the public sector, inclusive of the five (5) Regional Health Authorities. Pharmacists at times failed to follow a doctor's advice, and some dispensed without a prescription. Pharmacists also dispensed quinolones and sulfur-based antibiotics over the counter, which are registered under the Food and Drug Act. This corroborates the established narrative in this study, that over-the-counter dispensing does occur, and the finding that private sector pharmacists believe that dual registration under the two Acts may be contributing to the misuse of antibiotics. However, all pharmacists displayed the attitude that all antibiotics should be covered by one Act of parliament.

Ventola (2015) further stated that the regulation of antibiotics is an issue in many countries, with over-the-counter (OTC) antibiotics being easily available. The OTC dispensing of antibiotics has been discussed in the introduction for Hungary, Tanzania, and Nepal [5]. Additionally, "antibiotics are thus accessible, plentiful, and cheap, which promotes overuse" in some countries, with antibiotics also being available online [5].

Alkadhimi et al. (2021) stated that pharmacists in Iraq had good knowledge of antimicrobial resistance but were still inclined to practice OTC dispensing, similar to this study [25]. In this study, it was uncovered that OTC dispensing does occur, and pharmacists had good knowledge and attitudes; however, their practices appear unchanged despite good knowledge. Thus, efforts must be made to change these practices, norms, and beliefs.

According to the Antimicrobial Resistance Collaborators (2022), 50,000 to 100,000 deaths in 2019 were attributed to bacteria resistant to antibiotics, such as quinolones [29]. Ayukekbong et al. (2017) emphasized that regulatory issues are a contributor to antimicrobial resistance [30]. In this study, these also appear to be similar practices. Interestingly, this study revealed that there is a similar problem with quinolones and sulfur-based antibiotics.

Malik and Bhattacharyya (2019) stated previously that with their model, "lack of awareness can also accelerate the emergence of resistant strains and impart a significant economic cost on the population" [31]. This is driven by the irrational use of antibiotics in the community, as stated before [31]. Conversely, the evidence of a concerning lack of knowledge is highlighted in the statement that "dual registration allows for lawful dispensing of some antibiotics without a prescription, but it should still be controlled and not dispensed freely because of the monetary benefit". This belongs to the theme of "belief that laws allow legal OTC dispensing" and again highlights the belief that it is legal to dispense certain antibiotics OTC. Thus, from the study, it can be deduced that the knowledge gap may be due to a misunderstanding of the regulatory issues in the Acts [13,14].

The practice in Trinidad and Tobago of dispensing quinolones and sulfur-based antibiotics because pharmacists perceive it to be lawful is indicative of the need for education. It is also congruent with findings from Jordan, Tanzania, Mozambique, Saudi Arabia, Iraq, Uganda, and Nepal that while regulations exist to control the dispensing of antibiotics, inappropriate dispensing patterns persist, such as in Trinidad and Tobago [22–25,32–34]. Similarly, Gebretekle and Serbessa's (2016) paper found that fluoroquinolones and sulfur-based antibiotics, such as ciprofloxacin and co-trimoxazole, were the most frequently prescribed and possibly dispensed antibiotics [35]. Saleem et al. (2021) found high usage of co-amoxiclav and ciprofloxacin in the community. This is interesting, as pharmacists named co-amoxiclav as an incorrect drug under the Food and Drug Act.

Gebretekle and Serbessa (2016) agreed that the practice of OTC dispensing is fueled by the need for profits, similar to the finding in our study [35]. Notably, there should be consideration for penalties or health promotion advice against errant behavior so as not to reinforce that behavior. Interestingly, similar to this study, Ayukekbong et al. (2017) indicated that regulatory factors drive antimicrobial resistance. They also indicated that community pharmacies offered unauthorized clinical consultations that suggested a diagnosis and may have contributed to unregulated dispensing [30]. The study also uncovered that pharmacists sometimes dispense without a prescription or doctors' advice and sometimes do not ask the patient to get a doctor's advice, uncovering similar issues.

3.3.3. Open-Ended Response Supporting Practices

The concept of illegal trade and antibiotic misuse was highlighted in the statement that the "availability of antibiotics via suitcase traders is a problem" under the theme of 'Suitcase Trade'. The issue of the suitcase trade of pharmaceuticals in Trinidad and Tobago has been highlighted previously [36]. This practice would be a breach of existing regulations. It is not directly related to OTC dispensing but may contribute by providing substandard medication.

It has been recommended that suppliers from different countries be approved, not just locally based suppliers. Foreign-based suppliers should be considered for registration. Additionally, companies should not have to use only intermediate distributors, as is the current practice. This helps expand access to cheaper drugs [37].

Kakkar (2020) highlights that factors hampering adequate or effective regulation include a lack of political will and relaxed regulatory mechanisms [26]. Thus, the errant practices could be fueled by regulatory deficiencies [26]. Kurdi et al. (2020) have shown that even with new antibiotic regulations for controlling the dispensing of antibiotics in Saudi Arabia, the practice of OTC dispensing persists [34]. The authors further state that "educational programs and campaigns" are recommended. Jacobs et al. (2019) also recommended a multi-faceted approach to tackle the inappropriate dispensing of antibiotics in a review of OTC sales of antibiotics. Thus, changing the dichotomy of laws may not be the only answer [38].

The practice of pharmacy assistants and other categories of staff other than pharmacists dispensing prescription drugs to patients also breaches national laws [32]. This is highlighted under the theme "suitcase trade" in the statement, "A lot of pharmacies dispense antibiotics without a pharmacist in the pharmacy and also operate without a pharmacist present in the pharmacy." This supports the point that OTC dispensing practices may be facilitated by giving staff other than pharmacists the authority to dispense [32].

3.4. Limitations

There may have been some degree of apprehension in the responses to the questionnaires that were administered with assistants compared to those that were self-administered. This also led to removing the requirement for emails. This removal meant that the "only one response per participant" feature in Google Forms was removed. This may have led to duplicate responses and bias. The non-structured method of collecting data, including the convenience method of collecting data, means that the findings cannot be generalizable to the population. It was uncovered, however, that a problem with OTC dispensing does exist in Trinidad and Tobago. Some of the causes have been identified in this study.

3.5. Conclusions

Pharmacists appear to have significant and encouraging knowledge and attitudes regarding antimicrobial resistance and the effects of inappropriate dispensing of antibiotics. Over-the-counter dispensing still occurs in the private sector in Trinidad and Tobago. Additionally, practices were not congruent with positive knowledge and attitudes.

This is the first study examining the knowledge, attitudes, and practices of pharmacists, especially concerning over-the-counter dispensing with the two Acts of Parliament. This study is also unique in that it examines dispensing in a country with two laws governing antibiotic dispensing, inspections, and thus regulation. It uncovered that there was a deficiency in understanding the role of the various regulatory issues under each Act and that this dichotomy of laws may be contributing to inappropriate practices.

4. Materials and Methods

A quantitative, cross-sectional study was conducted. The study targeted pharmacies across the public and private sectors in Trinidad. Two populations were targeted in the study: public-sector pharmacists and pharmacists in the private sector.

In Trinidad and Tobago, public sector health services are split into five self-managed regions known as Regional Health Authorities (RHA). They are governed by the Regional Health Authorities Act, Chapter 29:05, Act 5 of 1994. (Ministry of The Attorney General and Legal Affairs, 2016).

The study was conducted from April to October 2021, over a seven-month period.

4.1. Study Sample

A stratified sampling of pharmacists from the Sangre Grande Hospital (SGH), St Andrews/St David (STAD), Nariva/Mayaro (NAMA), and private sector pharmacies was performed to obtain a sample of pharmacists from the public and private sectors.

The study initially targeted 145 pharmacists (across public and private-sector pharmacies); however, 104 were recruited from both the private and public sectors (~72% response rate). The public sector consisted of approximately 250 pharmacists out of a total of 641 pharmacists nationally (6). One RHA (the Eastern RHA) with 45 pharmacists was purposely selected to represent the public sector responses for this study. All the public-sector pharmacists at the Eastern RHA participated in the study. They represented pharmacists for: Biche Outreach Centre, Black Rock Outreach Centre, Brothers Road Outreach Centre, Coryal Outreach Centre, Cumuto Outreach Centre, Grande Riviere Outreach Centre,

Guayaguayare Outreach Centre, Manzanilla Outreach Centre, Matelot Outreach Centre, Matura Outreach Centre, Mayaro District Health Facility, Rio Claro Health Centre, San Souci Outreach Centre, Sangre Grande Enhanced Health Centre, Toco Health Centre, 24-h Accident and Emergency, the Valencia Outreach Centre, and the Sangre Grande Hospital. All public sector pharmacies and thus pharmacists follow the same regulations for public sector workers, which is why we chose a sample from one RHA rather than all. The COVID-19 pandemic also hindered movement and was a major consideration for the study design. There are approximately 375 registered private pharmacies in the country. Initially, the study sought to recruit 100 pharmacists from the private sector. It was noted that pharmacists in the private sector may work in public institutions and vice versa. A 95% confidence level was used, and a margin of error of 8.4% was assumed for this calculation. The response distribution was assumed to be 50%. This was performed because responses were obtained during a period of COVID-19 restrictions and due to the legal sensitivity of the topic.

4.2. Recruitment and Inclusion Criteria

Public Sector—All pharmacists with at least one year of dispensing experience in the in-patient and out-patient departments of the Sangre Grande Hospital, St. Andrews/St. David County Health Administration, and Nariva/Mayaro County Health Administration were eligible for inclusion in the survey and were given an equal chance of participation. Participation was voluntary, and all eligible public sector pharmacists in the inpatient and outpatient departments were offered a questionnaire from April 2021 to October 2021. Participants had the option of choosing the public sector or both the private and public sectors (they used the option "both" to do this). They chose both if they were captured in a public setting but worked privately also, and additionally if they were captured in a private setting but worked publicly also. No duplication was allowed when visiting pharmacies.

The survey was administered via email to the senior pharmacists at each facility. These senior pharmacists then distributed the survey via email to their junior colleagues. The respondents accessed the consent form and survey via a link using Google Forms (settings were adjusted to "responses required").

Private Sector: The private pharmacies were engaged via referral from colleagues and encompassed pharmacies throughout the country. Pharmacists were recruited by snowballing in the private sector. Three pre-trained assistants helped with administering the questionnaire via telephone, gathering data, and recruiting participants by snowballing (for the private sector pharmacists). Participation in the study was also voluntary.

4.3. Data Collection

The questionnaire was administered via Google Forms, and data was collected using a structured questionnaire with two open-ended questions. Data were collected for 7 months (up until the point of saturation and no more referrals from colleagues) from pharmacists in the private and public sectors.

Participants were emailed the Google Form (settings were adjusted to "responses required"). In some cases, WhatsApp private messenger was used, and a link to the Google form was sent to the respondents. Initially, participants were sent Google Forms with a feature for the collection of email addresses. This was removed a month into the study to improve the confidentiality of the respondents and increase confidence in the anonymity of the study.

4.4. Exclusion Criteria

Persons employed at pharmacies who were not pharmacists and pharmacists with less than one year of dispensing experience were excluded from the study.

4.5. Data Analysis

The collected data was inputted and analyzed using IBM SPPSv22 and Microsoft Excel software. Descriptive statistics were used in analyzing the data collected. The Chi-squared (X^2) test was used to measure the observed and expected variables of the categorical demographic variables versus the questioner's items. The study looked at whether relationships existed between age, sex, years of experience, or sector and the participant's knowledge, attitudes, and perceptions based on the questions asked in the questionnaire. This assumes that there are dependent and independent variables, and they are categorical. The significance level was set at $p < 0.05$ for all tests. Fisher's exact t-test was also used for fields with numbers less than or equal to 5. We avoided adjusting further for alpha to avoid Type 2 errors (39). Ranganathan (2016) further confirms that studies should not rely overly on alpha adjustments, as this may also lead to erroneous results. This was also given that we accepted an increased margin of error due to the sensitive nature of the study and the COVID-19 environment. Instead, we focused on the primary outcome of the presence or absence of over-the-counter dispensing (39). Two open-ended questions were used. These were: "Can you name an antibiotic under the Food and Drug Act?" and "Is there anything else you would like to say about dual registration of antibiotics and dispensing? Open-ended responses to the second question were analyzed and grouped into emerging themes.

4.6. Privacy and Confidentiality of Participant Information and Research Data

All participant identifiers were removed. No participant's personal information was required for this study, nor was patient information needed. To ensure privacy, no names were collected. Only electronic forms with no identifiers were used. Informed consent was obtained. The consent forms contained no addresses, email addresses, or phone numbers that could be used to trace the responses back to specific participants. Any personal data obtained from the use of WhatsApp and Google Forms was stored on a password-protected computer, with any hardcopy information kept in a locked cupboard. Most of the data for this study was stored electronically on a password-protected computer.

4.7. Ethical Considerations

Ethical permission was sought and granted from the University of Trinidad and Tobago (UTT) and the Eastern Regional Health Authority's (ERHA) Ethics Committee.

Author Contributions: Conceptualization, R.P.N. and A.C.; methodology, R.P.N., A.C. and D.K.D.; software, R.J.B.-N. and K.D.; validation, R.P.N., R.J.B.-N., A.C. and K.D.; formal analysis, R.P.N. and K.D.; investigation, R.P.N., R.J.B.-N. and D.K.D.; resources, R.P.N. and A.C.; writing—original draft preparation, R.P.N. and A.C.; writing—review and editing, R.P.N., A.C., R.J.B.-N., K.D. and D.K.D.; supervision, A.C. All authors have read and agreed to the published version of the manuscript.

Funding: This research received no external funding. It was self-funded.

Institutional Review Board Statement: Institutional Review Board approval was granted by the University of Trinidad and Tobago on March 23, 2021 by the IRB (reference: UTTO/15/21). Ethics committee approval was given by the Eastern Regional Health Authority on April 7, 2021 (reference number: ERHA-REC.004/04/2021).

Informed Consent Statement: The participants participated after giving informed consent. All participants were guaranteed that their personal data would not be shared.

Data Availability Statement: Data sharing not applicable. No new data were created or analyzed in this study. Data sharing is not applicable to this article.

Conflicts of Interest: R.P.N. is a past speaker for pharmaceutical houses.

References

1. Dache, A.; Dona, A.; Ejeso, A. Inappropriate use of antibiotics, its reasons and contributing factors among communities of Yirgalem town, Sidama regional state, Ethiopia: A cross-sectional study. *SAGE Open Med.* **2021**, *9*. [CrossRef] [PubMed]
2. Tangcharoensathien, V.; Chanvatik, S.; Sommanustweechai, A. Complex determinants of inappropriate use of antibiotics. *Bull. World Health Organ.* **2018**, *96*, 141–144. [CrossRef] [PubMed]
3. Browne, A.J.; Chipeta, M.G.; Haines-Woodhouse, G.; Kumaran, E.P.A.; Kashef Hamadani, B.H.; Zaraa, S.; Henry, N.J.; Deshpande, A.; Reiner, R.C.; Day, N.P.J.; et al. Global antibiotic consumption and usage in humans, 2000–18: A spatial modelling study. *Lancet* **2021**, *5*, e893–e904. [CrossRef] [PubMed]
4. Pearson, M.; Doble, A.; Glogowski, R.; Ibezim, S.; Lazenby, T.; Haile-Redai, A.; Shaikh, N.; Treharne, A.; Yardakul, S.; Yemanaberhan, R.; et al. Antibiotic Dispensing and Resistance: Views from LMIC Dispensing and Dispensing Professionals. Report to the World Health Organisation AMR Secretariat. 2018. Available online: http://www.who.int/antimicrobial-resistance/LSHTMAntibiotic-Dispensing-LMIC-Dispensing-and-Dispensing-2017.pdf (accessed on 20 February 2023).
5. Ventola, C.L. The antibiotic resistance crisis: Part 1: Causes and threats. P & T: A peer-reviewed. *J. Formul. Manag.* **2015**, *40*, 277–283.
6. Ministry of Health and Pan American Health Organisation. Republic of Trinidad and Tobago Pharmaceutical Country Profile. 2012. Available online: https://www.who.int/medicines/areas/coordination/PSCP_TRT_en.pdf?ua=1 (accessed on 17 July 2021).
7. Persaud, S.; Sukhraj, R.; Goetz, L. Knowledge, Attitude and Practices Towards Antibiotic Use Among Patients at a Tertiary Urology Centre in Trinidad and Tobago. *Caribb. Med. J.* **2020**. Available online: https://www.caribbeanmedicaljournal.org/2020/11/02/knowledge-attitude-and-practices-towards-antibiotic-use-among-patients-at-a-tertiary-urology-centre-in-trinidad-and-tobago/ (accessed on 23 January 2022). [CrossRef]
8. World Health Organisation. *WHO Policy Guidance on Integrated Antimicrobial Stewardship Activities*; Licence: CCBY-NC-SA 3.0 IGO; World Health Organisation: Geneva, Switzerland, 2021.
9. World Health Organisation (WHO). Global Action Plan on Antimicrobial Resistance. 2016. Available online: https://apps.who.int/gb/ebwha/pdf_files/WHA69/A69_24-en.pdf#:~:text=The%20global%20action%20plan%20on%20antimicrobial%20resistance%20was,which%20is%20submitted%20separately%20in%20document%20A69%2F24%20Add.1 (accessed on 23 January 2022).
10. World Health Organisation (WHO). Global Antimicrobial Resistance and Use Surveillance System (GLASS) Report: 2021. *World Health Organisation.* 2021. Available online: https://apps.who.int/iris/handle/10665/341666 (accessed on 23 January 2022).
11. Ministry of Health. Chemistry, Food and Drugs Division: List of Drugs Registered (In Accordance with the F&D Act Reg Chap 30:01). Available online: https://health.gov.tt/services/chemistry-food-and-drugs-division (accessed on 19 August 2021).
12. Ministry of Attorney General and Legal Affairs. Regional Health Authorities Act. Ministry of Legal Affairs. 2020. Available online: https://rgd.legalaffairs.gov.tt/laws2/alphabetical_list/lawspdfs/29.05.pdf (accessed on 23 January 2022).
13. Ministry of Legal Affairs. Food and Drug Act. 2020. Available online: https://rgd.legalaffairs.gov.tt/laws2/alphabetical_list/lawspdfs/30.01.pdf (accessed on 31 December 2021).
14. Ministry of Legal Affairs. Antibiotics Act. Available online: https://rgd.legalaffairs.gov.tt/laws2/Alphabetical_List/lawspdfs/30.02.pdf (accessed on 31 December 2021).
15. Nagassar, R.; Bridgelal-Nagassar, R.; Harper, L. A Pilot Study to Delineate Factors Contributing to Multi-Drug Resistant Organism (MDRO) Outbreak and Control at the Sangre Grande Hospital. *Caribb. Med. J.* **2020**, *82*, 1–6. [CrossRef]
16. Gajdács, M.; Paulik, E.; Szabo, A. Knowledge, Attitude and Practice of Community Pharmacists Regarding Antibiotic Use and Infectious Diseases: A Cross-Sectional Survey in Hungary (KAPPhA-HU). *Antibiotics* **2020**, *9*, 41. [CrossRef]
17. Kosiyaporn, H.; Chanvatik, S.; Issaramalai, T.; Kosiyaporn, W.; Kulthanmanusorn, A.; Saengruang, N.; Witthayapipopsakul, W.; Viriyathorn, S.; Kirivan, S.; Kunpeuk, W.; et al. Surveys of knowledge and awareness of antibiotic use and antimicrobial resistance in general population: A systematic review. *PLoS ONE* **2020**, *15*, e0227973. [CrossRef]
18. Voidăzan, S.; Moldovan, G.; Voidăzan, L.; Zazgyva, A.; Moldovan, H. Knowledge, Attitudes and Practices Regarding the Use of Antibiotics. Study On the General Population of Mureş County, Romania. *Infect. Drug Resist.* **2019**, *12*, 3385–3396. [CrossRef]
19. Pham-Duc, P.; Sriparamananthan, K. Exploring gender differences in knowledge and practices related to antibiotic use in Southeast Asia: A scoping review. *PLoS ONE* **2021**, *16*, e0259069. [CrossRef]
20. Zahreddine, L.; Hallit, S.; Shakaroun, J.; Al-Hajje, A.; Awada, S.; Lahoud, N. Knowledge of pharmacists and parents towards antibiotic use in paediatrics: A cross-sectional study in Lebanon. *Pharm. Pract.* **2018**, *16*, 1194. [CrossRef]
21. M. Hamel-Smith & Co. Importing Pharmaceuticals into T&T: The Regulatory Regime. Available online: http://trinidadlaw.com/importing-pharmaceuticals-into-tt-the-regulatory-regime/ (accessed on 17 February 2021).
22. Mahmoud, M.A.; Aldhaeefi, M.; Sheikh, A.; Aljadhey, H. Community pharmacists' perspectives about reasons behind antibiotics dispensing without prescription: A qualitative study. *Biomed. Res.* **2018**, *29*, 1194. [CrossRef]
23. Mate, I.; Come, C.E.; Gonçalves, M.P.; Cliff, J.; Gudo, E.S. Knowledge, attitudes, and practices regarding antibiotic use in Maputo City, Mozambique. *PLoS ONE* **2019**, *14*, e0221452. [CrossRef]
24. Adhikari, B.; Pokharel, S.; Raut, S.; Adhikari, J.; Thapa, S.; Paudel, K.; Narayan, G.C.; Neupane, S.; Neupane, S.R.; Yadav, R.; et al. Why do people purchase antibiotics over the counter? A qualitative study with patients, clinicians, and dispensers in central, eastern, and western Nepal. *BMJ Glob. Health* **2021**, *6*, e005829. [CrossRef]
25. Alkadhimi, A.; Dawood, O.T.; Hassali, M.A. Dispensing of antibiotics in community pharmacy in Iraq: A qualitative study. *Pharm. Pract.* **2020**, *18*, 2095. [CrossRef]

26. Kakkar, A.K.; Shafiq, N.; Singh, G.; Ray, P.; Gautam, V.; Agarwal, R.; Muralidharan, J.; Arora, P. Antimicrobial Stewardship Programs in Resource Constrained Environments: Understanding and Addressing the Need of the Systems. *Front. Public Health* **2020**, *8*, 140. [CrossRef] [PubMed]
27. Khan, T.M.; Azhar, S. A study investigating the community pharmacist knowledge about the appropriate use of inhaler, Eastern Region Al Ahsa, Saudi Arabia. *Saudi Pharm. J.* **2013**, *21*, 153–157. [CrossRef]
28. Torres, N.; Solomon, V.; Middleton, L. Pharmacists' practices for non-prescribed antibiotic dispensing in Mozambique. *Pharm. Pract.* **2020**, *18*, 1965. [CrossRef] [PubMed]
29. Antimicrobial Resistance Collaborators. Global burden of bacterial antimicrobial resistance in 2019: A systematic analysis. *Lancet* **2022**, *399*, 629–655. [CrossRef]
30. Ayukekbong, J.A.; Ntemgwa, M.; Atabe, A.N. The threat of antimicrobial resistance in developing countries causes and control strategies. *Antimicrob. Resist. Infect. Control* **2017**, *6*, 47. [CrossRef] [PubMed]
31. Malik, B.; Bhattacharyya, S. Antibiotic drug-resistance as a complex system driven by socio-economic growth and antibiotic misuse. *Sci. Rep.* **2019**, *9*, 9788. [CrossRef]
32. Haddadin, R.N.; Alsous, M.; Wazaify, M.; Tahaineh, L. Evaluation of antibiotic dispensing practice in community pharmacies in Jordan: A cross sectional study. *PLoS ONE* **2019**, *14*, e0216159. [CrossRef] [PubMed]
33. Jerving, S. The Pharmacist's Role in Fighting Antimicrobial Resistance. 2021. Available online: https://www.devex.com/news/the-pharmacist-s-role-in-fighting-antimicrobial-resistance-100537 (accessed on 20 August 2021).
34. Kurdi, S.; Faran, A.; Eareeni, E.; Alhalal, N.; Joseph, R.; Wali, H.; Alshayban, D. Assessment of knowledge and attitude toward the new antibiotic dispensing law and its effect on antibiotic use in Saudi Arabia. *J. Saudi Pharm. Soc.* **2020**, *28*, 58–67. [CrossRef]
35. Gebretekle, G.B.; Serbessa, M.K. Exploration of over-the-counter sales of antibiotics in community pharmacies of Addis Ababa, Ethiopia: Pharmacy professionals' perspective. *Antimicrob. Resist. Infect. Control* **2016**, *5*, 2. [CrossRef] [PubMed]
36. Maharaj, S.; Ramsewak, S.; Pooransingh, S.; Shah, Z.; Abdul, K.; Benasrie, T.; Manick, M.; Ramdin, D. Suitcase Trading and The Pharmaceutical Industry in Trinidad. *Int. J. Pharm. Res. BioScience* **2012**, *1*, 406–419.
37. Scheckel, C.J.; Rajkumar, S.V. Drug importation: Limitations of current proposals and opportunities for improvement. *Blood Cancer J.* **2021**, *11*, 132. [CrossRef] [PubMed]
38. Jacobs, T.G.; Robertson, J.; van den Ham, H.A.; Iwamoto, K.; Bak Pederson, H.; Mantel-Teeuwisse, A.K. Assessing the impact of law enforcement to reduce over the counter (OTC) sales of antibiotics in low- and middle-income countries; a systematic literature review. *BMC Health Serv. Res.* **2019**, *19*, 536. [CrossRef] [PubMed]

Disclaimer/Publisher's Note: The statements, opinions and data contained in all publications are solely those of the individual author(s) and contributor(s) and not of MDPI and/or the editor(s). MDPI and/or the editor(s) disclaim responsibility for any injury to people or property resulting from any ideas, methods, instructions or products referred to in the content.

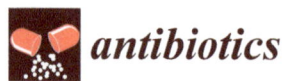

Article

Factors Influencing Antibiotic Consumption in Adult Population of Kazakhstan

Nazym Iskakova [1], Zaituna Khismetova [1], Dana Suleymenova [1], Zhanat Kozhekenova [2], Zaituna Khamidullina [3], Umutzhan Samarova [1], Natalya Glushkova [4,*] and Yuliya Semenova [5,*]

[1] Department of Public Health, Semey Medical University, Semey 070000, Kazakhstan
[2] Department of Public Health, Asfendiyarov Kazakh National Medical University, Almaty 050000, Kazakhstan
[3] Department of Obstetrics and Gynecology #1, NpJSC "Astana Medical University", Astana 010000, Kazakhstan
[4] Department of Epidemiology, Biostatistics and Evidence-Based Medicine, Al-Farabi Kazakh National University, Almaty 050010, Kazakhstan
[5] School of Medicine, Nazarbayev University, Astana 010000, Kazakhstan
* Correspondence: glushkovanatalyae@gmail.com (N.G.); yuliya.semenova@nu.edu.kz (Y.S.)

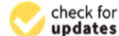

Citation: Iskakova, N.; Khismetova, Z.; Suleymenova, D.; Kozhekenova, Z.; Khamidullina, I.; Samarova, U.; Glushkova, N.; Semenova, Y. Factors Influencing Antibiotic Consumption in Adult Population of Kazakhstan. *Antibiotics* 2023, 12, 560. https://doi.org/10.3390/antibiotics12030560

Academic Editors: Juan Manuel Vázquez-Lago, Ana Estany-Gestal, Angel Salgado-Barreira and Masafumi Seki

Received: 4 February 2023
Revised: 7 March 2023
Accepted: 9 March 2023
Published: 11 March 2023

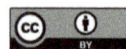

Copyright: © 2023 by the authors. Licensee MDPI, Basel, Switzerland. This article is an open access article distributed under the terms and conditions of the Creative Commons Attribution (CC BY) license (https://creativecommons.org/licenses/by/4.0/).

Abstract: Poor or suboptimal knowledge of appropriate antibiotic use is a cause for global concern and little is known about Central Asian countries. Therefore, this survey is aimed at evaluating awareness about antibiotic use and resistance among the adult population of Kazakhstan. A cross-sectional study of a random sample was conducted between October 2021 and February 2022 among 727 individuals without medical education and followed the methodology described in the WHO report "Antibiotic Resistance: Multi-country public awareness survey". Half of the respondents (50.4%) received antibiotic therapy within the last 12 months, 40.1% had no prescription for this and 40.4% received no advice from a medical professional. Nearly two-thirds of respondents (65.3%) never heard about antibiotic resistance and 57.2% believed that it is worth requesting the same antibiotic if it helped to treat a similar condition previously. In general, knowledge about antibiotic use proved to be low in 82.1% of respondents and 91.9% agreed with the statement that a common cold requires antibiotics. There is a need for awareness-raising campaigns to improve the knowledge about antibiotic use and resistance in the population of Kazakhstan.

Keywords: antibiotics; antibiotic resistance; awareness

1. Introduction

Since the discovery of the first antibiotic (penicillin) by Alexander Fleming in 1928, antibiotics have revolutionized modern medicine by making previously incurable infections and conditions, including pneumonia and other life-threatening bacterial infections, treatable. Today, many routine medical procedures, such as cesarean section, appendix removal, and chemotherapy, rely on effective antibiotics to prevent common infections from becoming fatal. However, decades of misuse of antibiotics and abuse by doctors and patients (to treat mild ailments) and farmers (to promote growth in agriculture and aquaculture) have led to the emergence of antimicrobial/antibiotic resistance (AMR or ABR), which seriously threatens the health of humans, animals, and the environment [1]. In recent years, numerous awareness-raising activities have been undertaken to educate both the public and medical professionals on the issue of unjustified antibiotic consumption, which remains a major public health concern.

Despite a slight reduction in the consumption of antibiotics for systemic use, the irrational use of these drugs remains prevalent in Kazakhstan. This is due to the over-the-counter availability of 27.5% of antibiotics and excessive prescription by medical professionals, where 29.9% of all medications prescribed are antibiotics [2]. The World Health Organization (WHO) recommends a decrease in global antibiotic prescriptions by 20% to combat the development of antibiotic resistance [1]. Additionally, the actual consumption of antibiotics in Kazakhstan is thought to be higher, given the widespread empirical use during the COVID-19 pandemic [3].

The excessive prescription of antibiotics can have significant financial implications for individuals and healthcare systems. When antibiotics are over-prescribed, not only can they become less effective due to the development of antibiotic resistance, but they can also cause side effects that lead to further medical expenses. As antibiotic resistance grows, the cost of treating infections increases, as more expensive and effective drugs are required. This can put a strain on health insurance providers and government healthcare programs, which may struggle to cover the cost of these treatments. The bulk of healthcare provided to the population of Kazakhstan is reimbursed from the state-owned social health insurance fund. Out-of-pocket payments contribute to over-the-counter sales and unnecessary prescriptions may affect the financial stability of the poorest population stratum [1].

Being concerned about the growing trend of antibiotic consumption, the WHO developed a global action plan to combat antibiotic resistance which urges all countries to increase public knowledge about antibiotics and antibiotic resistance through effective information and communication campaigns [4]. Thus, in order to develop effective intervention strategies, it is important to understand the level of awareness, attitudes, and perceptions of the population about antibiotics and antibiotic resistance [5]. We therefore conducted a cross-sectional study to evaluate awareness about antibiotic use and resistance among the adult population of Kazakhstan. In our study, we examined the following hypotheses: (i) there may be age and gender-based differences in awareness about antibiotic use; (ii) rural and urban residents may have different attitudes towards antibiotic use; and (iii) education and income levels may influence the pattern of antibiotic use.

2. Results

Table 1 presents an overview of the population under study, detailing their key characteristics. Out of the total sample, 542 individuals (74.6%) identified as female, while 185 (25.4%) identified as male. The majority of participants were under 25 years of age (60.2%) and resided in urban areas (53.6%). Over half of respondents held undergraduate or postgraduate degrees (55.5%). The most common household type was comprised of multiple adults aged > 16 years and at least one child under 16 (40.4% of all households). The median household income was 150,000 Tenge, which is equivalent to 350 US dollars [6].

Table 2 illustrates the level of awareness regarding antibiotic use and resistance by gender. Notably, there was a significant difference in the duration since respondents last received antibiotics between male and female participants. Specifically, 33.1% of females reported receiving antibiotics within the last month, compared to 28.8% of males who reported receiving antibiotics within the last 6 months. Moreover, 55.0% of males believed that they should stop taking antibiotics once they have taken all the prescribed medicine, in contrast to 70.5% of females. Regarding prescription patterns, the majority of females (64.1%) reported having a prescription for the antibiotics they last took, while the majority of males (52.1%) did not.

Furthermore, a greater proportion of females (83.2%) disagreed with the notion that it is advisable to use the same antibiotics as a friend or family member who previously treated similar symptoms or disease, compared to males (65.7%). It is noteworthy that while the vast majority of both males and females obtain antibiotics from a medical store or pharmacy, none of the females and 1.8% of males stored antibiotics from a previous time. Lastly, there was a significant difference between genders in seeking advice from healthcare professionals regarding antibiotic use. Specifically, 63.7% of females sought advice from healthcare professionals, while only 46.8% of males did so.

Between-group comparisons of individuals aged 24 years and younger and their older counterparts (Table 3) are of interest. Individuals aged 24 years and younger were more likely to disagree with the statement that it is good to use the same antibiotic if a friend or family member used it to treat the same symptoms or disease before than individuals 25 years and older (81.9% vs. 73.9%). In our study, younger participants reported hearing about antibiotic resistance significantly more often (68.7%) than older participants did (60.2%). However, individuals aged 25 years and older were more likely to seek advice from a doctor, nurse, or pharmacist on how to take antibiotics than their younger counterparts (65.7% vs. 55.6%). In addition, a significant difference was observed in the time of the last antibiotic intake, with most younger individuals (28.3%) receiving antibiotics in the last month. In contrast, the majority of older individuals (32.2%) received antibiotics in the past 6 months.

Table 1. General characteristics of the study participants.

General Characteristics (n = 727)		n	%
Sex	Males	185	25.4
	Females	542	74.6
Age	18–24	438	60.2
	25–34	114	15.7
	35–44	72	9.9
	45–54	36	5.0
	55–64	48	6.6
	65+	19	2.6
Location	Urban	390	53.6
	Suburban	200	27.5
	Rural	137	18.8
Education	No schooling completed	31	4.3
	Only school completed	151	20.8
	Some college credit, no degree	41	5.6
	Technical/Vocational training	101	13.9
	Bachelor's degree	343	47.2
	Master's degree	53	7.3
	Doctorate (Ph.D.) degree	7	1.0
Household composition	Single adult only	144	19.8
	Single adult and at least 1 child under 16	15	2.1
	Married adults only	22	3.0
	Married and at least 1 child under 16	132	18.2
	Multiple adults aged 16+ only	120	16.5
	Multiple adults aged 16+ only and at least 1 child under 16	294	40.4
Household income, median, 25–75 percentiles		150,000	(100,000–300,000)

According to Table 4, individuals with tertiary education had a prescription for the antibiotics they consumed significantly more often than those with pre-tertiary education (64.6% vs. 53.8%). Most individuals with pre-tertiary education had consumed antibiotics in the past month (30.3%), while the majority of those with tertiary education had taken antibiotics in the past six months (28.9%), which was significant ($p = 0.039$). Individuals with higher education heard about antibiotic resistance insignificantly more often than those with lower education (37.5% vs. 31.2%).

Table 2. Awareness about antibiotic use and resistance by sex.

Questions		Male		Female		p-Value
		n	%	n	%	
When do you think you should stop taking the antibiotics? (n = 620)	When you feel better	67	45.0	139	29.5	<0.001
	When you've taken all of the antibiotics as directed	82	55.0	332	70.5	
Do you think it is good to use the same antibiotic if a friend or family member used to treat same symptoms or disease before? (n = 548)	True	47	34.3	69	16.8	<0.001
	False	90	65.7	342	83.2	
Do you think it is good to ask/request the same antibiotic if it helped to treat the same symptoms/disease previously? (n = 516)	True	75	57.7	220	57.0	0.889
	False	55	42.3	166	43.0	
Have you heard term "Antibiotic resistance"? (n = 727)	Yes	67	36.2	185	34.1	0.607
	No	118	63.8	357	65.9	
When did you last take antibiotics? (571)	In the last month	49	33.1	109	25.8	0.014
	In the last 6 months	25	16.9	122	28.8	
	In the last year	12	8.1	50	11.8	
	More than a year ago	28	18.9	58	13.7	
	Never	34	23.0	84	19.9	
Did you have a prescription for this antibiotic? (n = 636)	Yes	78	47.9	303	64.1	<0.001
	No	85	52.1	170	35.9	
Did you get advice from a doctor, nurse or pharmacist on how to take them? (n = 628)	Yes	72	46.8	302	63.7	<0.001
	No	82	53.2	172	36.3	
Where did you get the antibiotics? (n = 650)	Medical store or pharmacy	156	95.7	479	98.4	0.009
	The internet	3	1.8	2	0.4	
	Friend or family member	1	0.6	6	1.2	
	I had them saved up from a previous time	3	1.8	0	0.0	

Table 5 presents the between-group comparisons based on the place of residence. The only significant difference was observed in the time of the last intake of antibiotics. Specifically, the majority of rural respondents (36.9%) took antibiotics in the past month, while only a quarter (25.6%) of urban and suburban residents did so. Nearly equal proportions of rural and urban/suburban residents consumed antibiotics within the past 6 months (25.2% vs. 25.9%).

The between-group comparisons based on income level are presented in Table 6. Respondents with income below the median ($\leq$150,000 Tenge) believed significantly less often than their wealthier counterparts that it is advisable to request the same antibiotic if it had previously helped to treat the same symptoms or disease (53.1% vs. 62.6%). Furthermore, they had a lower level of awareness about antibiotic resistance, with only 30.4% of them having ever heard the term "antibiotic resistance", compared to 40.3% of individuals with income above the study median. Additionally, there were significant differences in the time since the last intake of antibiotics, as the majority of individuals with lower income had consumed antibiotics in the past month, while the majority of individuals with higher income had consumed antibiotics in the past six months.

In general, the level of knowledge regarding antibiotic use was found to be inadequate. A total of 12 questions were asked, and respondents' knowledge was considered low if they answered six or fewer questions correctly, and good if they answered seven or more correctly. The vast majority of study participants (82.1%) had low knowledge about health problems that can be treated with antibiotics, with only 17.9% answering seven or more questions correctly.

Figure 1 presents the responses to questions about conditions that can be treated with antibiotics. More than half of the respondents (57.4%) believed that headaches can be treated with antibiotics, and 48.1% believed that antibiotics can relieve body aches. Notably, 67.9% of respondents were not aware that measles is a condition that can be managed with antibiotics. Additionally, 69.9% replied that they would use antibiotics in case of fever, and a high percentage of 91.9% agreed with the statement that antibiotics are required for the common flu.

Table 3. Awareness about antibiotic use and resistance by age.

Questions		18–24 Years of Age		25 Years and Older		p-Value
		n	%	n	%	
When do you think you should stop taking the antibiotics? (n = 620)	When you feel better	123	34.0	83	32.2	0.638
	When you've taken all of the antibiotics as directed	239	66.0	175	67.8	
Do you think it is good to use the same antibiotic if a friend or family member used to treat same symptoms or disease before? (n = 548)	True	61	18.1	55	26.1	0.026
	False	276	81.9	156	73.9	
Do you think it is good to ask/request the same antibiotic if it helped to treat the same symptoms/disease previously? (n = 516)	True	165	53.9	130	61.9	0.072
	False	141	46.1	80	38.1	
Have you heard term "Antibiotic resistance"? (n = 727)	Yes	137	31.3	115	39.8	0.018
	No	301	68.7	174	60.2	
When did you last take antibiotics? (571)	In the last month	92	28.3	66	26.8	<0.001
	In the last 6 months	68	20.9	79	32.2	
	In the last year	29	8.9	33	13.4	
	More than a year ago	41	12.6	45	18.3	
	Never	95	29.3	23	9.3	
Did you have a prescription for this antibiotic? (n = 636)	Yes	222	58.4	159	62.1	0.352
	No	158	41.6	97	37.9	
Did you get advice from a doctor, nurse or pharmacist on how to take them? (n = 628)	Yes	213	55.6	161	65.7	0.012
	No	170	44.4	84	34.3	
Where did you get the antibiotics? (n = 650)	Medical store or pharmacy	378	97.7	257	97.8	0.272
	The internet	2	0.5	3	1.1	
	Friend or family member	4	1.0	3	1.1	
	I had them saved up from a previous time	3	0.8	0	0.0	

Table 4. Awareness about antibiotic use and resistance by education level.

Questions		Pre-Tertiary Education		Tertiary Education		p-Value
		n	%	n	%	
When do you think you should stop taking the antibiotics? (n = 620)	When you feel better	99	35.6	107	31.3	0.256
	When you've taken all of the antibiotics as directed	179	64.4	235	68.7	
Do you think it is good to use the same antibiotic if a friend or family member used to treat same symptoms or disease before? (n = 548)	True	57	24.8	59	18.6	0.078
	False	173	75.2	259	81.4	
Do you think it is good to ask/request the same antibiotic if it helped to treat the same symptoms/disease previously? (n = 516)	True	123	54.4	172	59.3	0.266
	False	103	45.6	118	40.7	
Have you heard term "Antibiotic resistance"? (n = 727)	Yes	101	31.2	151	37.5	0.076
	No	223	68.8	252	62.5	

Table 4. Cont.

Questions		Pre-Tertiary Education		Tertiary Education		p-Value
		n	%	n	%	
When did you last take antibiotics? (571)	In the last month	81	30.3	77	25.3	0.039
	In the last 6 months	59	22.1	88	28.9	
	In the last year	22	8.2	40	13.2	
	More than a year ago	48	18.0	38	12.5	
	Never	57	21.3	61	20.1	
Did you have a prescription for this antibiotic? (n = 636)	Yes	149	53.8	232	64.6	0.006
	No	128	46.2	127	32.4	
Did you get advice from a doctor, nurse or pharmacist on how to take them? (n = 628)	Yes	156	58.6	218	60.2	0.691
	No	110	41.4	144	39.8	
Where did you get the antibiotics? (n = 650)	Medical store or pharmacy	274	96.5	361	98.6	0.172
	The internet	3	1.1	2	0.5	
	Friend or family member	4	1.4	3	0.8	
	I had them saved up from a previous time	3	1.1	0	0.0	

Table 5. Awareness about antibiotic use and resistance by the place of residence.

Questions		Urban and Suburban Residents		Rural Residents		p-Value
		n	%	n	%	
When do you think you should stop taking the antibiotics? (n = 620)	When you feel better	164	32.4	42	36.8	0.364
	When you've taken all of the antibiotics as directed	342	67.6	72	63.2	
Do you think it is good to use the same antibiotic if a friend or family member used to treat same symptoms or disease before? (n = 548)	True	99	22.4	17	16.0	0.150
	False	343	77.6	89	84.0	
Do you think it is good to ask/request the same antibiotic if it helped to treat the same symptoms/disease previously? (n = 516)	True	239	57.0	56	57.7	0.901
	False	180	43.0	41	42.3	
Have you heard term "Antibiotic resistance"? (n = 727)	Yes	208	35.3	44	32.1	0.487
	No	382	64.7	93	67.9	
When did you last take antibiotics? (571)	In the last month	120	25.6	38	36.9	0.010
	In the last 6 months	121	25.9	26	25.2	
	In the last year	58	12.4	4	3.9	
	More than a year ago	66	14.1	20	19.4	
	Never	103	22.0	15	14.6	
Did you have a prescription for this antibiotic? (n = 636)	Yes	309	58.7	72	65.5	0.192
	No	217	41.3	38	34.5	
Did you get advice from a doctor, nurse or pharmacist on how to take them? (n = 628)	Yes	309	59.8	65	58.6	0.814
	No	208	40.2	46	41.4	
Where did you get the antibiotics? (n = 650)	Medical store or pharmacy	527	98.0	108	96.4	0.273
	The internet	4	0.7	1	0.9	
	Friend or family member	4	0.7	3	2.7	
	I had them saved up from a previous time	3	0.6	0	0.0	

Table 6. Awareness about antibiotic use and resistance by the level of income.

Questions		Lower Income		Higher Income		p-Value
		n	%	n	%	
When do you think you should stop taking the antibiotics? (n = 620)	When you feel better	117	34.7	89	31.4	0.389
	When you've taken all of the antibiotics as directed	220	65.3	194	68.6	
Do you think it is good to use the same antibiotic if a friend or family member used to treat same symptoms or disease before? (n = 548)	True	61	20.8	55	21.6	0.830
	False	232	79.2	200	78.4	
Do you think it is good to ask/request the same antibiotic if it helped to treat the same symptoms/disease previously? (n = 516)	True	156	53.1	139	62.6	0.030
	False	138	46.9	83	37.4	
Have you heard term "Antibiotic resistance"? (n = 727)	Yes	126	30.4	126	40.3	0.006
	No	288	69.6	187	59.7	
When did you last take antibiotics? (571)	In the last month	90	28.8	68	26.4	0.004
	In the last 6 months	63	20.1	84	32.6	
	In the last year	34	10.9	28	10.9	
	More than a year ago	59	18.8	27	10.5	
	Never	67	21.4	51	19.8	
Did you have a prescription for this antibiotic? (n = 636)	Yes	203	59.0	178	61.0	0.618
	No	141	41.0	114	39.0	
Did you get advice from a doctor, nurse or pharmacist on how to take them? (n = 628)	Yes	200	58.8	174	60.4	0.685
	No	140	41.2	114	39.6	
Where did you get the antibiotics? (n = 650)	Medical store or pharmacy	341	97.4	294	98.0	0.092
	The internet	3	0.9	2	0.7	
	Friend or family member	6	1.7	1	0.3	
	I had them saved up from a previous time	0	0.0	3	1.0	

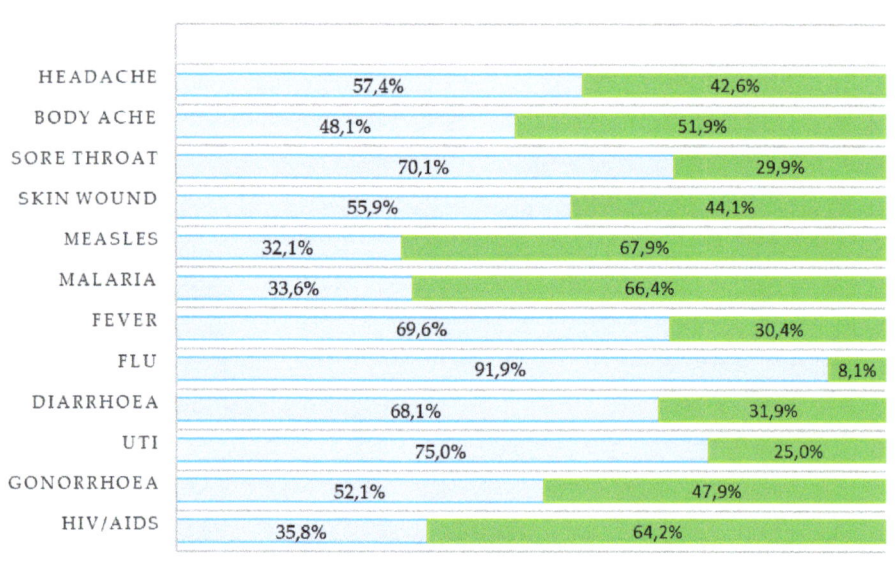

Figure 1. Knowledge of conditions that can be treated with antibiotics.

3. Discussion

This survey aimed to evaluate the level of awareness regarding antibiotic use and resistance among the adult population of Kazakhstan. Half of the respondents (50.4%) received antibiotic therapy within the last 12 months, of which 40.1% had no prescription and 40.4% did not receive advice from a medical professional on how to take them. Nearly two-thirds of respondents (65.3%) had never heard of antibiotic resistance, and 57.2% believed that it is acceptable to request the same antibiotic if it had helped to treat the same symptoms previously. In general, knowledge about antibiotic use for specific health conditions was found to be low in 82.1% of the study participants.

Our study findings are consistent with reports from other Eastern European countries. A study by Zajmi et al. in Kosovo showed that more than half of the respondents (58.7%) used antibiotics in the past year, and a quarter (25.0%) took them without a physician's prescription. Notably, 42.5% of respondents believed that viral infections could be effectively treated with antibiotics [7]. In Georgia, over half (55%) of adults received antibiotics without consulting a medical professional, and 62% bought antibiotics without a prescription [8]. A study in Lithuania revealed that 61.1% of respondents had poor knowledge of antibiotics, and 26.0% believed that antibiotics are effective against viral infections [9]. In Serbia, 58.4% of respondents considered antibiotics to be effective against the common cold [10]. In Romania, more than half (61.45%) of the general public received antibiotics at least once in the past year, and only 57.43% reported consulting a physician before taking them [11]. However, a study from Poland reported lower rates of antibiotic consumption in the previous year (38.0%). Unlike the findings of other Eastern European studies, the majority of antibiotics (90%) were prescribed by a doctor [12].

To mitigate the problem of antibiotic resistance, the sale of antibiotics without a prescription should be prohibited, and self-medication should be discouraged. Nevertheless, it is a common practice in many developing countries to sell antibiotics upon a patient's request. A qualitative study from India confirmed that pharmacists readily admitted to selling antibiotics over the counter and were generally unaware of the issue of antibiotic resistance [13]. In Damascus, Syria, 87% of pharmacy workers easily agreed to sell antibiotics without a prescription, and 97% sold antibiotics if a patient insisted [14]. Another study from the Middle East reported high rates of over-the-counter sales of antibiotics (63.6%) in Saudi Arabia [15]. Both online and community pharmacies sell antibiotics without a valid prescription, as a study from China showed. However, community pharmacies were more likely to sell antibiotics over the counter and provide no necessary information to patients [16].

Poor or suboptimal knowledge of appropriate antibiotic use is another cause for global concern, as it significantly contributes to antibiotic resistance. This includes awareness of the spectrum of diseases that can be treated with antibiotics, the duration of therapy, and understanding when it is appropriate to stop taking them. Akhund et al. conducted an online survey in Pakistan and found that out of 1132 participants, 837 (73.9%) believed that it is possible to stop the course of antibiotics whenever they feel better, and 505 (44.6%) were convinced that frequent and unnecessary use of antibiotics reduces their effectiveness. Notably, 157 (13.9%) of the participants did not adhere to the duration of treatment recommended by a doctor. As many as 467 (41.3%) of the respondents reused antibiotics left over from a previous prescription when experiencing similar symptoms [17]. In our study, 33.2% of respondents stopped their intake of antibiotics when they felt better. Inadequate knowledge concerning the time to stop antibiotic therapy was also reported by other researchers [14–16].

Self-medication with antibiotics is becoming widespread, and many people are convinced that they can use the same antibiotic for a condition with similar symptoms. In this study, more than half of the participants (57.2%) thought it is acceptable to buy the same antibiotic or request it from a doctor if it helped them to get better when the same symptoms were present before. In a study from Romania, 10.34% of respondents took antibiotics following recommendations of a family member or friend, and 22.9% used the same antibiotic prescribed by a doctor at the last visit [11]. In general, the population of Eastern Europe has higher rates of self-medication with antibiotics as compared to the population of Western Europe. This could be attributed to cultural differences and law enforcement efforts to prohibit the over-the-counter sale of prescription drugs [18].

A striking finding of this study is that a high proportion of the population (91.9%) is ready to take antibiotics for a common cold. This is probably best explained by the incorrect identification of bacteria as the most common cause of upper respiratory tract infections. The same misconception is shared by the populations of other countries, although to a lesser extent. In Germany, 10.5% of patients asked for antibiotics to treat common colds [19], and 14% of patients in Denmark requested a prescription of antibiotics for upper respiratory tract infections [20]. This proportion is declining in Romania, where as many as 51% of respondents considered antibiotics effective against flu in 2009 [21], compared to 39% in 2016 [22]. Indeed, our findings are comparable to data from Myanmar, where 72.6% of respondents believed that antibiotics can eliminate viruses and 73.5% considered antibiotics effective against the flu. Interestingly, these beliefs were more prevalent among younger individuals and those residing in urban areas [23].

Another commonly shared misbelief is that antibiotics can be used to treat non-bloody diarrhea. According to a systematic review by Carter et al., low- and middle-income countries tend to over-rely on antibiotics in the treatment of childhood diarrhea as they are prescribed in 10–77% of cases [24]. Another meta-analysis by Edessa et al. showed that the rate of non-prescribed antibiotics in pediatric practice at the community level in low- and middle-income countries constitute 45% [25].

There is a need for awareness-raising campaigns to improve knowledge about antibiotic use and resistance in the population of Kazakhstan. This could be done via social media, and the importance of seeking professional advice before initiating antibacterial therapy has to be emphasized. The country's medical community, in particular the primary healthcare sector, should adopt the best health education strategies, and policymakers have to reinforce their efforts to control the over-the-counter sale of prescription medications. Currently, there is a lack of recognition of antibiotic misuse in Kazakhstan, and therefore it is important to sensitize all stakeholders. The country's stakeholders can benefit from the strategies proposed by World Antimicrobial Awareness Week, which was designed to enable communication with a focus on effective approaches to prevent and mitigate antimicrobial resistance [26].

The current study has several limitations primarily stemming from its cross-sectional design. One of the main limitations is the inability to establish causal relationships between knowledge and practice of antibiotic use and individual participant characteristics. Originally, our intention was to sample healthy individuals visiting outpatient facilities for routine check-ups or accompanying their diseased relatives. However, we quickly realized that few adults attend healthcare facilities for preventive purposes. As a result, the majority of participants in our study were accompanying persons, leading to observed shifts in gender and age. Therefore, this sample is not representative of the entire population of Kazakhstan and should be considered as a pilot study. Despite these limitations, our study has many strengths. It is based on a reasonably large sample of the adult population enrolled from a typical region of the country. Furthermore, it is the first study to investigate awareness about antibiotic use and resistance among the population of Kazakhstan and can serve as a benchmark for future research.

4. Materials and Methods

4.1. Study Design and Procedures

A cross-sectional study was conducted between October 2021 and February 2022, using a random sample of adult residents without medical education in the East Kazakhstan region. This region was selected as a representative area of the country, based on socio-economic indicators, and had an estimated population of 1,349,400 in 2022 [27]. The sample size was calculated using the Sample XS calculator from Brixton Health [28], for a population size of 13 million (the adult population of Kazakhstan), 80% power, an estimated prevalence of 20%, and a design effect of 1.0. The resulting sample size was 683 individuals, but we enrolled 750 participants to allow for potential dropouts. Ultimately, 727 individuals agreed to participate, resulting in a response rate of 96.9%.

We recruited healthy individuals attending regional outpatient facilities for routine check-ups or as accompanying persons, using a systematic random sampling method. Out of 35 outpatient polyclinic organizations located on the territory of the East Kazakhstan region, 15 were sampled to represent two cities—Ust-Kamenogorsk and Semey (5 facilities from each city) and rural territories. We sampled 5 rural outpatient facilities located in the region's north-west (Beskaragay district), north-east (Altai district), center (Zharma district), south-west (Ayagoz district), and south-east (Tarbagatay district). A maximum of 15–20 individuals were recruited from each clinic per day. The full WHO questionnaire was administered through face-to-face interviews. Age below 18 years, presence of medical education, and unwillingness to participate in the study served as the exclusion criteria.

4.2. The Tool and Data Collection Techniques

This survey followed the methodology described in the WHO report "Antibiotic Resistance: Multi-country public awareness survey" [29]. The questionnaire consisted of four sections. The first section included questions related to the social and demographic characteristics of respondents, while the second and third sections focused on the knowledge and use of antibiotics. Knowledge about antibiotic resistance was assessed in the fourth section. The questionnaire was administered in the Kazakh and Russian languages and it took approximately 10–15 min to complete it. The study aim was clearly explained to the participants before the data collection and informed consent was obtained. To keep confidentiality, identity information was not collected. All data were encrypted and stored electronically in a secure location and a password was solely available to the principal investigator (N.I.) to ensure the privacy of study participants.

4.3. Statistical Analysis

The study data were analyzed using the Statistical Package for Social Sciences (SPSS) version 20. As a first step of statistical analysis, the type of data distribution was evaluated for continuous variables by the Kolmogorov-Smirnov test. As the distribution of data proved to be different from normal, the continuous variables were presented as the median with interquartile ranges and non-parametric tests were used to compare differences between the groups. Categorical variables were presented as the frequency with percentage and Pearson's chi-square test was utilized for between-group comparisons. A p-value of 0.05 and below was considered statistically significant.

To facilitate educational level comparisons, we classified educational attainments into two categories: pre-tertiary (including no schooling, completed school, some college credit, and non-degree technical/vocational training) and tertiary (comprising bachelor's, master's, and doctoral (Ph.D.) degrees). To elucidate the differences between groups based on place of residence, we compared individuals living in urban and suburban areas with individuals living in rural areas. To compare responses from different income groups, we divided all respondents into two groups based on their monthly income levels: a lower income group (monthly income $\leq$150,000 Tenge) and a higher income group (monthly income exceeding 150,000 Tenge). At the time of the survey in 2021, 150,000 Tenge was approximately equivalent to 350 US dollars [30].

4.4. Ethical Considerations

This study has been approved by the Ethics Committee of Semey Medical University with registration code 2, dated 28 October 2020.

5. Conclusions

This study sheds light on the level of awareness and behavior regarding antibiotic use and resistance in Kazakhstan, with a focus on gender, age, education, place of residence, and income level. The findings reveal significant differences in the duration since respondents last received antibiotics, prescription patterns, beliefs about antibiotic use, and seeking advice from healthcare professionals between males and females. Moreover, age, education, and income level were associated with differences in antibiotic use and awareness. Our study highlights the importance of increasing awareness and promoting the appropriate use of antibiotics among different population groups in Kazakhstan. Further research and interventions are needed to address the identified differences and improve antibiotic use practices in the country.

Author Contributions: Conceptualization, N.I. and Z.K. (Zaituna Khismetova); Data curation, N.G.; Formal analysis, N.G.; Funding acquisition, Z.K. (Zaituna Khismetova); Investigation, Y.S.; Methodology, N.G.; Project administration, Z.K. (Zhanat Kozhekenova); Resources, Z.K. (Zaituna Khamidullina) and U.S.; Software, N.G. and Y.S.; Supervision, D.S.; Validation, D.S., Z.K. (Zhanat Kozhekenova) and U.S.; Visualization, N.G.; Writing—original draft, N.I.; Writing—review & editing, Y.S. All authors have read and agreed to the published version of the manuscript.

Funding: This research received no external funding.

Institutional Review Board Statement: The study was conducted in accordance with the Declaration of Helsinki, and approved by the Ethics Committee of Semey Medical University (protocol code 2, dated 28 October 2020).

Informed Consent Statement: Informed consent was obtained from all subjects involved in the study.

Data Availability Statement: The data presented in this study are available on a reasonable request from the corresponding author.

Acknowledgments: The authors would like to thank all individuals who participated in this survey.

Conflicts of Interest: The authors declare no conflict of interest.

References

1. The World Health Organization. Antibiotic Resistance. Available online: https://www.who.int/news-room/fact-sheets/detail/antibiotic-resistance (accessed on 8 January 2023).
2. Zhussupova, G.; Zhaldybayeva, S.; Utepova, D. Improving the use of medicines in healthcare organizations to solve the problem of irrational use of medicines in the Republic of Kazakhstan. *J. Health Dev.* **2020**, *36*, 84–100. [CrossRef]
3. Semenova, Y.; Pivina, L.; Khismetova, Z.; Auyezova, A.; Nurbakyt, A.; Kaysheva, A.; Ospanova, D.; Kuziyeva, G.; Kushkarova, A.; Ivankov, A.; et al. Anticipating the Need for Healthcare Resources Following the Escalation of the COVID-19 Outbreak in the Republic of Kazakhstan. *J. Prev. Med. Public Health* **2020**, *53*, 387–396. [CrossRef] [PubMed]
4. The World Health Organization. Global Action Plan on Antimicrobial Resistance. Available online: https://www.who.int/publications/i/item/9789241509763 (accessed on 8 January 2023).
5. King, R.; Hicks, J.; Rassi, C.; Shafique, M.; Barua, D.; Bhowmik, P.; Das, M.; Elsey, H.; Questa, K.; Fieroze, F.; et al. A process for developing a sustainable and scalable approach to community engagement: Community dialogue approach for addressing the drivers of antibiotic resistance in Bangladesh. *BMC Public Health* **2020**, *20*, 950. [CrossRef] [PubMed]
6. The Average Weighted Exchange Rate of the Dollar at the Cash Is 431.67 Tenge Capital. Available online: https://kapital.kz/finance/101590/srednevzveshennyy-kurs-dollara-na-kase-431-67-tenge.html (accessed on 8 January 2023).
7. Zajmi, D.; Berisha, M.; Begolli, I.; Hoxha, R.; Mehmeti, R.; Mulliqi-Osmani, G.; Kurti, A.; Loku, A.; Raka, L. Public knowledge, attitudes and practices regarding antibiotic use in Kosovo. *Pharm. Pract.* **2017**, *15*, 827. [CrossRef] [PubMed]
8. Kandelaki, K.; Lundborg, C.S.; Marrone, G. Antibiotic use and resistance: A cross-sectional study exploring knowledge and attitudes among school and institution personnel in Tbilisi, Republic of Georgia. *BMC Res. Notes* **2015**, *8*, 495. [CrossRef] [PubMed]
9. Pavydė, E.; Veikutis, V.; Mačiulienė, A.; Mačiulis, V.; Petrikonis, K.; Stankevičius, E. Public Knowledge, Beliefs and Behavior on Antibiotic Use and Self-Medication in Lithuania. *Int. J. Environ. Res. Public Health* **2015**, *12*, 7002–7016. [CrossRef] [PubMed]
10. Horvat, O.J.; Tomas, A.D.; Paut Kusturica, M.M.; Savkov, A.V.; Bukumirić, D.U.; Tomić, Z.S.; Sabo, A.J. Is the level of knowledge a predictor of rational antibiotic use in Serbia? *PLoS ONE* **2017**, *12*, e0180799. [CrossRef] [PubMed]

11. Voidăzan, S.; Moldovan, G.; Voidăzan, L.; Zazgyva, A.; Moldovan, H. Knowledge, Attitudes and Practices Regarding the Use Of Antibiotics. Study on The General Population of Mureş County, Romania. *Infect. Drug Resist.* **2019**, *12*, 3385–3396. [CrossRef] [PubMed]
12. Mazińska, B.; Strużycka, I.; Hryniewicz, W. Surveys of public knowledge and attitudes with regard to antibiotics in Poland: Did the European Antibiotic Awareness Day campaigns change attitudes? *PLoS ONE* **2017**, *12*, e0172146. [CrossRef] [PubMed]
13. Chandran, D.S.; Manickavasagam, P.P. Sale of antibiotics without prescription in stand-alone pharmacies in Tamil Nadu. *J. Fam. Med. Prim. Care* **2022**, *11*, 5516–5520. [CrossRef] [PubMed]
14. Al-Faham, Z.; Habboub, G.; Takriti, F. The sale of antibiotics without prescription in pharmacies in Damascus, Syria. *J. Infect. Dev. Ctries.* **2011**, *5*, 396–399. [CrossRef] [PubMed]
15. El Zowalaty, M.E.; Belkina, T.; Bahashwan, S.A.; El Zowalaty, A.E.; Tebbens, J.D.; Abdel-Salam, H.A.; Khalil, A.I.; Daghriry, S.I.; Gahtani, M.A.; Madkhaly, F.M.; et al. Knowledge, awareness, and attitudes toward antibiotic use and antimicrobial resistance among Saudi population. *Int. J. Clin. Pharm.* **2016**, *38*, 1261–1268. [CrossRef] [PubMed]
16. Gong, Y.; Jiang, N.; Chen, Z.; Wang, J.; Zhang, J.; Feng, J.; Lu, Z.; Yin, X. Over-the-counter antibiotic sales in community and online pharmacies, China. *Bull. World Health Organ.* **2020**, *98*, 449–457. [CrossRef] [PubMed]
17. Akhund, R.; Jamshed, F.; Jaffry, H.A.; Hanif, H.; Fareed, S. Knowledge and Attitude of General Pakistani Population Towards Antibiotic Resistance. *Cureus* **2019**, *11*, e4266. [CrossRef] [PubMed]
18. Paget, J.; Lescure, D.; Versporten, A.; Goossens, H.; Schellevis, F.; van Dijk, L. *Antimicrobial Resistance and Causes of Non-Prudent Use of Antibiotics in Human Medicine in the EU*; European Commission: Brussels, Belgium, 2017; pp. 8–156.
19. Faber, M.S.; Heckenbach, K.; Velasco, E.; Eckmanns, T. Antibiotics for the common cold: Expectations of Germany's general population. *Euro Surveill. Bull. Eur. Sur Les Mal. Transm. Eur. Commun. Dis. Bull.* **2010**, *15*, 19655. [CrossRef]
20. Bagger, K.; Nielsen, A.B.; Siersma, V.; Bjerrum, L. Inappropriate antibiotic prescribing and demand for antibiotics in patients with upper respiratory tract infections is hardly different in female versus male patients as seen in primary care. *Eur. J. Gen. Pract.* **2015**, *21*, 118–123. [CrossRef] [PubMed]
21. European Commission. European Commission Special Eurobarometer 338. Wave EB85.1—TNS Opinion & Social. Available online: https://www.efsa.europa.eu/sites/default/files/corporate_publications/files/Eurobarometer2019_Food-safety-in-the-EU_Full-report.pdf (accessed on 8 January 2023).
22. European Commission. European Commission Special Eurobarometer 445. Wave EB85.1—TNS Opinion & Social. Available online: https://deputyprimeminister.gov.mt/en/nac/Documents/Eurobarometers/2016_eb445_amr_generalreport_en.pdf (accessed on 8 January 2023).
23. Miyano, S.; Htoon, T.T.; Nozaki, I.; Pe, E.H.; Tin, H.H. Public knowledge, practices, and awareness of antibiotics and antibiotic resistance in Myanmar: The first national mobile phone panel survey. *PLoS ONE* **2022**, *17*, e0273380. [CrossRef] [PubMed]
24. Carter, E.; Bryce, J.; Perin, J.; Newby, H. Harmful practices in the management of childhood diarrhea in low- and middle-income countries: A systematic review. *BMC Public Health* **2015**, *15*, 788. [CrossRef] [PubMed]
25. Edessa, D.; Assefa, N.; Dessie, Y.; Asefa, F.; Dinsa, G.; Oljira, L. Non-prescribed antibiotic use for children at community levels in low- and middle-income countries: A systematic review and meta-analysis. *J. Pharm. Policy Pract.* **2022**, *15*, 57. [CrossRef] [PubMed]
26. Langford, B.J.; Matson, K.L.; Eljaaly, K.; Apisarnthanarak, A.; Bailey, P.L.; MacMurray, L.; Marra, A.R.; Simonsen, K.A.; Sreeramoju, P.; Nori, P.; et al. Ten ways to make the most of World Antimicrobial Awareness Week. *Antimicrob. Steward. Healthc. Epidemiol.* **2022**, *2*, e187. [CrossRef] [PubMed]
27. Bureau of National Statistics. Available online: https://new.stat.gov.kz/ru/ (accessed on 8 January 2023).
28. Brixton Health. SampleXS. Available online: http://www.brixtonhealth.com/ (accessed on 8 January 2023).
29. The World Health Organization. *Antibiotic Resistance. Multy-Country Public Awareness Survey*; World Health Organization: Geneva, Switzerland, 2015; pp. 4–51.
30. Media Holding "Atameken Business". Available online: https://inbusiness.kz/ru/news/kak-tenge-prozhil-2021-god (accessed on 16 February 2023).

Disclaimer/Publisher's Note: The statements, opinions and data contained in all publications are solely those of the individual author(s) and contributor(s) and not of MDPI and/or the editor(s). MDPI and/or the editor(s) disclaim responsibility for any injury to people or property resulting from any ideas, methods, instructions or products referred to in the content.

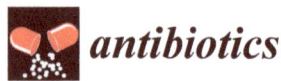

Review

Antimicrobial Resistance in Papua New Guinea: A Narrative Scoping Review

Brady Page [1,2,*] and Simeon Adiunegiya [3]

1. Department of Infectious Diseases and Global Public Health, University of California, San Diego (UCSD), La Jolla, CA 92103, USA
2. Scripps Research Institute, La Jolla, CA 92037, USA
3. School of Public Health, University of Washington, Seattle, WA 98195, USA
* Correspondence: bpage@ucsd.edu

Abstract: Antimicrobial-resistant bacterial infections are a known threat to the public health of low-income countries and are undercharacterized in Papua New Guinea. A scoping literature review of scientific peer-reviewed publications on antimicrobial resistance in Papua New Guinea was conducted, and their results were summarized. Many of the available data on resistant bacteria in Papua New Guinea have come from Port Moresby and Goroka and have been focused on *Staphylococcus aureus*, as well as important pediatric pathogens such as *Streptococcus pneumoniae* and *Haemophilus influenzae*. Progressive resistance to the commonly used antibiotics penicillin and chloramphenicol among most clinically important bacterial pathogens has prompted healthcare workers to adopt expensive broad-spectrum antibiotics. There is already evidence of resistance to newly adopted antibiotics among several Gram-negative organisms. Drivers of antimicrobial resistance in Papua New Guinea include a high burden of infectious diseases, inappropriate antibiotic prescription practices, poor regulation of antibiotics, incomplete adherence, substandard drug quality, and overcrowding of healthcare facilities. There is a lack of information on antimicrobial resistance among priority pathogens and from several important regions of Papua New Guinea.

Keywords: antimicrobial resistance; Papua New Guinea; antibiotics; Oceania; Melanesia

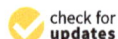

Citation: Page, B.; Adiunegiya, S. Antimicrobial Resistance in Papua New Guinea: A Narrative Scoping Review. *Antibiotics* **2023**, *12*, 1679. https://doi.org/10.3390/antibiotics12121679

Academic Editors: Juan Manuel Vázquez-Lago, Ana Estany-Gestal and Angel Salgado-Barreira

Received: 13 October 2023
Revised: 26 November 2023
Accepted: 27 November 2023
Published: 29 November 2023

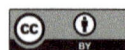

Copyright: © 2023 by the authors. Licensee MDPI, Basel, Switzerland. This article is an open access article distributed under the terms and conditions of the Creative Commons Attribution (CC BY) license (https://creativecommons.org/licenses/by/4.0/).

1. Introduction

Papua New Guinea (PNG) is a Melanesian country in Oceania with a population of over 7 million that is composed of the eastern half of the island of New Guinea as well as hundreds of smaller islands scattered throughout the Solomon and Bismarck Seas [1]. The country is predominantly mountainous, with a tropical rainforest climate and densely populated central highlands. As a consequence of its dramatic geography, human communities in PNG have historically remained relatively isolated from one another, making it among the most culturally and biologically diverse regions on Earth (Figure 1).

As of 2020, the population of PNG is primarily rural, with only around 13% of Papuans living in urban settings and the remainder residing in villages—often in extremely remote locations. PNG is classified as a lower–middle-income country by the World Bank [2]. Its human development index is 155th in the world, and the life expectancy at birth is 67.8 years [3]. Infections are widespread in PNG—endemic and emerging infectious diseases are implicated in half of childhood deaths and over 40% of all mortality in the country [4,5].

The modern antibiotic era began in 1928 with the discovery of penicillin by Alexander Fleming [6]. Since then, antibiotics have transformed the medical field and saved countless lives; however, by the 1950s, penicillin resistance had already become a serious global problem [7]. Thus began the ongoing *contradanse* of new antibiotic development in the face of intensifying resistance.

The recognition and characterization of antimicrobial resistance (AMR) in high-income countries is well established, and data have emerged showing that the problem is more prevalent and, indeed, of higher magnitude in low-income countries, heralding a true global public health emergency [8,9]. Given the pervasiveness of infectious diseases and antibiotic use in PNG—coupled with the relative paucity of health infrastructure and resource capacity—it is worth examining the history and current state of AMR in the country.

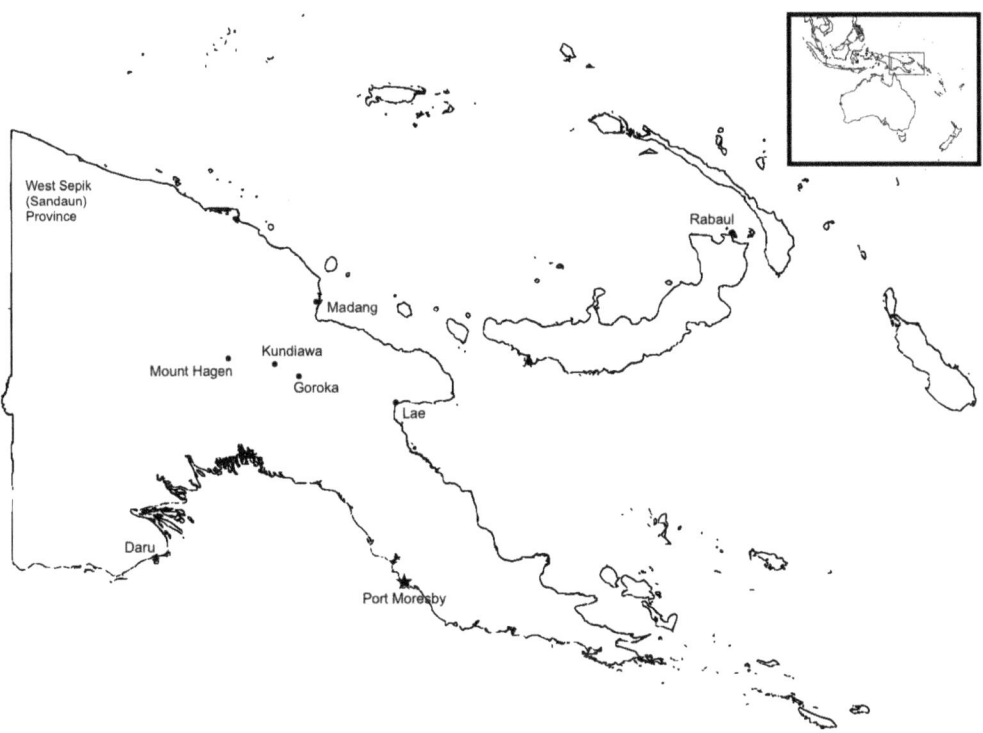

Figure 1. Map of Papua New Guinea and selected cities.

To achieve these ends, this comprehensive scoping review will summarize knowledge and epidemiological trends with respect to AMR in PNG (as well as the former Australian-administered territory of Papua and New Guinea, prior to 1975) that have been disclosed in peer-reviewed surveys, case series, case reports, theses, or conference communications. Prevalence and sample size data pertaining to resistance among bacterial species or genera against individual antibiotics or antibiotic classes are reported, when available. There will then be a discussion of factors that contribute to AMR in PNG. This review will not address resistance in *Mycobacterium tuberculosis*, *Plasmodium* spp., or HIV, as these topics have been reviewed elsewhere [8–10].

2. Methods

A literature review of scientific peer-reviewed publications was conducted following the Preferred Reporting Items for Systematic Reviews and Meta-Analyses Extension for Scoping Reviews (PRISMA-ScR) on the electronic databases PubMed and Web of Science. The search included combinations of the following keywords present in the title and/or abstract: "Papua", "New Guinea", "AMR", and "antimicrobial resistance". The format of publications could be prospective or retrospective studies, case reports, or case series, and they were evaluated to ensure that the contents represented commentary on antimicrobial susceptibility in what today constitutes the nation of Papua New Guinea. Antimicrobial susceptibility data were then extracted, and the AMR rates were calculated manually when not included in the publications (Figure 2).

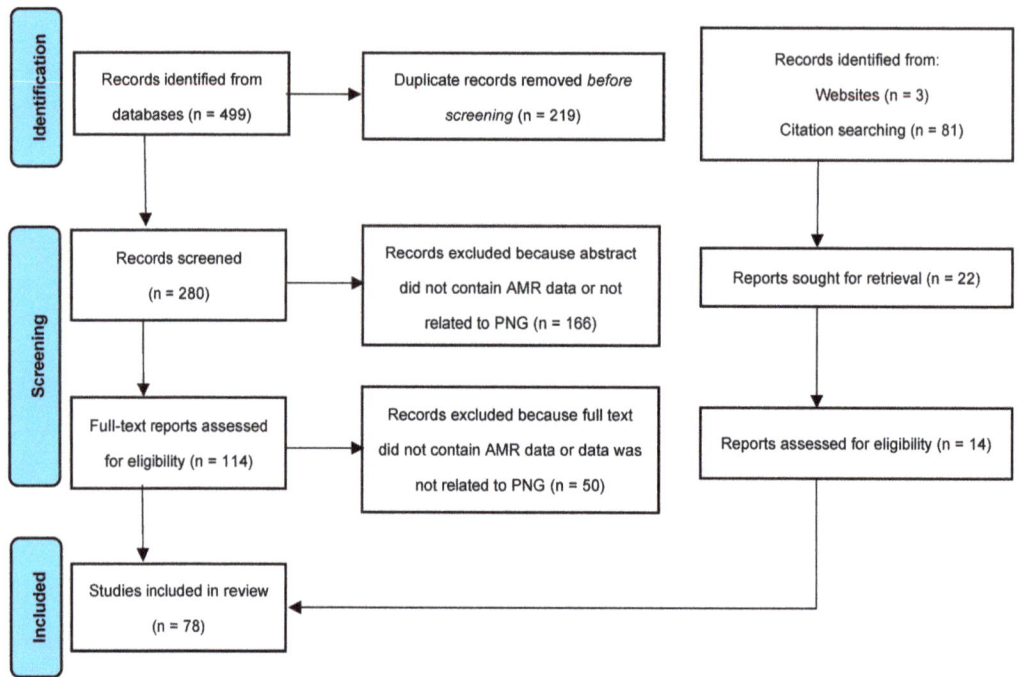

Figure 2. PRISMA chart of article identification and screening [11].

2.1. Antimicrobial Resistance among Gram-Positive Organisms

2.1.1. Staphylococcus aureus

S. aureus is an important cause of a multitude of both community-acquired and nosocomial infections worldwide [12]. Between 1971 and 1981—a period during which penicillin was the first-line therapy for staphylococcal pyomyositis, acute osteomyelitis, pneumonia, and bacteremia in PNG—over 90% of *S. aureus* isolated from pus specimens at Port Moresby General Hospital was already penicillin-resistant (Supplementary Materials Table S1; Figure 3) [13].

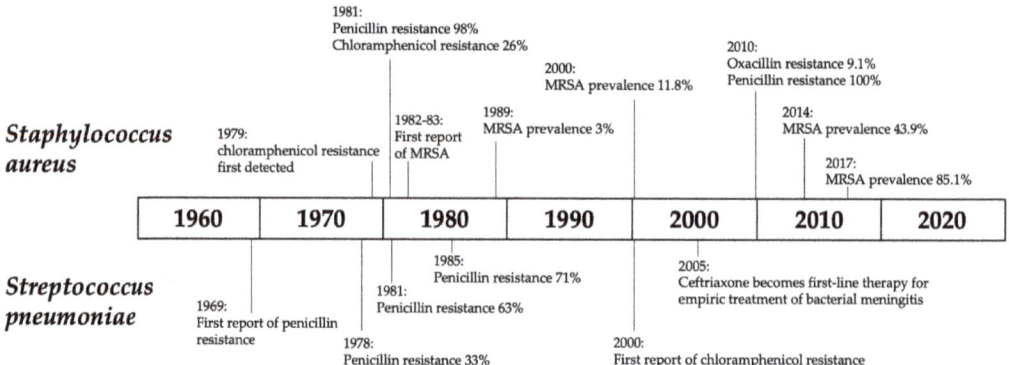

Figure 3. Timeline of antimicrobial resistance events for *Staphylococcus aureus* and *Streptococcus pneumoniae* in Papua New Guinea [9,10,12,14–24].

During the last 3 years of this period, penicillin resistance had risen to 98%; however, no methicillin or gentamicin resistance was detected. A penicillin-resistant *S. aureus* that was sensitive to cloxacillin and gentamicin was cultured in 1978 from the pus and sputum of a 33-year-old man in Rabaul, East New Britain with gluteal pyomyositis and hematogenously seeded pneumonia [25].

In 1979, the first incidence of chloramphenicol-resistant *S. aureus* in PNG was identified in Port Moresby, and from 1979 to 1981 chloramphenicol resistance was detected in 26% of isolates [13].

The first methicillin-resistant *S. aureus* (MRSA) reported in PNG was isolated from the infected skin lesion of a child in Goroka at some point between 1982 and 1983, and it was thought to be community-acquired [15]. During the same period, MRSA was detected in a total of 0.75% (3/399) of *S. aureus* cultured from skin swabs from unrelated children in Goroka with infected skin lesions. These 3 MRSA isolates were also resistant to chloramphenicol, tetracycline, and erythromycin, while 98.2% (392/399) of all *S. aureus* isolates produced β-lactamase and were resistant to penicillin.

Also in Goroka, a survey of 73 *S. aureus* isolates from blood, CSF, urine, skin lesions, stool, joint aspirates, and lung tissue from patients of all ages between 1982 and 1986 found 97% (71/73) penicillin resistance, 7% (5/73) chloramphenicol resistance, 3% (2/66) tetracycline resistance, 1% (1/73) cotrimoxazole resistance, 1% (1/73) erythromycin resistance, and no resistance to gentamicin [16]. A survey of the bacteriology of children's untreated skin sores in Goroka, Eastern Highlands in 1984 found that 92% (23/25) of *S. aureus* isolates were penicillin-resistant [26]. MRSA was cultured from one blood sample and one sputum sample, representing 3% (2/73) of all *S. aureus* isolates and the first report of MRSA in a hospitalized patient in PNG. MRSA was again isolated from the lung tissue of a 9-month-old with community-acquired pneumonia in Goroka in 1989 [27].

By the year 2000 there has been 3 deaths among children in Goroka from community-acquired MRSA infections that were also resistant to chloramphenicol, as well as reports of methicillin resistance in 11.8% (2/17) of *S. aureus* isolated from cases of fatal pediatric infection [14,28]. Oxacillin resistance was detected in 75% (3/4) of *S. aureus* isolated from the blood of surgical patients in Madang, Morobe Province from 2008 to 2009 [29]. All 3 isolates were susceptible to chloramphenicol and considered to have been community-acquired.

In 2010, a cross-sectional survey of *S. aureus* nasal colonization in Madang found oxacillin resistance in 9.1% (4/44) of isolates [17]. All of the isolates were penicillin-resistant (*n* = 44), 2.3% (1/44) were erythromycin-resistant, 2.3% (1/44) were trimethoprim–sulfamethoxazole-resistant, 4.6% (2/44) were tetracycline-resistant, and none were resistant to either rifampicin or clindamycin (*n* = 44).

In a 2013 report from Kundiawa, Simbu Province, more than 90% of *Staphylococcus* isolates from patients with osteomyelitis were resistant to flucloxacillin and chloramphenicol but retained universal susceptibility to ciprofloxacin [30].

By 2014, national data reported that 43.9% (72/164) of *S. aureus* cultured from blood, urine, and wounds was MRSA [18]. A prospective analysis of *S. aureus* isolates from the blood, joints, bone, or surrounding soft tissues of children from the community presenting with osteomyelitis in Kundiawa from 2012 to 2017 found that 85.1% (40/47) were methicillin-resistant, 89.4% (12/17) were oxacillin-resistant, 91.5% (43/47) were penicillin-resistant, 93.6% (44/47) were ampicillin-resistant, and 80.9% (38/47) were ceftriaxone-resistant [19]. There was also 8.5% (4/47) gentamicin resistance, 6.4% (3/47) erythromycin resistance, 6.4% (3/47) tetracycline resistance, 6.4% (3/47) clindamycin resistance, and 4.3% (2/47) cotrimoxazole resistance.

2.1.2. *Streptococcus pneumoniae*

S. pneumoniae is a highly invasive encapsulated bacterial pathogen and the most common cause of pneumonia, meningitis, bloodstream infections, and middle-ear infections in children [31]. The first known penicillin-resistant *S. pneumoniae* was detected in 1967 in the sputum of a patient with hypogammaglobulinemia and bronchiectasis in Sydney,

Australia [20]. In April of 1969, the first penicillin-resistant *S. pneumoniae* in PNG was isolated from a throat swab collected from a healthy 3-year-old boy in Anguganak, West Sepik who had been given penicillin the previous year for pneumonia [32]. As part of a regional survey of Anguganak conducted during the same year, penicillin-resistant *S. pneumoniae* isolates from 15 more individuals that also demonstrated decreased susceptibility to cephaloridine, cephalothin, and methicillin while maintaining susceptibility to ampicillin were identified [33]. Ultimately, surveys conducted from 1968 to 1970 in West Sepik found that 12% (n = 530) of *S. pneumoniae* isolates were resistant to penicillin, with MICs (minimum inhibitory concentrations) that could be overcome in cases of pneumococcal pneumonia but posed a serious problem when attempting to achieve the therapeutic levels required to treat pneumococcal meningitis [34].

From 1971 to 1974, 14% (42/292) of *S. pneumoniae* isolates evaluated in PNG were penicillin-insensitive [32]. By 1978, 33% (19/57) of *S. pneumoniae* isolates from 23 children and 34 adults in Port Moresby with bacteremic pneumonia, meningitis, or bacteremia were resistant to penicillin [21]. No resistance to chloramphenicol, erythromycin, or tetracycline was detected at that time. By 1981, a prospective collection of lung aspirates and blood from children admitted to Goroka Hospital with pneumonia between 1978 and 1981 found 63% (15/24) of *S. pneumoniae* isolates to be penicillin-resistant [21]. In a subsequent survey taking place between 1980 and 1984 of CSF from children under 10 years old with purulent meningitis in Goroka Hospital, penicillin resistance in *S. pneumoniae* was 22% (15/67), and there was no resistance to chloramphenicol [35]. *S. pneumoniae* isolated from infected skin lesions of children in Goroka between 1982 and 1983 found 60% (3/5) penicillin resistance and preserved universal susceptibility to chloramphenicol [15].

In a large cohort of samples collected between 1980 and 1985 from the blood, CSF, joint aspirates, stool, lung tissue, urine, and skin lesions of patients of all ages in Goroka (with a small number of samples from Port Moresby), intermediate resistance to penicillin was detected in 56% (1701/3018) of *S. pneumoniae* isolates [16]. The prevalence of penicillin resistance was found to have increased throughout the duration of the survey, from 38% in 1980 to 71% in 1985. Among carriage and invasive isolates of *S. pneumoniae*, penicillin resistance was detected in 60% and 27% of isolates, respectively. Of 1047 isolates analyzed, all remained susceptible to chloramphenicol. From 1983 to 1984, 46% (13/28) of *S. pneumoniae* isolates from the blood of children with lower respiratory infections in Goroka were relatively penicillin-resistant, with MICs greater than 0.05 µg/mL, but remained sensitive to chloramphenicol [36].

Isolates of *S. pneumoniae* cultured from blood and lung aspirates collected from children with acute respiratory infections in Eastern Highlands between 1978 and 1987 demonstrated 52% (38/73) penicillin resistance [37]. Among carriage isolates from children between 1980 and 1982, there was 63% (602/956) resistance to penicillin, which had risen to nearly 75% by 1987 [38,39]. Analysis of a further 655 invasive isolates from lung aspirates or blood in the same region between 1985 and 1987 found no resistance to chloramphenicol, erythromycin, tetracycline, or cotrimoxazole [37].

In a survey carried out between 1980 and 1987 to compare the epidemiology and resistance patterns of carriage and invasive *S. pneumoniae* in Eastern Highlands, insensitivity to penicillin was detected in 67% (605/898) of isolates [40]. There was no significant change in the prevalence of penicillin insensitivity between the periods from 1980 to 1984 and from 1985 to 1987. Between 1989 and 1992, a prospective analysis of blood and CSF from children in Goroka with suspected bacterial meningitis found 22% (10/46) oxacillin resistance and 74% (45/61) cotrimoxazole resistance, as well as insensitivity to penicillin and trimethoprim in 23% (7/31) and 65% (20/32) of isolates, respectively [41]. In the same cohort, there was no resistance in *S. pneumoniae* to either chloramphenicol or erythromycin. Between 1998 and 2000, there was a single report in Eastern Highlands of a pediatric death from infection by penicillin-resistant *S. pneumoniae* that remained susceptible to chloramphenicol [14]. Between 1996 and 2000, the median MIC of chloramphenicol for *S. pneumoniae* was 3 µg/mL, and by 2000 chloramphenicol resistance was finally identified in 2 isolates of *S. pneumoniae* from children with bacterial meningitis in Goroka [22,23].

Between 1996 and 2005, prospective antimicrobial sensitivity testing of *S. pneumoniae* cultured from the CSF of children with meningitis in Goroka identified penicillin resistance in 21.5% (38/177) of isolates as well as 2.3% (4/176) chloramphenicol resistance, 4.2% (4/96) tetracycline resistance, and 4% (7/176) cotrimoxazole resistance [42]. Over the course of the survey, penicillin resistance decreased from 25% (29/116) to 14.8% (9/61), chloramphenicol resistance increased from 0.9% (1/115) to 4.9% (3/61), tetracycline resistance increased from 2.9% (2/69) to 7.4% (2/27), and cotrimoxazole resistance increased from 7.8% (9/116) to 10% (6/60).

In 2005, based on elucidated resistance patterns in *S. pneumoniae* and *H. influenzae*, the antibiotic of choice for the empiric management of bacterial meningitis in PNG was officially changed from chloramphenicol to ceftriaxone [24]. Although frank resistance to ceftriaxone had never been identified in PNG, 0.8% (1/124) of *S. pneumoniae* isolates from the CSF of children in Goroka between 1996 and 2005 were already intermediately resistant [42].

From 2006 to 2009, when the breakpoint for chloramphenicol resistance in *S. pneumoniae* was 16 μg/mL, among isolates from the blood and CSF of children with bacterial meningitis in Madang the median MIC of chloramphenicol was 3 μg/mL, and 42.8% (6/14) had an MIC of ≥ 4 μg/mL [23]. The likelihood of achieving a therapeutic AUC_{0-24}/MIC with chloramphenicol against *S. pneumoniae* with an MIC of 4 was estimated to be 51–70%. This same survey detected 13.3% (2/15) penicillin resistance, 17.7% (3/17) trimethoprim–sulfamethoxazole resistance, 41% (7/17) trimethoprim–sulfamethoxazole insensitivity, 6.3% (1/16) tetracycline resistance, 25% (4/16) tetracycline insensitivity, and no resistance to ceftriaxone ($n = 15$).

In 2009, a retrospective analysis of invasive *S. pneumoniae* from patients with bacterial meningitis in Port Moresby identified chloramphenicol resistance in 8% (3/38) of isolates as well as 93.9% (31/33) gentamicin resistance, 16.7% (1/6) cotrimoxazole resistance, 7% (3/40) penicillin resistance, 4% (3/28) tetracycline resistance, and no resistance to ampicillin ($n = 13$), amoxicillin ($n = 3$), ceftriaxone ($n = 6$), erythromycin ($n = 40$), or cefaclor ($n = 28$) [43].

2.1.3. *Streptococcus pyogenes* (Group A *Streptococcus*)

S. pyogenes is a common colonizer of the pharynx and skin and can cause pharyngitis, skin infections, and toxic shock syndrome [44]. A 1983 survey of skin swabs from children in Goroka with infected skin lesions found that all 337 isolates of *S. pyogenes* were penicillin-sensitive [15]. A prospective analysis of several body tissues in Goroka between 1984 and 1986 found no evidence of resistance to penicillin, chloramphenicol, or tetracycline [16].

2.1.4. *Streptococcus agalactiae* (Group B *Streptococcus*)

Traditionally considered to be a neonatal pathogen, *S. agalactiae* is also associated with invasive disease in other high-risk groups [45]. Skin swabs collected as part of a prospective survey of children in Goroka with infected skin lesions from 1982 to 1983 found that 100% ($n = 2$) of *S. agalactiae* isolates were susceptible to penicillin [15]. Between 1998 and 2000, there was a report of a single pediatric death from pneumonia caused by multidrug-resistant *S. agalactiae* [14].

2.1.5. Other β-Hemolytic *Streptococcus* spp.

Other β-hemolytic streptococci are colonizers of animals and humans and are associated with invasive infection in rare instances [46]. Analysis of isolates from blood, CSF, urine, skin lesions, stool, and lung tissue from Eastern Highlands between 1984 and 1986 found that 5% (1/22) of β-hemolytic streptococci were chloramphenicol-resistant, 15% (3/20) were tetracycline-resistant, and none ($n = 22$) were resistant to penicillin [16]. Specifically, there was one Group C *Streptococcus* isolated from a leprous foot ulcer that was the first instance of chloramphenicol resistance in this group in PNG, as well as 3 isolates that were tetracycline-resistant.

2.1.6. *Corynebacterium* spp.

The corynebacteria are generally innocuous constituents of the human microflora that are occasionally implicated in skin and soft tissue, respiratory, genitourinary tract, or implanted device infections [47]. Most notable among them is *C. diphtheriae*, which causes diphtheria. In a survey of infected skin lesions collected between 1984 and 1986 in Eastern Highlands, no evidence of resistance to penicillin, chloramphenicol, erythromycin, or tetracycline was detected among 8 isolates of *C. diphtheriae* and *C. haemolyticum* (now *Arcanobacterium haemolyticum*) [16].

2.2. Antimicrobial Resistance among Gram-Negative Organisms

2.2.1. Haemophilus influenzae

Prior to the introduction of a vaccine, *H. influenzae* type b was a common cause of invasive bacterial infection and bacterial meningitis in children [48]. Penicillin resistance in *H. influenzae* in PNG was first detected in 1981 in isolates from one CSF sample and one nasopharyngeal aspirate from 2 infants in Goroka as part of larger prospective analyses of children with meningitis or pneumonia [49,50]. Both isolates produced β-lactamase and were susceptible to chloramphenicol. During the same survey, the overall rate of penicillin-resistant *H. influenzae* was found to be only 0.7% (2/293). A survey of CSF from children with purulent meningitis in Goroka conducted between 1980 and 1984 found that only 1.8% (1/56) of *H. influenzae* isolates (83% of which were type b) were insensitive to penicillin and all isolates were susceptible to both chloramphenicol and ampicillin (Supplementary Materials Table S2) [35].

Among *H. influenzae* isolates from a number of bodily fluids and tissue types between 1981 and 1986 in Eastern Highlands, only 0.3% (4/1516) were resistant to penicillin and ampicillin [16]. The same survey found 100% susceptibility to chloramphenicol in 839 isolates analyzed from 1983 to 1986.

Between 1983 and 1984, all isolates of *H. influenzae* from the blood of 30 children with lower respiratory infections in the same region were susceptible to ampicillin and chloramphenicol [36]. From 1989 to 1992, 13% (3/24) of *H. influenzae* type b isolates from the blood or CSF of children in Goroka with suspected bacterial meningitis were ampicillin-resistant, although none of the isolates produced β-lactamase (n = 32) [41]. In the same cohort, 28% (7/25) of isolates were cotrimoxazole-resistant, 44% (4/9) were trimethoprim-resistant, and there was still no resistance to either chloramphenicol or tetracycline.

Despite reliable efficacy throughout most of the twentieth century, in 1998 chloramphenicol resistance was detected in 25% of invasive *H. influenzae* type b isolates from children with bacterial meningitis in Lae, Goroka, and Port Moresby [51]. By 2000, chloramphenicol resistance in the same cohort was 21% [39]. Later that same year, resistance to chloramphenicol was similarly detected in 22.7% of *H. influenzae* isolates in Goroka, including 36.4% (4/11) of cases of fatal pediatric meningitis in the region [4,20].

During a survey conducted from 1996 to 2005, *H. influenzae* isolates from the CSF of children in Goroka with meningitis were 31.5% (51/162) chloramphenicol-resistant, 28.4% (46/162) ampicillin-resistant, and 34% (55/162) cotrimoxazole resistant, with 28% (38/165) of isolates demonstrating resistance to all three antibiotics [42]. Over the survey period, chloramphenicol resistance increased significantly from 26% (27/104) to 41.4% (24/58), ampicillin resistance increased significantly from 26% (27/104) to 46.6% (27/58), and cotrimoxazole resistance increased from 33.7% (35/104) to 48.3% (28/58). From this same cohort, 5% (4/80) of isolates were found to be non-susceptible to ceftriaxone. The observation of increasing chloramphenicol resistance in *H. influenzae* prompted the adoption of ceftriaxone for the empiric management of meningitis in PNG in 2005, with subsequent improvements in mortality [22,52].

From 2006 to 2009, 100% ($n = 14$) of *H. influenzae* isolates from the blood or CSF of children with bacterial meningitis in Madang were resistant to chloramphenicol [23]. Additionally, 93.3% (14/15) were penicillin-resistant, 100% ($n = 15$) were resistant to trimethoprim–sulfamethoxazole, 93.3% (14/15) were tetracycline-resistant, and there was no resistance to ceftriaxone ($n = 10$).

2.2.2. *Escherichia coli*

E. coli is an environmental bacterium that commensally composes part of the normal mammalian gut microflora but can become pathogenic, most frequently implicated in genitourinary infections and gastroenteritis as well as pneumonia and meningitis [53]. Some strains are toxigenic, such as the enterohemorrhagic *E. coli* responsible for causing hemolytic uremic syndrome. Penicillin- and methicillin-resistant *E. coli* that was susceptible to chloramphenicol and gentamicin was isolated from the sputum of a man with *S. aureus* pneumonia in East New Britain in 1978 [25]. During a prospective survey of blood, urine, stool, CSF, lung tissue, and joint aspirates in Eastern Highlands from 1984 to 1986, ampicillin resistance was present in 46% (17/37) of isolates while 32% (12/27) were resistant to chloramphenicol, 11% (3/27) were resistant to tetracycline, 8% (3/37) were resistant to cotrimoxazole, 8% (1/13) were resistant to kanamycin, and 3% (1/37) were resistant to gentamicin [16]. *E. coli* isolates from children in Goroka with sepsis in 1997 and 1998 were 88% (7/8) chloramphenicol-resistant and 38% (3/8) gentamicin-resistant [54].

National data in 2012 reported that *E. coli* cultured from a variety of tissues demonstrated 24.1% (42/174) resistance to third-generation cephalosporins and 13.3% (70/526) resistance to fluoroquinolones [18].

2.2.3. *Klebsiella* spp.

The *Klebsiella* are opportunistic pathogens implicated most frequently in nosocomial infections of the genitourinary tract, bloodstream, and respiratory system [55]. In 1978, a penicillin- and methicillin-resistant *Klebsiella* that remained susceptible to chloramphenicol and gentamicin was isolated from the sputum of a man with *S. aureus* pneumonia in Rabaul [25]. Among *Klebsiella* and *Enterobacter* isolates from blood, stool, urine, and lung tissue in Goroka between 1984 and 1986, 95% (21/22) were resistant to ampicillin while 45% (10/22) were resistant to chloramphenicol, 36% (4/11) were resistant to tetracycline, 32% (7/22) were resistant to cotrimoxazole, 6% (1/17) were kanamycin-resistant, and 5% (1/22) were gentamicin-resistant [16].

In 1992, there were 3 isolates of multidrug-resistant *Klebsiella* identified at Port Moresby General Hospital, including a single hospital-acquired *K. oxytoca* cultured from the blood of a 23-year-old man with pneumococcal pneumonia that was tetracycline-susceptible but resistant to penicillin, carbenicillin, ampicillin, chloramphenicol, gentamicin, cotrimoxazole, and streptomycin [56]. At that time, there was 54% (15/28) resistance to chloramphenicol, 61% (17/28) resistance to cotrimoxazole, and 29% (8/28) resistance to tetracycline in *K. pneumoniae* and *K. oxytoca* isolated from blood collected at the same hospital.

Klebsiella collected in 1997 and 1998 from various sites of infection among children with sepsis in Goroka showed 100% ($n = 14$) resistance to chloramphenicol and 76% (11/14) resistance to gentamicin [54]

From October 2007 to October 2008, there was an outbreak of nosocomial sepsis due to multidrug-resistant *K. pneumoniae* in the special care nursery at Port Moresby General Hospital. During the first 3 months of the outbreak, 20% (4/20) of *K. pneumoniae* isolates cultured from blood were found to be resistant to cephalosporins [57]. Over the ensuing 10 months, cephalosporin resistance increased to 73% (27/37), with 19% (6/31) of isolates demonstrating resistance to all available antibiotics.

From 2008 to 2009 in Madang, *K. pneumoniae* that was isolated from bacteremic surgical patients was 100% ($n = 2$) resistant to ampicillin, chloramphenicol, cotrimoxazole, and tetracycline, 50% (1/2) resistant to gentamicin, and completely susceptible to ciprofloxacin

(n = 2) [29]. By 2012, 63.5% (160/252) of *Klebsiella* isolates from blood, urine, stool, wounds, and pus from around PNG were resistant to third-generation cephalosporins [18].

2.2.4. *Enterobacter* spp.

Enterobacter spp. are responsible for nosocomial infections of the genitourinary tract, bloodstream, and respiratory system and are naturally resistant to penicillins, first- and second-generation cephalosporins, and amoxicillin–clavulanic acid [58]. Resistance in *Enterobacter* and *Klebsiella* spp. to ampicillin, chloramphenicol, tetracycline, cotrimoxazole, and aminoglycosides was detected in Eastern Highlands from 1984 to 1986, as above. From 1997 to 1998, again in Eastern Highlands, chloramphenicol resistance was detected in 100% (7/7) and gentamicin resistance in 57% (4/7) of isolates from children with severe sepsis [54].

2.2.5. *Proteus* spp.

Proteus spp. are urease-producing bacilli that are uncommonly implicated in catheter-associated urinary-tract and wound infections that can invade to cause nosocomial bacteremia [59]. Resistance to ampicillin was present in 45% (5/11) of *Proteus* spp. and *Providencia* spp. isolated from urine, blood, stool, CSF, and skin lesions in Goroka between 1984 and 1986 [16]. This same survey detected resistance to chloramphenicol in 82% (9/11), resistance to tetracycline in 100% (n = 10), resistance to cotrimoxazole in 55% (6/11), resistance to gentamicin in 18% (2/11), and resistance to kanamycin in 33% (3/9) of isolates. Chloramphenicol resistance was present in 100% (n = 3) and gentamicin resistance in 33% (1/3) of *P. mirabilis* isolated from children in Goroka with sepsis between 1997 and 1998 [54].

2.2.6. *Providencia* spp.

Providencia spp. are environmental organisms that are an uncommon cause of catheter-associated urinary-tract infections and a rare cause of nosocomial bacteremia [60]. Between 1984 and 1986, a prospective analysis of isolates from urine, blood, stool, and skin lesions in Goroka found resistance to ampicillin, chloramphenicol, tetracycline, cotrimoxazole, and aminoglycosides in *Providencia* spp. and *Proteus* spp., as above. A single isolate of *Providencia* from a child in Goroka with sepsis between 1997 and 1998 was susceptible to both gentamicin and chloramphenicol [54].

2.2.7. *Morganella morganii*

M. morganii is commensal in the gastrointestinal flora of many animals and is rarely implicated in nosocomial urinary-tract and wound infections [61]. There was no evidence of gentamicin resistance (n = 2) or chloramphenicol resistance (n = 2) in isolates of *M. morganii* cultured from children with sepsis in 1997 and 1998 in Goroka [54].

2.2.8. *Pseudomonas* spp.

The *Pseudomonas* spp., particularly *P. aeruginosa*, are environmental organisms with high levels of AMR that can cause severe opportunistic infections of many different organ systems, especially in immunocompromised hosts [62]. In a prospective analysis of blood, skin lesions, urine, CSF, joint fluid, and lung tissue from Goroka between 1984 and 1986, isolates of *Pseudomonas* spp. demonstrated 83% (10/12) resistance to chloramphenicol, 55% (6/11) resistance to ampicillin, 50% (4/8) resistance to tetracycline, 67% (8/12) resistance to cotrimoxazole, 30% (3/10) resistance to kanamycin, and no resistance (n = 12) to gentamicin [16]. Isolates of *P. aeruginosa* were 100% resistant to ampicillin, chloramphenicol, tetracycline, and cotrimoxazole. Isolates of *P. aeruginosa* from several sites of infection among children with severe sepsis in Goroka between 1997 and 1998 were 100% (n = 11) resistant to chloramphenicol and 82% (9/11) resistant to gentamicin [54].

A single *P. aeruginosa* cultured from the blood of a bacteremic surgical patient in Madang between 2008 and 2009 was resistant to ampicillin, tetracycline, cotrimoxazole, and chloramphenicol but remained susceptible to ciprofloxacin and gentamicin [29].

2.2.9. Acinetobacter spp.

Acinetobacter spp. are multidrug-resistant environmental organisms and an important emerging cause of nosocomial urinary-tract, respiratory, bloodstream, and wound infections in critically ill patients [63]. In a case series of 5 community-acquired pneumonia cases in Port Moresby from 1986 to 1987, A. calcoaceticus was isolated from four percutaneous pulmonary aspirates and one blood culture [64]. Penicillin insensitivity was suggested, as the 2 patients who received only penicillin died and the 3 who received additional gentamicin survived their illnesses.

A single isolate of Acinetobacter from a child in Goroka with sepsis between 1997 and 1998 was resistant to chloramphenicol but susceptible to gentamicin [54].

2.2.10. Burkholderia spp.

B. cepacia is an emerging cause of multidrug-resistant pneumonia in cystic fibrosis patients, while B. pseudomallei causes a severe multiorgan infection known as melioidosis [65,66]. B. cepacia cultured from children with sepsis in Goroka from 1997 to 1998 was 100% resistant to gentamicin and 67% (2/3) resistant to chloramphenicol [54]. A retrospective analysis of clinical and environmental isolates of B. pseudomallei from Balimo, Western Province between 1995 and 2005 identified 48.7% (19/39) chloramphenicol resistance and universal susceptibility to tetracycline, amoxicillin–clavulanate, and meropenem ($n = 39$) [67].

2.2.11. Aeromonas spp.

The Aeromonas spp. are environmental organisms of fresh or brackish water that are rarely implicated in intraabdominal, respiratory, gastrointestinal, genitourinary, bloodstream, and traumatic skin and soft-tissue infections—especially those associated with animal bites [68]. Among isolates of A. hydrophila cultured from stool and skin lesions in Eastern Highlands between 1984 and 1986, ampicillin resistance was 75% (6/8), chloramphenicol resistance was 13% (1/8), and there was no resistance to gentamicin ($n = 8$), cotrimoxazole ($n = 8$), or tetracycline ($n = 5$) [16]. A lone isolate of Aeromonas from a child with sepsis in Goroka between 1997 and 1998 was sensitive to gentamicin but resistant to chloramphenicol [54].

2.2.12. Citrobacter freundii

C. freundii is an environmental and human intestinal commensal organism that is an uncommon cause of gastroenteritis as well as nosocomial urinary-tract infections, pneumonia, and bacteremia [69]. A prospective observational study over 16 months from 1997 to 1998 among children with sepsis in Goroka found that C. freundii isolates from multiple tissue types were 100% (3/3) gentamicin-resistant and 67% (2/3) chloramphenicol-resistant [54].

2.2.13. Alcaligenes spp.

Bacteria in the genus Alcaligenes are multidrug-resistant environmental organisms that are rarely implicated in a multitude of opportunistic infections [70]. A single isolate of Alcaligenes from a child with sepsis in Goroka between 1997 and 1998 was susceptible to gentamicin and resistant to chloramphenicol [54]. A second Alcaligenes cultured from the blood of a bacteremic surgical patient in Madang between 2008 and 2009 was resistant to ampicillin and tetracycline, intermediately resistant to gentamicin and ciprofloxacin, and susceptible to chloramphenicol and cotrimoxazole [29].

2.2.14. Shigella spp.

There are four major species of Shigella, which are highly virulent pathogens that carry a significant burden of gastrointestinal illness worldwide, especially in resource-limited settings [71]. Toxin-producing subtypes of S. dysenteriae can cause hemolytic uremic syndrome. A prospective analysis of 851 stool samples from patients with acute gastroenteritis in Port Moresby between 1962 and 1963 identified 75% (120/160) as S. flexneri and 15.6% (25/160) as S. sonnei [72]. Of the Shigella spp. isolates that were tested, 12.9%

(9/70) were resistant to streptomycin and 8.6% (6/70) were resistant to oxytetracycline. Resistance to sulfonamides was found in 38.9% (14/36) of isolates, all of which were *S. flexneri*.

An analysis of stool samples in Eastern Highlands from 1984 to 1986 detected ampicillin resistance in 86% (81/94) of *Shigella* isolates, while tetracycline and cotrimoxazole resistance was found in 91% (49/54) and 1% (1/94) of isolates, respectively [16]. Among the 94 isolates tested, there was no resistance to either kanamycin or gentamicin. Resistance to chloramphenicol was detected in 83% (78/94) of *Shigella* spp. isolates, all of which were *S. flexneri* serotypes 1 or 3. Among these *S. flexneri* isolates, 35% were resistant to 2 antibiotics, 48% were resistant to 3 antibiotics, and 1% were resistant to 4 antibiotics.

Between 2000 and 2009, the antibiotic susceptibilities of *Shigella* isolated from the stool of patients with severe diarrhea in Port Moresby—composed of 90.4% *S. flexneri*, 3.7% *S. boydii*, 2.9% *S. dysenteriae*, and 1.5% *S. sonnei*—were analyzed [73]. Among all combined *Shigella* spp. tested, 96% (94/98) were resistant to amoxicillin, 86% (65/76) were resistant to cotrimoxazole, 60% (68/114) were resistant to chloramphenicol, 27% (31/114) were intermediately resistant to chloramphenicol, and 15% (2/13) were resistant to nalidixic acid. No isolates were resistant to ciprofloxacin or cephalexin, but one isolate was intermediately resistant to ciprofloxacin and another was intermediately resistant to cephalexin.

Among 30 *S. flexneri*, 2 *S. dysenteriae*, and 15 non-typed *Shigella* spp. isolates from Eastern Highlands between 2010 and 2011, 91.5% (43/47) were ampicillin-resistant, 76.6% (36/47) were tetracycline-resistant, 70.2% (33/47) were resistant to trimethoprim–sulfamethoxazole, and 55.3% (26/47) were chloramphenicol-resistant [74]. There was no resistance to ceftriaxone or ciprofloxacin ($n = 47$). Resistance to 4 antibiotics was detected in 55.3% (26/47) of isolates, while resistance to 3 antibiotics was detected in 21.3% (10/47) of isolates. As of 2014, there was no resistance to fluoroquinolones ($n = 53$) among *Shigella* isolates from several sites in PNG [18].

A retrospective analysis in 2018 of archived stool from throughout Oceania—which included 60 samples from PNG—found that among isolates of *S. flexneri*, 77% (41/53) were ampicillin-resistant, 74% (39/53) were tetracycline-resistant, 60% (32/53) were chloramphenicol-resistant, and 49% (26/53) were trimethoprim–sulfamethoxazole-resistant [75]. Among isolates of *S. sonnei*, there was 56% (9/16) resistance to ampicillin, 19% (3/16) resistance to tetracycline, 75% (12/16) resistance to trimethoprim–sulfamethoxazole, and 6% (1/16) resistance to nalidixic acid. *S. dysenteriae* isolates were 33% (1/3) ampicillin-resistant, 33% (1/3) tetracycline-resistant, and 33% (1/3) trimethoprim–sulfamethoxazole-resistant. There was a significant increase in resistance to several antibiotics among *Shigella* spp. isolates when comparing isolates collected before and after 2010. Specifically, ampicillin resistance increased from 14% to 58%, chloramphenicol resistance increased from 10% to 35%, tetracycline resistance increased from 14% to 46%, and trimethoprim–sulfamethoxazole resistance increased from 8% to 48%. There was no resistance to ceftriaxone or ciprofloxacin identified.

2.2.15. *Salmonella* spp.

Salmonella spp. are associated with acute gastroenteritis, usually caused by the consumption of contaminated water and food, or through contact with colonized animals [76]. Invasive disease—known as typhoid fever—is caused by *S. enterica* subsp. enterica serovar Typhi and can be life-threatening. From 1984 to 1986, a prospective analysis of blood and stool from Eastern Highlands demonstrated that 58% (22/38) of *Salmonella* spp. isolates were chloramphenicol-resistant, 53% (20/38) were ampicillin-resistant, 37% (14/38) were kanamycin-resistant, 6% (2/33) were tetracycline-resistant, 3% (1/38) were cotrimoxazole-resistant, and all ($n = 38$) were susceptible to gentamicin [16]. There was no resistance in *S. typhi*. Of the isolates tested, 11% were resistant to 2 antibiotics, 40% were resistant to 3 antibiotics, and 8% were resistant to 4 antibiotics. By the year 2000, *S. typhi* was broadly considered to be chloramphenicol-resistant in PNG [28].

A small number of *S. typhi* isolates from children and adults in Eastern Highlands in 2010 and 2011 found that 80% (4/5) were ampicillin-resistant, 60% (3/5) were tetracycline-resistant, 60% (3/5) were trimethoprim–sulfamethoxazole-resistant, and 40% (2/5) were chloramphenicol-resistant [74]. There was no resistance to ceftriaxone or ciprofloxacin (n = 5). In 2014, 33.3% (5/15) of non-typhoidal *Salmonella* isolates from around the country were resistant to fluoroquinolones [18].

2.2.16. *Campylobacter* spp.

Campylobacter is an important cause of foodborne diarrheal illness in the highlands of PNG [77]. Among 22 *C. jejuni* and 33 *C. coli* isolates from stool in Eastern Highlands between 1984 and 1986, there was 24% (13/55) resistance to ampicillin, 100% (n = 55) resistance to cotrimoxazole, and no resistance to gentamicin, chloramphenicol, or tetracycline (n = 55) [16].

2.2.17. *Vibrio cholerae*

Toxigenic *V. cholerae* is an outbreak-prone environmental organism of brackish water whose transmission via the fecal–oral route in areas of poor sanitation and poverty can elicit a disease characterized by devastating watery diarrhea and rapid dehydration, known as cholera [78]. An outbreak of *V. cholerae* serogroup O1, biotype El Tor, serotype Ogawa began in Morobe Province in 2009 and then spread to nearly half of the provinces of PNG by 2011. Among stool samples and rectal swabs collected during the outbreak between 2009 and 2011, 75.8% (229/302) of *V. cholerae* isolates were resistant to amoxicillin, and 17.2% (52/302) were intermediately resistant [79]. Chloramphenicol resistance was detected in 3.1% (8/255) of isolates, and 1.6% (4/244) were intermediately resistant. There was no resistance to norfloxacin (n = 296), but 0.7% (2/296) of isolates were intermediately resistant. Ciprofloxacin resistance was present in 1% (3/305) of isolates, and 3.2% (9/282) of isolates were resistant to cotrimoxazole. Similarly, 0.7% (2/305) of isolates were intermediately resistant to ciprofloxacin, and 1.4% (4/282) were intermediately resistant to cotrimoxazole. There was 0.3% (1/300) resistance to nalidixic acid.

In 2009, the first year of the cholera outbreak, 27.8% (10/36) of isolates demonstrated at least intermediate resistance to tetracycline [79]. By 2010, this figure had risen to 50.5% (107/212), and it had decreased to 11.8% (6/51) by 2011. The overall rate of resistance to tetracycline during the outbreak was 9.7% (29/299). Erythromycin resistance was detected in 38.2% (97/254) of isolates, with the percentage of *V. cholerae* isolates that were at least intermediately resistant to erythromycin increasing from 92.1% (187/203) in 2010 to 96.1% (49/51) by 2011.

2.2.18. *Neisseria meningitidis*

N. meningitidis—or meningococcus—is a strictly human pathogen that causes significant morbidity and mortality among non-immunized children and young adults through epidemic or sporadic meningitis with bacteremia [80]. A prospective survey from 1980 to 1984 in Goroka isolated *N. meningitidis* from 5.2% (8/155) of CSF samples from children with purulent meningitis [81]. A survey from 1984 to 1986, also in Goroka, found no evidence of resistance to penicillin or chloramphenicol in 5 isolates of *N. meningitidis* from CSF or blood [16]. In 2009, a small retrospective analysis of *N. meningitidis* isolates from patients with bacterial meningitis in Port Moresby identified 33% (1/3) resistance to ceftazidime, 33% (1/3) resistance to tetracycline, and no resistance to penicillin or ceftriaxone [43].

2.2.19. *Neisseria gonorrhoeae*

N. gonorrhoeae, or gonococcus, is a common cause of sexually transmitted urethritis and cervicitis that can progress into pelvic inflammatory disease or disseminate to other organ systems [82]. Certain strains of *N. gonorrhoeae* have rapidly developed resistance to all antibiotic classes except for extended-spectrum cephalosporins, with some regions already grappling with ceftriaxone-resistant strains [83]. Penicillinase-producing *N. gonorrhoeae* represented 44% of all gonococcal isolates from sexually transmitted infection clinics in 5 towns across PNG in 1989 and 1990 [81]. Beginning in 1992, low but consistent levels of spectinomycin resistance began to be detected in the country [84]. In 1993, national data described penicillin resistance in 12.5% (5/40), tetracycline resistance in 7.5% (3/40), and spectinomycin resistance in 3.3% (1/30) of isolates with no evidence of fluoroquinolone resistance (n = 40) [85]. By 1994, penicillin resistance was 8.7% (19/218), tetracycline resistance was 4.1% (9/218), spectinomycin resistance was 1.8% (1/57), and resistance to fluoroquinolones was detected in 5% (11/218) of isolates. As of 1994, no resistance to third-generation cephalosporins had been detected in PNG [84].

By 2005, ceftriaxone resistance was detected at an extremely low level in Port Moresby, with only 0.7% of several hundred isolates demonstrating reduced susceptibility [86]. That same year, 1.2% ciprofloxacin resistance, 61.1% penicillin resistance, 49% tetracycline resistance, 0.7% spectinomycin resistance, and 5% nalidixic acid resistance were recognized. In 2006, ciprofloxacin resistance was 1.5%, penicillin resistance was 64.7%, tetracycline resistance was 17.7%, nalidixic acid resistance was 2.9%, and there was no evidence of resistance to either ceftriaxone or spectinomycin in Port Moresby.

A further 52 isolates collected from STI clinics in Port Moresby, Lae, Mount Hagen, and Goroka in 2004 and 2005 were all susceptible to amoxicillin–clavulanate, spectinomycin, erythromycin, azithromycin, and ceftriaxone [87]. However, 19% (10/52) of isolates were resistant to tetracycline, and 2% (1/52)—isolated in Lae—were resistant to ciprofloxacin. Penicillin resistance due to penicillinase was detected in 40% (21/52) of isolates.

2.3. Drivers of Antimicrobial Resistance in Papua New Guinea

There has historically been a high burden of infectious diseases in PNG that warrant antibiotic treatment, as well as a pervasive presence of risk factors for infection including malnutrition, home birth, and prolonged hospitalization [28]. However, antibiotic misuse is a known cause of the development of AMR. Initially, penicillin was widely employed in PNG after World War II, with the establishment of the aid post system of primary healthcare [37]. It was used liberally, perhaps indiscriminately, at the village level for respiratory infections and for the eradication of yaws, even in remote areas [33]. In fact, data suggest that in the 10 years following 1961 the amount of penicillin used by the PNG Department of Health was equivalent to 10,670,000 5-day courses of the antibiotic [88].

Given the lack of robust microbiological laboratory capacity at many centers in PNG, practitioners sometimes resort to the empiric administration of broad or redundant antibiotics, as is the case with the management of genital discharge in PNG [89,90]. In healthcare facilities without the capacity to perform bacterial cultures or antimicrobial sensitivity testing, the only clue to AMR may be an increase in clinical failure in appropriately treated infections [22]. In the absence of routinely generated clinical microbiological data, deliberate research efforts have often been necessary in order to uncover the true state of resistance patterns in PNG [91].

Unofficial use of antibiotics has emerged as an important driver of AMR in PNG. Nonprescription dispensing of amoxicillin, chloramphenicol, and trimethoprim–sulfamethoxazole is common in the PNG highlands, where infection due to multidrug-resistant Gram-negative organisms has become a common cause of death [54]. In Popondetta, nearly all children with the common cold receive empiric antibiotics, with 30% of healthcare workers believing that antibiotics were indicated in this setting [92]. A significant number of patients in PNG have already received antibiotics by the time they present to a healthcare facility, indicating a need to regulate commercial pharmacies and provide education to health workers about appropriate antibiotic use [28,91].

Poor adherence to oral antibiotics can foster AMR [93]. The development of ampicillin resistance among Gram-negative organisms may be related to difficulties in adhering to newer dosing schedules that are more complicated compared to older approaches to the outpatient management of pneumonia [28]. Resistance to gentamicin amongst Gramnegative organisms has remained relatively low, probably due to the difficulty in the non-prescription dispensing and administration of intravenous medication. Throughout the twentieth century, third-generation cephalosporin use in PNG was extremely limited, minimizing opportunities for the development of resistance [94].

Even in the context of responsible antibiotic prescription practices and patient adherence, the circulation of poor-quality drugs in under-resourced regions has the potential to generate AMR [95]. Substandard or falsified drugs with inappropriate reductions in active pharmaceutical ingredients have been detected throughout the PNG supply chain and have been associated with inadequate manufacturing, quality control, and regulatory practices [96,97].

There is growing awareness amidst intensifying globalization that the emergence of resistant organisms in one part of the world can lead to an international problem [98]. Even if PNG manages to address the issues described above, growing interconnectedness with Asia and Australia—particularly through PNG's productive extractive industries—raises the possibility that AMR could enter from abroad [99].

Other factors contributing to the spread of resistant organisms in PNG include overcrowding with low nurse-to-patient ratios and the absence of effective hygiene practices, both within hospitals and in the community [57].

3. Discussion and Conclusions

This is the first comprehensive review to specifically address the problem of AMR in PNG. Much of the effort on AMR in PNG has focused on *S. pneumoniae* and *H. influenzae*, as these agents were responsible for a high degree of mortality in childhood meningitis and pneumonia in the pre-vaccine age [35].

Historically, penicillin was the drug of choice for the treatment of infections caused by *S. pneumoniae* in PNG [100]. Resistance developed early and quickly, but susceptibility to chloramphenicol persisted throughout the twentieth century, prompting its adoption as the empiric treatment for childhood pneumonia and meningitis. Nonetheless, evolving resistance patterns among *S. pneumoniae* and *H. influenzae* dictated a broadening of the empiric treatment of bacterial meningitis in PNG to ceftriaxone in 2005. In 2014, the 13-valent pneumococcal conjugate vaccine (PCV13) was introduced into PNG's national immunization program; however, coverage of the complete three-dose schedule in 2015 was estimated to be between 4% and 6.5% [42].

Chloramphenicol resistance among *H. influenzae* was absent for most of the twentieth century in PNG but became established quickly after it was initially detected in the late 1990s, generating concerns that expensive broad-spectrum antibiotics would soon be needed in order to empirically treat children with meningitis [22]. Fortunately, *H. influenzae* type b vaccination was included in PNG's expanded program of immunization in 2008 [52]. By 2016, between 43% and 47.7% of children surveyed in Eastern Highlands had received three doses of the DTPw-HepB-Hib vaccine [91]. The integration of available vaccines—especially against *S. pneumoniae* and *H. influenzae* type b—into routine childhood immunization schedules has since led to reductions in childhood mortality [42].

Over time, the country has seen a marked increase in resistance to penicillin, methicillin, and oxacillin among *S. aureus*. There is already considerable circulation of MRSA in the community in PNG [19].

Shigella and *Salmonella* spp. appear to remain susceptible to ceftriaxone, but fluoroquinolone resistance has developed in *Salmonella* [16,18]. Ampicillin, chloramphenicol, and tetracycline are not good options for the treatment of infections associated with these organisms in PNG.

There is widespread, high-level resistance among *N. gonorrhoeae* to penicillin, azithromycin, and ciprofloxacin in the Western Pacific, as well as increased MICs of ceftriaxone and other extended-spectrum cephalosporins [84,101]. There is sporadic low-level resistance to fluoroquinolones and ceftriaxone among *N. gonorrhoeae* in PNG.

Resistant Gram-negative organisms—especially extended-spectrum β-lactamase (ESBL)-producing Enterobacterales—have been identified as a serious threat to human health in the twenty-first century [102]. There is a high degree of known resistance among Gram-negative organisms to a number of common antibiotics in PNG, including significant resistance to third-generation cephalosporins among the Enterobacterales [14,28]. It is possible that there is also substantial undetected AMR among Gram-negative organisms to newly available antibiotics such as ciprofloxacin, second- and third-generation cephalosporins, and other broad-spectrum parenteral antibiotics that have entered into empiric use in PNG.

Broad-spectrum antibiotic resistance among Gram-negative organisms is concerning due to the high mortality rate associated with the progression of Gram-negative infections into sepsis [14]. Investigations of the prevalence of ESBL-producing organisms in PNG have been extremely limited, and the sample sizes in surveys of Gram-negative resistance have been small [29]. There is even more of a dearth of data from PNG on microbial susceptibility to carbapenems—which, along with other parenteral antibiotics such as vancomycin, daptomycin, lincomycin, linezolid, and ceftaroline, are not readily available in much of PNG [17,18]. It is likely that access to broader-spectrum antibiotics as a solution to growing AMR would only precipitate resistance to them [57].

There are no published data from PNG on AMR among *Enterococcus* spp., a genus of coliform bacteria associated with nosocomial infections and prone to plasmid-mediated resistance to vancomycin and beta-lactams [102].

The overwhelming majority of AMR data from PNG come from Port Moresby and Goroka, since these are the only centers where sufficient resources have traditionally existed to perform the required microbiological techniques [28]. As a result, little is known about patterns of resistance in other parts of the country. Ongoing sentinel surveillance for multidrug-resistant organisms should be continued in several carefully selected sites—including the Sepik, Daru, and outer insular regions, which have been largely excluded from AMR studies—that represent the extreme regional diversity within PNG [28,29].

Compared to the rest of the world, Oceania has reported more deaths associated with AMR than all regions except for southern Latin America, South Asia, and sub-Saharan Africa [103]. Among Pacific island countries, PNG boasts some of the best-characterized AMR and may harbor some of the highest rates of resistance [104].

As with any region, the increasing availability of newer and more powerful antibiotics in PNG will inevitably engender the development of broad and potentially novel AMR. With increasing connectivity to the world, it is easier than ever for resistant organisms or traits to spread to and from PNG [105,106]. Given these certitudes, further research should emphasize pathogens that have been identified as priorities by the WHO and for which there are currently scarce data from PNG, especially ESBL-producing and carbapenem-resistant Gram-negative organisms, cephalosporin- and fluoroquinolone-resistant *Neisseria gonorrhoeae*, and vancomycin-resistant *Enterococcus* [107].

Supplementary Materials: The following supporting information can be downloaded at: https://www.mdpi.com/article/10.3390/antibiotics12121679/s1, Table S1: Antimicrobial resistance among Gram-positive organisms in Papua New Guinea; Table S2: Antimicrobial resistance among Gram-negative organisms in Papua New Guinea.

Author Contributions: Conceptualization, B.P.; literature review, B.P. and S.A.; analysis, B.P.; original draft preparation, B.P.; review and editing, S.A. All authors have read and agreed to the published version of the manuscript.

Funding: This research received no external funding.

Institutional Review Board Statement: This work did not involve human subjects.

Informed Consent Statement: Not applicable.

Data Availability Statement: All data are available as outlined in the References.

Conflicts of Interest: The authors declare no conflict of interest.

References

1. Kitur, U.; Adair, T.; Riley, I.; Lopez, A.D. Estimating the pattern of causes of death in Papua New Guinea. *BMC Public. Health* **2019**, *19*, 1322. [CrossRef] [PubMed]
2. Sutherland, T.; Mpirimbanyi, C.; Nziyomaze, E.; Niyomugabo, J.-P.; Niyonsenga, Z.; Muvunyi, C.M.; Mueller, A.; Bebell, L.M.; Nkubana, T.; Musoni, E.; et al. Widespread antimicrobial resistance among bacterial infections in a Rwandan referral hospital. *PLoS ONE* **2019**, *14*, e0221121. [CrossRef] [PubMed]
3. Central Intelligence Agency. Papua New Guinea. In *The World Factbook 2020*; Central Intelligence Agency: Langley, VA, USA, 2020.
4. World Bank. Papua New Guinea. Available online: https://data.worldbank.org/country/papua-new-guinea (accessed on 19 May 2020).
5. United Nations Development Programme. Human Development Index (HDI). Available online: http://hdr.undp.org/en/content/human-development-index-hdi (accessed on 19 May 2020).
6. Ventola, C.L. The Antibiotic Resistance Crisis Part 1: Causes and Threats. *Pharm. Ther.* **2015**, *40*, 277–283.
7. Spellberg, B.; Gilbert, D.N. The Future of Antibiotics and Resistance: A Tribute to a Career of Leadership by John Bartlett. *Clin. Infect. Dis.* **2014**, *59* (Suppl. S2), 71–75. [CrossRef] [PubMed]
8. Aia, P.; Kal, M.; Lavu, E.; Lucy, N.; Johnson, K. The Burden of Drug-Resistant Tuberculosis in Papua New Guinea: Results of a Large Population-Based Survey. *PLoS ONE* **2016**, *11*, e0149806. [CrossRef] [PubMed]
9. Cleary, E.; Hetzel, M.W.; Clements, A.C.A. A review of malaria epidemiology and control in Papua New Guinea 1900 to 2021: Progress made and future directions. *Front. Epidemiol.* **2022**, *2*, 980795. [CrossRef]
10. Gare, J.; Toto, B.; Pokeya, P.; Le, L.-V.; Dala, N.; Lote, N.; John, B.; Yamba, A.; Soli, K.; DeVos, J.; et al. High prevalence of pre-treatment HIV drug resistance in Papua New Guinea: Findings from the first nationally representative pre-treatment HIV drug resistance study. *BMC Infect. Dis.* **2022**, *22*, 266. [CrossRef]
11. Page, M.J.; McKenzie, J.E.; Bossuyt, P.M.; Boutron, I.; Hoffmann, T.C.; Mulrow, C.D.; Shamseer, L.; Tetzlaff, J.M.; Akl, E.A.; Brennan, S.E.; et al. The PRISMA 2020 statement: An updated guideline for reporting systematic reviews. *BMJ* **2021**, *372*, n71. [CrossRef]
12. von Eiff, C.; Becker, K.; Machka, K.; Stammer, H.; Peters, G. Nasal carriage as a source of *Staphylococcus aureus* bacteremia. *N. Engl. J. Med.* **2001**, *344*, 11–16. [CrossRef]
13. Scrimgeour, E.; Igo, J. Penicillin resistant *Staphylococcus aureus* in Port Moresby. *PNG Med. J.* **1981**, *24*, 261–263.
14. Duke, T.; Michael, A.; Mgone, J.; Frank, D.; Wal, T.; Sehuko, R. Etiology of child mortality in Goroka, Papua New Guinea: A prospective two-year study. *Bull. World Health Organ.* **2002**, *80*, 16–25.
15. Montgomery, J. The Aerobic Bacteriology of Infected Skin Lesions in Children of the Eastern Highlands Province. *PNG Med. J.* **1985**, *28*, 93–103.
16. Montgomery, J.; West, B.; Michael, A.; Kadivaion, B. Bacterial Resistance in the Eastern Highlands Province. *PNG Med. J.* **1987**, *30*, 11–19.
17. Laman, M.; Greenhill, A.; Coombs, G.W.; Robinson, O.; Pearson, J.; Davis, T.M.E.; Manning, L. Methicillin-resistant *Staphylococcus aureus* in Papua New Guinea: A community nasal colonization prevalence study. *Trans. R. Soc. Trop. Med. Hyg.* **2017**, *111*, 360–362. [CrossRef] [PubMed]
18. World Health Organization. *Antimicrobial Resistance: Global Report on Surveillance*; World Health Organization: Geneva, Switzerland, 2014.
19. Aglua, I.; Jaworski, J.; Drekore, J. Methicillin-Resistant *Staphylococcus aureus* in Melanesian Children with Haematogenous Osteomyelitis from the Central Highlands of Papua New Guinea. *Int. J. Pediatr.* **2018**, *6*, 8361–8370.
20. Hansman, D.; Bullen, M. A resistant pneumococcus. *Lancet* **1967**, *290*, 264–265. [CrossRef]
21. Gratten, M.; Naraqi, S.; Hansman, D. High prevalence of penicillin-insensitive pneumococci in Port Moresby, Papua New Guinea. *Lancet* **1980**, *316*, 192–195. [CrossRef] [PubMed]
22. Duke, T.; Michael, A.; Mokela, D.; Wal, T.; Reeder, J. Chloramphenicol or ceftriaxone, or both, as treatment for meningitis in developing countries? *Arch. Dis. Child.* **2003**, *88*, 536–539. [CrossRef]
23. Manning, L.; Laman, M.; Greenhill, A.R.; Michael, A.; Siba, P.; Mueller, I.; Davis, T.M.E. Increasing chloramphenicol resistance in Streptococcus pneumoniae isolates from Papua New Guinean Children with acute bacterial meningitis. *Antimicrob. Agents Chemother.* **2011**, *55*, 4454–4456. [CrossRef]
24. Laman, M.; Manning, L. Acute bacterial meningitis in Papua New Guinea: New treatment guidelines in response to increasing antibiotic resistance. *PNG Med. J.* **2011**, *54*, 1–3.
25. Scrimgeour, E.M.; Kaven, J. Severe staphylococcal pneumonia complicating pyomyositis. *Am. J. Trop. Med. Hyg.* **1982**, *31*, 822–826. [CrossRef] [PubMed]
26. Browness, P.; Bower, M.; Montgomery, J.; Lupiwa, T.; Gratten, M.; Shann, F. The bacteriology of skin sores in Goroka children. *PNG Med. J.* **1984**, *27*, 83–87.
27. Brian, M.J.; Michael, A. Community-acquired infection with methicillin-resistant *Staphylococcus aureus* in Papua New Guinea. *Pediatr. Infect. Dis. J.* **1989**, *8*, 807–808. [CrossRef] [PubMed]
28. Duke, T. Antibiotic-resistant bacterial sepsis in Papua New Guinea. *PNG Med. J.* **2000**, *43*, 82–90.
29. Asa, H.; Laman, M.; Greenhill, A.R.; Siba, P.M.; Davis, T.M.E.; Maihua, J.; Manning, L. Bloodstream infections caused by resistant bacteria in surgical patients admitted to Modilon Hospital, Madang. *PNG Med. J.* **2012**, *55*, 5–11.

30. Poka, H.; Duke, T. Clinical management of diarrhoea in children. *PNG Med. J.* **2013**, *56*, 156–161.
31. Henriques-Normark, B.; Tuomanen, E.I. The Pneumococcus: Epidemiology, Microbiology, and Pathogenesis. *Cold Spring Harb. Perspect. Med.* **2013**, *3*, a010215. [CrossRef]
32. Hansman, D.; Glasgow, H.; Sturt, J.; Devitt, L.; Douglas, R. Increased resistance to penicillin of pneumococci isolated from man. *N. Engl. J. Med.* **1971**, *284*, 175–177. [CrossRef]
33. Hansman, D. Pneumococci insensitive to Penicillin. *Nature* **1971**, *230*, 407–408. [CrossRef]
34. Hansman, D.; Devitt, L.; Riley, I. Pneumococci with increased resistance to penicillin. *Br. Med. J. (Clin. Res. Ed.)* **1973**, *3*, 405. [CrossRef] [PubMed]
35. Gratten, M.; Barker, J.; Shann, F.; Gerega, G.; Montgomery, J.; Kajoi, M.; Lupiwa, T. The Aetiology of Purulent Meningitis in Highland Children: A Bacteriological Study. *PNG Med. J.* **1985**, *28*, 233–240.
36. Barker, J.; Gratten, M.; Riley, I.; Lehmann, D.; Montgomery, J.; Kajoi, M.; Gratten, H.; Smith, D.; Marshall, T.F.D.C.; Alpers, M.P. Pneumonia in Children in the Eastern Highlands of Papua New Guinea: A Bacteriologic Study of Patients Selected by Standard Clinical Criteria. *J. Infect. Dis.* **1989**, *159*, 348–352. [CrossRef]
37. Gratten, M.; Montgomery, J. The bacteriology of acute pneumonia and meningitis in children in Papua New Guinea: Assumptions, facts and technical strategies. *PNG Med. J.* **1991**, *34*, 185–198.
38. Gratten, M. Carriage and Invasion of Respiratory Bacterial Pathogens in Melanesian Children. MSc Thesis, University of Papua New Guinea, Port Moresby, Papua New Guinea, 1984.
39. Montgomery, J. A Longitudinal Study of Upper Respiratory Tract Bacterial Carriage and Its Association with Acute Lower Respiratory Infections in Children in the Highlands of Papua New Guinea. MSc Thesis, University of Papua New Guinea, Port Moresby, Papua New Guinea, 1989.
40. Lehmann, D.; Gratten, M.; Montgomery, J. Susceptibility of pneumococcal carriage isolates to penicillin provides a conservative estimate of susceptibility of invasive pneumococci. *Pediatr. Infect. Dis. J.* **1997**, *16*, 297–305. [CrossRef]
41. Lehmann, D.; Yeka, W.; Rongap, T.; Javati, A.; Saleu, G.; Clegg, A.; Michael, A.; Lupiwa, T.; Omena, M.; Alpers, M.P. Aetiology and clinical signs of bacterial meningitis in children admitted to Goroka Base Hospital, Papua New Guinea, 1989–1992. *Ann. Trop. Paediatr.* **1999**, *19*, 21–32. [CrossRef]
42. Greenhill, A.R.; Phuanukoonnon, S.; Michael, A.; Yoannes, M.; Orami, T.; Smith, H.; Murphy, D.; Blyth, C.; Reeder, J.; Siba, P.; et al. *Streptococcus pneumoniae* and *Haemophilus influenzae* in paediatric meningitis patients at Goroka General Hospital, Papua New Guinea: Serotype distribution and antimicrobial susceptibility in the pre-vaccine era. *BMC Infect. Dis.* **2015**, *15*, 485. [CrossRef]
43. Daimen, M. Acute bacterial meningitis in adult patients at the Port Moresby General Hospital 1998–2008. In *Public Private Partnership in Health Care, 45th Annual Medical Symposium, 30 August–4 September 2009*; Medical Society of Papua New Guinea: Port Moresby, Papua New Guinea, 2009.
44. Martin, J.; Green, M. Group A Streptococcus. *Semin. Pediatr. Infect. Dis.* **2006**, *17*, 140–148. [CrossRef]
45. Raabe, V.N.; Shane, A.L. Group B Streptococcus (*Streptococcus agalactiae*). *Microbiol. Spectr.* **2019**, *7*, 1–21. [CrossRef]
46. Shah, M.; Centor, R.M.; Jennings, M. Severe acute pharyngitis caused by group C Streptococcus. *J. Gen. Intern. Med.* **2007**, *22*, 272–274. [CrossRef]
47. Kalt, F.; Schulthess, B.; Sidler, F.; Herren, S.; Fucentese, S.F.; Zingg, P.O.; Berli, M.; Zinkernagel, A.S.; Zbinden, R.; Achermann, Y. Corynebacterium Species Rarely Cause Orthopedic Infections. *J. Clin. Microbiol.* **2018**, *56*, 1–8. [CrossRef]
48. Agrawal, A.; Murphy, T.F. *Haemophilus influenzae* infections in the *H. influenzae* type b conjugate vaccine era. *J. Clin. Microbiol.* **2011**, *49*, 3728–3732. [CrossRef]
49. Shann, F.; Germer, S.; Hazlett, D.; Gratten, M.; Linnemann, V.; Payne, R. Aetiology of pneumonia in children in Goroka Hospital, Papua New Guinea. *Lancet* **1984**, *324*, 537–541. [CrossRef]
50. Shann, F.; Gratten, M.; Montgomery, J.; Lupiwa, T.; Polume, H. *Haemophilus influenzae* Resistant to Penicillin in Goroka. *PNG Med. J.* **1982**, *25*, 23–24.
51. Duke, T.; Mokela, D.; Frank, D.; Michael, A.; Paulo, T.; Mgone, J.; Kurubi, J. Management of meningitis in children with oral fluid restriction or intravenous fluid at maintenance volumes: A randomised trial. *Ann. Trop. Paediatr.* **2002**, *22*, 145–157. [CrossRef]
52. Paediatric Society of Papua New Guinea. *Standard Treatment for Common Illnesses of Children in Papua New Guinea*, 10th ed.; Paediatric Society of Papua New Guinea: Port Moresby, Papua New Guinea, 2016.
53. Packham, D.; Sorrell, T. Pneumonia with bacteraemia due to *Escherichia coli*. *Aust. N. Z. J. Med.* **1981**, *11*, 669–672. [CrossRef]
54. Duke, T.; Michael, A. Increase in sepsis due to multi-resistant enteric gram-negative bacilli in Papua New Guinea. *PNG Med. J.* **1999**, *353*, 2210–2211. [CrossRef]
55. Podschun, R.; Ullmann, U. *Klebsiella* spp. as nosocomial pathogens: Epidemiology, taxonomy, typing methods, and pathogenicity factors. *Clin. Microbiol. Rev.* **1998**, *11*, 589–603. [CrossRef]
56. Trevett, A.; SenGupta, S. Gentamicin resistance in fatal Klebsiella septicaemia. *PNG Med. J.* **1992**, *35*, 202–204.
57. Lithgow, A.E.; Kilalang, C. Outbreak of nosocomial sepsis in the Special Care Nursery at Port Moresby General Hospital due to multiresistant Klebsiella pneumoniae: High impact on mortality. *PNG Med. J.* **2009**, *52*, 28–34.
58. Hilty, M.; Sendi, P.; Seiffert, S.N.; Droz, S.; Perreten, V.; Hujer, A.M.; Bonomo, R.A.; Mühlemann, K.; Endimiani, A. Characterisation and clinical features of Enterobacter cloacae bloodstream infections occurring at a tertiary care university hospital in Switzerland: Is cefepime adequate therapy? *Int. J. Antimicrob. Agents.* **2013**, *41*, 236–249. [CrossRef] [PubMed]

59. Endimiani, A.; Luzzaro, F.; Brigante, G.; Perilli, M.; Lombardi, G.; Amicosante, G.; Rossolini, G.M.; Toniolo, A. Proteus mirabilis bloodstream infections: Risk factors and treatment outcome related to the expression of extended-spectrum beta-lactamases. *Antimicrob. Agents Chemother.* **2005**, *49*, 2598–2605. [CrossRef]
60. Choi, H.K.; Kim, Y.K.; Kim, H.Y.; Park, J.E.; Uh, Y. Clinical and microbiological features of Providencia bacteremia: Experience at a tertiary care hospital. *Korean J. Intern. Med.* **2015**, *30*, 219–225. [CrossRef]
61. Liu, H.; Zhu, J.; Hu, Q.; Rao, X. Morganella Morganii, a non-negligent opportunistic pathogen. *Int. J. Infect. Dis.* **2016**, *50*, 10–17. [CrossRef]
62. de Bentzmann, S.; Plésiat, P. The Pseudomonas aeruginosa opportunistic pathogen and human infections. *Environ. Microbiol.* **2011**, *13*, 1655–1665. [CrossRef]
63. Howard, A.; O'Donoghue, M.; Feeney, A.; Sleator, R.D. Acinetobacter baumannii: An emerging opportunistic pathogen. *Virulence* **2012**, *3*, 243–250. [CrossRef]
64. Barnes, D.J.; Naraqi, S.; Igo, J.D. Community-Acquired Acinetobacter Pneumonia in Adults in Papua New Guinea. *Rev. Infect. Dis.* **1988**, *10*, 636–639. [CrossRef]
65. Sfeir, M.M. *Burkholderia cepacia* Complex Infections: More Complex Than the Bacterium Name Suggest. *J. Infect.* **2018**, *77*, 166–170. [CrossRef]
66. Wiersinga, W.J.; Virk, H.S.; Torres, A.G.; Currie, B.J.; Peacock, S.J.; Dance, D.A.B. Melioidosis. *Nat. Rev. Dis. Prim.* **2018**, *4*, 17107. [CrossRef]
67. Baker, A.; Pearson, T.; Price, E.P.; Dale, J.; Keim, P.; Hornstra, H.; Greenhill, A.; Padilla, G.; Warner, J. Molecular Phylogeny of *Burkholderia pseudomallei* from a Remote Region of Papua New Guinea. *PLoS ONE* **2011**, *6*, e18343. [CrossRef]
68. Janda, J.M.; Abbott, S.L. The genus Aeromonas: Taxonomy, pathogenicity, and infection. *Clin. Microbiol. Rev.* **2010**, *23*, 35–73. [CrossRef] [PubMed]
69. Ranjan, K.P.; Ranjan, N. Citrobacter: An emerging health care associated urinary pathogen. *Urol. Ann.* **2013**, *5*, 313–314. [CrossRef] [PubMed]
70. Hasan, M.J.; Nizhu, L.N.; Rabbani, R. Bloodstream infection with pandrug-resistant *Alcaligenes faecalis* treated with double-dose of tigecycline. *IDCases* **2019**, *18*, e00600. [CrossRef]
71. Zaidi, M.B.; Estrada-García, T. Shigella: A Highly Virulent and Elusive Pathogen. *Curr. Trop. Med. Rep.* **2014**, *1*, 81–87. [CrossRef]
72. Curtis, P. The isolation, incidence and sensitivity of Shigella organisms. *PNG Med. J.* **1964**, *7*, 23–26.
73. Rosewell, A.; Ropa, B.; Posanai, E.; Dutta, S.R.; Mola, G.; Zwi, A.; MacIntyre, C.R. Shigella spp. Antimicrobial Drug Resistance, Papua New Guinea, 2000–2009. *Emerg. Infect. Dis.* **2010**, *16*, 8–10. [CrossRef]
74. Greenhill, A.R.; Guwada, C.; Siba, V.; Michael, A.; Yoannes, M.; Wawarie, Y.; Ford, R.; Siba, P.M.; Horwood, P.F. Antibiotic resistant Shigella is a major cause of diarrhoea in the Highlands of Papua New Guinea. *J. Infect. Dev. Ctries.* **2014**, *8*, 1391–1397. [CrossRef]
75. Malau, E.; Ford, R.; Valcanis, M.; Jennison, A.V.; Mosse, J.; Bean, D.; Yoannes, M.; Pomat, W.; Horwood, P.F.; Greenhill, A.R. Antimicrobial sensitivity trends and virulence genes in *Shigella* spp. from the Oceania region. *Infect. Genet. Evol.* **2018**, *64*, 52–56. [CrossRef]
76. Kurtz, J.R.; Goggins, J.A.; McLachlan, J.B. Salmonella infection: Interplay between the bacteria and host immune system. *Immunol. Lett.* **2017**, *190*, 42–50. [CrossRef]
77. Howard, P.; Alexander, N.D.; Atkinson, A.; Clegg, A.; Gerega, G.; Javati, A.; Kajoi, M.; Lupiwa, S.; Lupiwa, T.; Mens, M.; et al. Bacterial, Viral and Parasitic Aetiology of Paediatric Diarrhoea in the Highlands of Papua New Guinea. *J. Trop. Pediatr.* **2000**, *46*, 10–14. [CrossRef]
78. Faruque, S.; Albert, M.; Mekalanos, J. Epidemiology, genetics, and ecology of toxigenic Vibrio cholerae. *Microbiol. Mol. Biol. Rev.* **1998**, *62*, 1301–1314. [CrossRef]
79. Murhekar, M.; Dutta, S.; Ropa, B.; Dagina, R.; Posanaic, E.; Rosewell, A. Vibrio cholerae antimicrobial drug resistance, Papua New Guinea, 2009–2011. *West. Pac. Surveill. Response J. WSPAR* **2013**, *4*, 2009–2011. [CrossRef]
80. Rouphael, N.G.; Stephens, D.S. Neisseria meningitidis: Biology, microbiology, and epidemiology. *Methods Mol. Biol.* **2012**, *799*, 1–20.
81. Hudson, B.; van der Meijden, W.; Lupiwa, T.; Howard, P.; Tabua, T.; Tapsall, J.W.; Phillips, E.A.; Lennox, V.A.; Backhouse, J.L.; Pyakalyia, T. A survey of sexually transmitted diseases in five STD clinics in Papua New Guinea. *PNG Med. J.* **1994**, *37*, 152–160.
82. Piszczek, J.; St Jean, R.; Khaliq, Y. Gonorrhea: Treatment update for an increasingly resistant organism. *Can. Pharm. J.* **2015**, *148*, 82–89. [CrossRef]
83. Unemo, M.; Shafer, W.M. Antimicrobial resistance in Neisseria gonorrhoeae in the 21st century: Past, evolution, and future. *Clin. Microbiol. Rev.* **2014**, *27*, 587–613. [CrossRef]
84. Lahra, M.M.; Lo, Y.R.; Whiley, D.M. Gonococcal antimicrobial resistance in the Western Pacific Region. *Sex. Transm. Infect.* **2013**, *89* (Suppl. S4), 19–23. [CrossRef]
85. WHO Western Pacific Region Gonococcal Antimicrobial Surveillance Programme. Surveillance of antibiotic susceptibility of Neisseria gonorrhoeae in the WHO Western Pacific Region. *Genitourin. Med.* **1997**, *73*, 355–361.
86. Pusahai-Riman, P.; Soepol, N. A retrospective assessment of antibiotic susceptibility pattern of Neisseria gonorrhoeae and prevalence rate of gonorrhoea in Port Moresby General Hospital from 2005 to 2006. *Pac. J. Med. Sci.* **2008**, *5*, 82–90.
87. Toliman, P.J.; Lupiwa, T.; Law, G.J.; Reeder, J.C.; Siba, P.M. Neisseria gonorrhoeae isolates from four centres in Papua New Guinea remain susceptible to amoxycillin-clavulanate therapy. *PNG Med. J.* **2010**, *53*, 15–20.

88. Riley, I. Pneumonia in Papua New Guinea. Bachelor's Thesis, University of Sydney, Sydney, Australia, 1979.
89. Peacock, S.; Newton, P. Public health impact of establishing the cause of bacterial infections in rural Asia. *Trans. R. Soc. Trop. Med. Hyg.* **2008**, *102*, 5–6. [CrossRef] [PubMed]
90. *Standard Management of Sexually Transmitted Infections Genital Conditions in Papua New Guinea: A Manual for Health Workers in PNG*; Papua New Guinea Department of Health: Port Moresby, Papua New Guinea, 2006.
91. Blyth, C.C.; Ford, R.; Sapura, J.; Kumani, T.; Masiria, G.; Kave, J.; Yuasi, L.; Greenhill, A.; Hwaihwanje, I. Childhood pneumonia and meningitis in the Eastern Highlands Province, Papua New Guinea in the era of conjugate vaccines: Study methods and challenges. *Pneumonia* **2017**, *9*, 1–10. [CrossRef]
92. Zamunu, A.; Pameh, W.; Ripa, P.; Vince, J.; Duke, T. Antibiotic use in the management of children with the common cold at a provincial hospital in Papua New Guinea: A point-prevalence study. *Paediatr. Int. Child. Health.* **2018**, *38*, 261–265. [CrossRef]
93. Eells, S.J.; Nguyen, M.; Jung, J.; Macias-Gil, R.; May, L.; Miller, L.G. Relationship between adherence to oral antibiotics and postdischarge clinical outcomes among patients hospitalized with *Staphylococcus aureus* skin infections. *Antimicrob. Agents Chemother.* **2016**, *60*, 2941–2948. [CrossRef]
94. Wandi, F.; Kiagi, G.; Duke, T. Long-term outcome for children with bacterial meningitis in rural Papua New Guinea. *J. Trop. Pediatr.* **2005**, *51*, 51–53. [CrossRef]
95. Weinstein, Z.B.; Zaman, M.H. Evolution of rifampin resistance in Escherichia coli and Mycobacterium smegmatis due to substandard drugs. *Antimicrob. Agents Chemother.* **2018**, *63*, e01243-18. [CrossRef]
96. Hetzel, M.W.; Page-Sharp, M.; Bala, N.; Pulford, J.; Betuela, I.; Davis, T.M.E.; Lavu, E.K. Quality of antimalarial drugs and antibiotics in Papua New Guinea: A survey of the health facility supply chain. *PLoS ONE* **2014**, *9*, e96810. [CrossRef]
97. Papua New Guinea Department of Health, World Health Organization. *Papua New Guinea Pharmaceutical Country Profile*. 2012. Available online: https://www.who.int/countries/png/ (accessed on 19 May 2020).
98. Berndtson, A.E. Increasing Globalization and the Movement of Antimicrobial Resistance between Countries. *Surg. Infect.* **2020**, *21*, 579–585. [CrossRef] [PubMed]
99. Banks, G. Globalization, poverty, and hyperdevelopment in Papua New Guinea's mining sector. *Focaal* **2005**, *2005*, 128–144. [CrossRef]
100. John, B.; Bowler, D.; Gooch, P.; Lawson, J. Purulent meningitis in Papuan children. *PNG Med. J.* **1968**, *11*, 23–29.
101. World Health Organization, Gonococcal Antimicrobial Surveillance Programme. Gonococcal antimicrobial susceptibility. In *Report on Global Sexually Transmitted Infection Surveillance, 2018*; WHO: Geneva, Switzerland, 2018.
102. Centers for Disease Control and Prevention. *Antibiotic Resistant Threats in the United States*; U.S. Department of Health and Human Services: Atlanta, GA, USA, 2019.
103. Antimicrobial Resistance Collaborators. Global burden of bacterial antimicrobial resistance in 2019: A systematic analysis. *Lancet* **2022**, *399*, 10325.
104. Foxlee, N.D.; Townell, N.; McIver, L.; Lau, C.L. Antibiotic Resistance in Pacific Island Countries and Territories: A Systematic Scoping Review. *Antibiotics* **2019**, *8*, 29. [CrossRef]
105. Observatory of Economic Complexity. Papua New Guinea Country Profile. Available online: https://oec.world/en/profile/country/png/ (accessed on 19 May 2020).
106. Bainomugisa, A.; Pandey, S.; Donnan, E.; Simpson, G.; Foster, J.; Lavu, E.; Hiasihri, S.; McBryde, E.S.; Moke, R.; Vincent, S.; et al. Cross-border movement of highly drug-resistant Mycobacterium tuberculosis from Papua New Guinea to Australia through Torres Strait Protected Zone, 2010–2015. *Emerg. Infect. Dis.* **2019**, *25*, 406–415. [CrossRef]
107. World Health Organization. *Global Priority List of Antibiotic-Resistant Bacteria to Guide Research, Discovery, and Development of New Antibiotics*; World Health Organization: Geneva, Switzerland, 2017.

Disclaimer/Publisher's Note: The statements, opinions and data contained in all publications are solely those of the individual author(s) and contributor(s) and not of MDPI and/or the editor(s). MDPI and/or the editor(s) disclaim responsibility for any injury to people or property resulting from any ideas, methods, instructions or products referred to in the content.

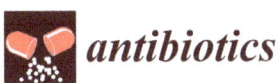

Article

Prevalence and Predictors of Antibiotic Self-Medication in Sudan: A Descriptive Cross-Sectional Study

Mohamed A. Hussain [1], Ahmed O. Mohamed [1,*], Omalhassan A. Abdelkarim [2], Bashir A. Yousef [3], Asma A. Babikir [4], Maysoon M. Mirghani [4], Entsar A. Mohamed [4], Wadah Osman [5], Ramzi A. Mothana [6] and Rashid Elhag [7]

1 Department of Pharmaceutical Microbiology, Faculty of Pharmacy, International University of Africa, Khartoum P.O. Box 2469, Sudan
2 Department of Pharmacy Practice and Clinical Pharmacy, Faculty of Pharmacy, International University of Africa, Khartoum P.O. Box 2469, Sudan
3 Department of Pharmacology, Faculty of Pharmacy, University of Khartoum, Khartoum P.O. Box 1996, Sudan
4 Department of Pharmaceutical Microbiology, Pharmacy Program, Al-Yarmouk College, Khartoum P.O. Box 11111, Sudan
5 Department of Pharmacognosy, Faculty of Pharmacy, University of Khartoum, Khartoum P.O. Box 1996, Sudan
6 Department of Pharmacognosy, College of Pharmacy, King Saud University, Riyadh 11451, Saudi Arabia
7 Department of Biology, College of Science and Technology, Florida A & M University, Tallahassee, FL 32307, USA
* Correspondence: ahmedkunna93@hotmail.com or ahmedkunna@iua.edu.sd

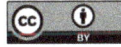

Abstract: Background: Self-medication with antibiotics (SMA) is one of the common factors which precipitate antimicrobial resistance, yet if effective implementations are amended it can be effortlessly controlled. The present study aimed to estimate the prevalence and predictors of SMA in Sudan. Methods: The study adopted a cross-sectional study design conducted in all Sudan states between June and December 2021. Multi-stage stratified cluster sampling was used. A semi-structured questionnaire was used for data collection. Descriptive statistics were used to present the data. Binary logistic regression was computed to investigate the possible factors which associated with SMA. Results: Out of 1492 participants surveyed, 71.3% utilize antibiotics as self-medication. The derived reasons for SMA were convenience (63.3%) and cost-saving (34.8%). Tonsillitis was the most common ailment behind SMA (55.5%). Log-binominal regression revealed that non-insured and low level of education participants were more likely to predict SMA. Regarding the practice, 40% changed the dose and/or antibiotics mainly owing to improvement (53.7%) or worsening of the condition (37.9%). The most commonly used antibiotic was amoxicillin/clavulanic acid (32.5%). Conclusions: Two out of three individuals in Sudan practice SMA mainly to manage upper respiratory tract ailments. Thus, the necessity of implementing an antimicrobial stewardship program throughout the country, as well as implementing effective legislation to prohibit dispensing antibiotics without prescription is urgently required.

Keywords: antibiotic self-medication; Sudan; antimicrobial resistance

1. Introduction

The behaviors of patients toward different medical conditions vary considerably, from immediately seeking medical advice, relying on self-medication (SM), or neglecting the condition [1]. The World Health Organization (WHO) described self-medication (SM) as the use of medicinal products or herbs to manage self-diagnosed disorders or symptoms; moreover, SM also comprises repeated or continued use of a prescribed drug for chronic, recurrent diseases or symptoms. This generally occurs through obtaining medicines without a prescription, sharing medicines, or using leftover medicines stored at home [2].

Even though SM might have some positive outcomes when used properly such as reducing the cost of the treatment [3], numerous pitfalls are associated with the inappropriate use of SM including: delay in the treatment, drug–drug interactions, masking of symptoms, adverse drug reactions (ADR), and most importantly antimicrobial resistance (AMR) [3,4]. AMR was affirmed by the WHO as one of the major problems facing humanity [5]. Overuse and misuse of antibiotics through inadequate dosing, incomplete dose, extensive veterinary use, public beliefs that antibiotics can cure any conditions, overprescribing, non-prescription, and self-medication with antibiotics (SMA) are common factors that are associated with the development of AMR [6,7]. SMA in low to middle-income countries (LMICs) is thought to be more prevalent, mainly owing to the combined effect of external factors such as dispensing antibiotics without prescription and internal factors like economic status [6,8].

Worldwide, effective implementation of rational antibiotic prescription is lacking despite the availability of issued legislation. This is quite understandable when you come to know that two-thirds of antibiotics are available without prescription in the pharmaceutical sector as stated by WHO [9]. Additionally, a recent study estimated that half of the antibiotics were purchased without prescription globally, the same study outlined that non-prescription use of antibiotics reached 82% in some middle-eastern countries [10]. In LMICs, the SM and inappropriate antibiotic practice was declared to be more intensive, according to a meta-analysis published in 2021, in which SMA was outlined to be ranging between 50–93.8% [8]. Another meta-analysis review reported 55.7% as an overall median prevalence of SM with antibiotics in Africa [11]. The same study pointed to the highest prevalence of SMA identified in the west and north African sub-regions [11].

Antibiotics in Sudan are listed under prescription only medicine, albeit the presence of clear regulations, which prohibit dispensing of antibiotics as over the counter drug, antibiotics in Sudan like its counterpart from developing countries can be accessed easily. Most of the antibiotics were purchased from pharmacies in several regions in Sudan [12–14]. This is compatible with the preceding report which revealed that more than 80% of the pharmacists in Sudan frequently dispense antibiotics without prescription [15].

A study conducted in Khartoum state showed that more than 80% of the communities were self-medicated, among them approximately one-third (28.7%) were antibiotic utilizers [13]. The prevalence of SMA in Khartoum state has been described by Abdelmoneim Awad et al. to be 73.9% in 2005 [16]. Another recent study reported a prevalence of 60.3% among Sudanese undergraduate medical students [17]. Most of the studies which were carried out in Sudan pointed toward the association of SMA with age, gender, income, and level of education [13,16–18]. It is worth mentioning that penicillin antibiotics were declared to be the most commonly prescribed antibiotics in most of the studies [17,19].

Given the above backdrop, the present study aimed at providing an updated and comprehensive nationwide estimation of the prevalence of SMA in general Sudanese communities and its association with socio-demographic factors, also the study investigated predictors of SMA including the most common reasons and ailments behind SMA and the most frequently self-medicated antibiotics.

2. Results

2.1. Demographic Characteristics of the Included Participants

Out of 1492 participants surveyed in this study from all Sudan states (The distribution of the participants according to their states is provided in Supplementary Materials Table S1), 53.4% (796) were female. The majority of the participants were aged from 18 to 24 (36.3%) and 25 to 39 (38.7%). More than half (54.3%) of the participants had a low monthly income, however, more than two-thirds (69.3) were medically insured. Regarding the level of education, more than half (55.9%) of the participants completed their university studentship. The demographic characteristics of the included participants are presented in Table 1.

Table 1. Demographic characteristics of the included participants and their association with the use of antibiotic as self-medications.

Demographic Characteristics	Frequency (%)	I Use Antibiotic as Self-Medication (%)	χ^2 p-Value
Gender			
Male	695 (46.6)	523 (72)	0.71
Female	796 (53.4)	590 (71)	
Age (years)			
18–24	542 (36.3)	374 (69)	0.438
25–39	577 (38.7)	422 (73)	
40–59	303 (20.3)	221 (73)	
More than 60	70 (4.7)	45 (64)	
Monthly income ($)			
Less than 50	810 (54.3)	575 (71)	0.089
50–99	297 (19.9)	220 (74)	
100–149	149 (10)	104 (70)	
More than 150	236 (15.8)	182 (77)	
Insurance status			
Insured	1034 (69.3)	745 (72)	>0.00
Non-insured	458 (30.7)	285 (62.3)	
Level of education			
Primary school	146 (9.8)	114 (78)	>0.00
Secondary school	352 (23.6)	243 (69)	
Graduate	834 (55.9)	617 (74)	
Post-graduate	160 (10.7)	91 (57)	
Total	1492 (100)	1059 (71.3)	

Legends: (1 United State Dollars = 250 Sudanese Pounds, all conversion were made based on the central bank of Sudan).

2.2. Prevalence, Sources, and Reasons behind SMA

More than two-thirds (71.3%) of the participants used antibiotics as SM. The Chi-square test revealed that, the participants level of education was significantly associated with antibiotic SM. The vast majority of the participants obtained antibiotics from the pharmacy (92.1%). Additionally, graduate (93.9%) and post-graduate (94.4%) participants obtained antibiotics from pharmacies in higher proportions than primary (89.2%) and secondary school (86.5%) participants, Table 2.

Table 2. Relation between demographical characteristic of the included participants and common sources and reasons behind SMA.

	Source of Antibiotics		Reason behind SMA		
Demographic Characteristics	Pharmacy (%)	Left-Over (%)	Cost Saving (%)	Convenience (%)	Lack of Trust in Prescribing Doctor (%)
Gender					
Male	472 (94.8)	97 (19.5)	230 (46.2)	294 (59.0)	110 (22.1)
Female	505 (90.2)	150 (26.8)	204 (36.4)	379 (67.7)	93 (16.6)
Age (years)					
18–24	338 (90.1)	89 (23.7)	131 (34.9)	252 (67.2)	70 (18.7)
25–39	389 (93.1)	100 (23.9)	191 (45.7)	257 (61.5)	84 (20.1)
40–59	209 (94.6)	46 (20.8)	89 (40.3)	141 (63.8)	36 (16.3)
More than 60	41 (93.2)	12 (27.3)	23 (52.3)	23 (52.3)	13 (29.5)
Monthly income ($)					
Less than 50	516 (91.8)	129 (23.0)	245 (43.6)	356 (63.3)	92 (16.4)
50–99	202 (93.5)	63 (29.2)	88 (40.7)	131 (60.6)	48 (22.2)
100–149	95 (92.2)	23 (22.3)	33 (32.0)	71 (68.9)	24 (23.3)

Table 2. Cont.

	Source of Antibiotics		Reason behind SMA		
Demographic Characteristics	Pharmacy (%)	Left-Over (%)	Cost Saving (%)	Convenience (%)	Lack of Trust in Prescribing Doctor (%)
More than 150	164 (92.1)	32 (18.0)	68 (38.2)	115 (64.6)	39 (21.9)
Insurance status					
Insured	703 (92.3)	184 (24.1)	307 (40.3)	494 (64.8)	201 (26.4)
Non-insured	274 (92.3)	63 (21.2)	127 (42.8)	179 (60.3)	73 (24.6)
Level of education					
Primary school	102 (90.3)	33 (29.2)	64 (56.6)	61 (54.0)	22 (19.5)
Secondary school	205 (85.1)	64 (26.6)	116 (48.1)	147 (61.0)	41 (17.0)
Graduate	582 (94.8)	125 (20.4)	217 (35.3)	412 (67.1)	116 (18.9)
Post-graduate	88 (97.8)	25 (27.8)	37 (41.1)	53 (58.9)	24 (26.7)
Total	274 (92.3)	247 (23.3)	434 (41.0)	673 (63.6)	22 (19.5)

2.3. Common Ailments for Taking Antibiotic as SM

Tonsillitis was the most common aliment that drove participants to self-treatment. It was rated by more than half of the participants (55.5%). This was followed by cough (45%), while a small proportion of the participants used antibiotics for vomiting (10%) (Table 3).

Table 3. Relation between common ailments of SMA and demographic characteristic of the included participants.

	Tonsillitis	Cough	Runny Nose	Nasal Congestion	Fever	Pain	Diarrhea	Wound Infection	Vomiting
Gender									
Male	274 (55)	222 (44.6)	207 (41.6)	166 (33.3)	147 (29.5)	127 (25.5)	109 (21.9)	85 (17.1)	48 (9.6)
Female	314 (56.1)	255 (45.5)	193 (34.5)	188 (33.6)	191 (34.1)	181 (32.3)	123 (22)	73 (13)	60 (10.7)
Age (years)									
18–24	180 (48)	161 (42.9)	126 (33.6)	126 (33.6)	127 (33.9)	110 (29.3)	67 (17.9)	41 (10.9)	35 (9.3)
25–39	263 (62.9)	189 (45.2)	157 (37.6)	133 (31.8)	122 (29.2)	109 (26.1)	85 (20.3)	73 (17.5)	37 (8.9)
40–59	123 (55.7)	104 (47.1)	94 (42.5)	77 (34.8)	67 (30.3)	67 (30.3)	58 (26.2)	35 (15.8)	24 (10.9)
More than 60	22 (50)	23 (52.3)	23 (52.3)	18 (40.9)	22 (50)	22 (50)	22 (50)	9 (20.5)	12 (27.3)
Monthly income ($)									
Less than 50	291 (51.8)	245 (43.6)	195 (34.7)	179 (31.9)	199 (35.4)	182 (32.4)	116 (20.6)	71 (12.6)	55 (9.8)
50–99	132 (61.1)	93 (43.1)	81 (37.5)	81 (37.5)	62 (28.7)	64 (29.6)	68 (31.5)	43 (19.9)	28 (13)
100–149	60 (55.3)	59 (57.3)	49 (47.6)	34 (33)	34 (33)	29 (28.2)	22 (21.4)	18 (17.5)	9 (8.7)
More than 150	105 (59)	80 (44.9)	75 (42.1)	60 (33.7)	43 (24.2)	33 (18.5)	26 (14.6)	26 (14.6)	16 (9)
Insurance status									
Insured	426 (55.9)	351 (46.1)	291 (38.2)	274 (36.0)	242 (31.7)	220 (28.9)	166 (21.8)	109 (14.3)	426 (55.9)
Non-insured	162 (54.7)	125 (42.2)	109 (36.7)	80 (26.9)	97 (32.5)	87 (29.4)	66 (22.1)	49 (16.6)	162 (54.7)
Level of education									
Primary school	46 (40.7)	53 (46.9)	54 (47.8)	40 (35.4)	49 (43.4)	23 (20.4)	40 (35.4)	16 (14.2)	16 (14.2)
Secondary school	132 (54.8)	102 (42.3)	95 (39.4)	88 (36.5)	80 (33.2)	66 (27.4)	50 (20.7)	34 (14.1)	35 (14.5)
Graduate	350 (57)	282 (45.9)	219 (35.7)	194 (31.6)	201 (32.7)	189 (30.8)	134 (21.8)	88 (14.3)	53 (8.6)
Post-graduate	60 (66.7)	40 (44.4)	32 (35.6)	32 (35.6)	8 (8.9)	30 (33.3)	9 (10)	20 (22.2)	4 (4.4)
Total	588 (55.5)	477 (45)	400 (37.8)	354 (33.4)	338 (31.9)	308 (29.1)	232 (21.9)	158 (14.9)	108 (10.2)

2.4. Factors Associated with the Use of Antibiotics as SM

At the bivariate level, medically insured (COR: 0.656; 95% CI (0.506–0.817)) were more likely to use antibiotics as SM. Individuals having secondary (COR: 0.61; 95% CI (0.39–0.97), and post-graduate (COR: 0.38; 95% CI (0.23–0.63)) levels of education were less likely to use antibiotics as SM, other factors were not statistically significant. Regarding the multivariate model, the model sensitivity was 70.2%, further, the model adequately fits the data since there were no differences between the observed and the predicted (Hosmer and Lemeshow test = 0.761). Medically non-insured (AOR: 0.645; 95% CI (0.487–0.855)) and post-graduates (AOR: 0.27; 95% CI (0.15–0.5)) were the only predictors for SMA. Complete logistic regression for the use of antibiotic as SM are presented in Table 4.

Table 4. Bivariate and multiple logistic regression of the demographic factors of SMA.

Demographic Characteristics	Crude Odds Ratio (95% CI)	p-Value	Adjusted Odds Ratio (95% CI)	p-Value
Gender				
Male	1 (baseline)		1 (baseline)	
Female	0.956 (0.761–1.20)	0.700	0.997 (0.758–1.321)	0.984
Age (years)				
18–24	1 (base line)		1 (baseline)	
25–39	1.178 (0.908–1.529)	0.217	1.067 (0.767–1.485)	0.669
40–59	1.184 (0.865–1.621)	0.293	1.04 (0.689–1.571)	0.852
More than 60	0.784 (0.465–1.323)	0.362	0.687 (0.353–1.337)	0.269
Monthly income ($)				
Less than 50	1 (baseline)		1 (baseline)	
50–99	1.195 (0.868–1.643)	0.274	1.3 (0.892–1.894)	0.172
100–149	0.959 (0.641–1.436)	0.840	0.952 (0/59–1.537)	0.841
More than 150	1.333 (0.932–1.907)	0.166	1.976 (1.244–3.14)	0.004 *
Insurance status				
Insured	1 (baseline)		1 (baseline)	
Non-insured	0.656 (0.506-0.817)	0.000 *	0.645 (0.487-0.855)	0.002 *
Level of education				
Primary school	1 (baseline)		1 (baseline)	
Secondary school	0.618 (0.393–0.972)	0.037 *	0.658 (0.39–1.111)	0.117
Graduate	0.786 (0.516–1.199)	0.264	0.721 (0.44–1.181)	0.193
Post-graduate	0.382 (0.23–0.633)	0.000 *	0.278 (0.152-0.508)	0.000 *

Legends: CI = confidence interval, * = significant p-Value.

2.5. Knowledge and Adherence to Antibiotic Dosage

More than half of the participants knew the dosage of antibiotics through pharmacist consultation (56.4%) and they fully understood the instructions (59.6%). About 40% of the participants sometimes changed the dosage and/or the antibiotics deliberately during treatment, while 10% always changed the dosage. The main reasons for changing the dosage were improvement (53.7%) or worsening of the condition (37.9%). Approximately two-thirds (67.1%) of the participants changed the former antibiotics if they weren't effective, on the other hand, more than half of the participants (55.1%) stopped taking the antibiotics when symptoms disappeared, and about 10% consulted the doctor or the pharmacist before stopping the antibiotics (Table 5).

Table 5. Knowledge, practice, and adherence to dosage of antibiotics and/or instructions.

Source and/or Adherence Practice	Practice	Frequency (%)
Did you ever check the instructions that come with the package insert of antibiotics for self-treatment	Always	514 (48.5)
	Sometimes	323 (30.5)
	Never	222 (21)

Table 5. Cont.

Source and/or Adherence Practice	Practice	Frequency (%)
How much did you understand the instructions that come with the package insert of antibiotics for self-treatment	Fully understood	631 (59.6)
	Partly understood	381 (36)
	Did not understand at all	47 (4.4)
How did you know the dosage of antibiotics [a]	By checking the package insert	371 (35)
	By consulting a doctor	304 (28.7)
	By consulting a pharmacist	597 (56.4)
	By consulting family members/friends	131 (12.4)
	From the Internet	93 (8.8)
	From my previous experience	210 (19.8)
	By guessing the dosage by myself	54 (5.1)
Did you ever change the dosage of antibiotics deliberately during the course of self-treatment	Always	114 (10)
	Sometimes	445 (42)
	Never	500 (47.2)
Why did you change the dosage of antibiotics during the course of self-treatment [a]	Improving conditions	300 (53.7)
	Worsening conditions	212 (37.9)
	To reduce adverse reactions	101 (18.1)
	Drug insufficient for complete treatment	100 (17.8)
Did you ever switch antibiotics during the course of self-treatment	Always	87 (8.2)
	Sometimes	430 (40.6)
	Never	542 (51.2)
Why did you switch antibiotics during the course of self-treatment [a]	The former antibiotics weren't effective	393 (67.1)
	The latter one was cheaper	85 (16.5)
	To reduce adverse reactions	121 (23.4)
	Based on my experience	64 (12.3)
Have you ever found out that you had taken the same antibiotics with different names at the same time	Yes	632 (59.7)
	No	427 (40.3)
When did you normally stop taking antibiotics	After a few days regardless of the outcome	212 (20)
	After symptoms disappeared	501 (55.1)
	A few days after the recovery	291 (29.1)
	At the completion of the course	401 (37.9)

Legends: [a] = more than one options is allowed.

2.6. Commonly Used Antibiotics and Common Adverse Reactions

The most commonly used antibiotics were amoxicillin/clavulanic acid combinations (32.5%), followed by amoxicillin (26.5%), metronidazole (25.3%), and azithromycin (25.3%). About one-fifth (21.8%) of the participants experienced ADR when they took antibiotics. The primary action taken by more than half (57%) of those who experienced ADR was to stop the antibiotics (Table 6). About half of the participants thought that SMA (51.9%) was not an acceptable practice, and more than one-third (37.4%) thought that they cannot treat the infectious disease on their own. Most of the participants (61%) selected antibiotics based on its indications, and about half of the participants used antibiotics when recommended by community pharmacists (47.9%) and according to their own experience (46.8%). The type of antibiotics was the main factor considered by the majority of the participants (45.4%), while the brand of the antibiotics was only considered by less than one-fifth of the participants (16.3%) (Table 6).

Table 6. Commonly used antibiotics and common adverse reactions.

Commonly Used Antibiotics and Adverse Reactions	Practice	Frequency (%)
Commonly used antibiotics	Amoxicillin and clavulanic acid	344 (32.5)
	Amoxicillin	281 (26.5)
	Metronidazole	268 (25.3)
	Azithromycin	268 (25.3)
	Don't remember	236 (22.3%)
Your selection of antibiotics was based on	Indications	646 (61)
	Recommendation by community pharmacists	507 (47.9)
	My own experience	496 (46.8)
	Opinion of family members	231 (21.8)
	Opinion of friends	230 (21.7)
	Previous doctor's prescription	205 (19.4)
What did you consider when selecting antibiotics	Type of antibiotics	481 (45.4)
	Price of antibiotics	229 (21.6)
	Brand of antibiotics	173 (16.3)
Have you ever had adverse drug reaction when taking antibiotics	Yes	231 (21.8)
	No	828 (78.2)
What did you do for adverse drug reaction	Stop taking the antibiotics	131 (57.7)
	Switch the antibiotics	48 (20.8)
	Consulted a pharmacist	64 (27.6)
	Consulted a doctor	55 (24)
	Consulted family members/friends	26 (11.3)
	No action	35 (13.2)
What do you think about self-medication with antibiotics for self-health care	Good practice	132 (12.5)
	Acceptable practice	377 (35.6)
	Not acceptable practice	550 (51.9)
Do you think you can treat common infectious diseases with antibiotics successfully by yourself	Yes	164 (15.5)
	No	396 (37.4)
	Not sure	499 (47)

3. Discussion

SMA is one of the common factors which precipitate AMR, yet if effective implementations are adopted it can be easily controlled. Tracking SM behaviors of public individuals are of paramount importance since it facilitates the development of preventable measures towards this condition. Moreover, it also uncovers the weakest domains in the health system. It was on these grounds that the current nationwide survey was conducted to determine the prevalence of SMA in different Sudanese states, as well as to provide an insight into the reasons, and factors associated with SMA.

The current cross-sectional survey indicated that the prevalence of SMA among the Sudanese community was 71.3%. The reported figure lies in the middle of local and regional figures in previous studies. For instance; locally, one of the earliest and most comprehensive surveys conducted by Abdelmoneim Awad et al. in 2005 reported a prevalence of 73.1% [16], while a recent study which included Sudanese university medical students reported that antibiotics were self-medicated by 60% of the students [17]. Regionally, a meta-analysis review pooled the prevalence of SMA in Africa using 40 studies from 19 countries and the computed prevalence ranged from 50–93.8% [11]. On the other hand, another systematic review outlined the proportion of SMA in middle-eastern countries to be in the range of 12.1–93.1% [10]. Our finding points towards a higher prevalence of SMA in Sudan, unfortunately, it also emphasizes the fact that the practice of SMA in Sudan has remained consistent throughout the last 20 years.

Different reasons behind SMA were mentioned previously, such as cost saving, previous experience, and convenience which were reported repeatedly. However, less frequently, the emergence of illness, and the long delays in clinic have been reported [1,20–22]. Likewise, participants in the present study cited convenience (63.3%) and cost-saving (41%) as common reasons for SMA (Table 2). The finding is consistent with the results reported previously in Sudan, Malaysia, India, and Ethiopia [14,23–25].

The present study illustrated the common ailments for SMA. Generally, SMA to manage upper respiratory tract infections (URT) such as tonsillitis (55.5%), cough (45%), runny nose (37.8%), and nasal decongestion (33.4%) were higher than other ailments which comprise fever (31.9%), pain (29.1%), diarrhea (21.9%), and wound infection (14.9%) (Table 3). This finding is in line with previous studies conducted in Sudan, Tanzania, and India [12,21,23]. Bearing in mind that most of the URT infections are of viral origin, and antibacterial agents must be preserved only for bacterial infections which indeed requires a series of investigations and diagnoses provided by health care specialists, and considering that this pattern remains consistent in Sudan through the last 20 years with a gradual increment, health authorities in Sudan should effectively implement an antimicrobial stewardship program to optimize the utilization of antimicrobial agents.

Health services in Sudan are provided by different bodies including: government, private sectors, army, police, universities, and civil society [26]. The national health insurance fund (NHIF) is an extension of social health insurance which was introduced in 1994, the finance of NHIF is based on cost sharing (national social system based on the cooperation between the government and community) [27]. The coverage in all states is around 50% (except Khartoum = 70%), and the out of pocket share in Sudan is reported to be 70% [27,28]. Nearly one third (30.7%) of the participants from the present study were not medically insured (Table 1). Further, insurance status was significantly associated with SMA (p-value < 0.00), binary logistic regression indicated that medically non-insured participants were less likely to use antibiotics as SM in comparison to insured participants (COR: 0.656; 95% CI (0.506–0.718), (AOR: 0.645; 95% CI (0.487–0.855) (Table 4). Similar findings have been reported previously in Pakistan [12]. Additionally, 41% declared cost saving as one of the main reasons behind SMA. On the other hand, participants with secondary school and post-graduates were less likely to take SMA compared to primary school levels of education (Table 4). This pattern is not limited to this study, and it has been observed in previous studies in Lebanon, Uganda, and Malaysia [18,29,30]. However, it contradicted studies carried out in Sudan, Eritrea, and Bangladesh [16,20,31]. Such a finding is best explained by the fact that educated individuals understand the difficulties in discriminating infectious diseases and knew the consequences of SMA, therefore, they prefer to visit doctors instead of self-medicating.

Previous studies outlined that the main focus of community pharmacists in Sudan is to efficiently prescribe medications [32,33]. A considerable proportion of the participants from the present study sought antibiotics mainly from the community pharmacies (90%), and the remaining participants obtain antibiotics from leftover medication (Table 5). Previous researchers in Sudan reported a similar pattern [14,17]. This finding indicated that the gap between the actual role of the community pharmacist which is extended to include patient counseling and education is a promising area for mitigating SMA.

Additionally, more than half of the participants in this study (51.9%) thought that SMA is not an acceptable practice (Tables 5 and 6). Paradoxically, the practice of the participants diverges from rationality, when you come to know that 41% of the participants change the dosage of the antibiotics deliberately (Table 5). Moreover, the fact that a high percentage of the enrolled participants switch antibiotics harmonizes with the finding that only 37% stop taking antibiotics after dosage completions. The abovementioned malpractice is consistent with previous studies conducted in India (24%), Malaysia (41%), and Egypt (71%) that participants change the dosage of antibiotics during usage [23,24,34]. In Afghanistan, 33% of the participants stop taking antibiotics [35], while in Malaysia 35.3% of university students switch the dosage of antibiotics [24]. Given the above backdrop, it is not surprising that at the national level multi drug resistant and extensively drug-resistant isolates detected from clinical specimens are increasingly reported [7,36,37].

Participants in the current study cited amoxicillin/clavulanic acid as the most common antibiotic used as SM (32.5%), followed by amoxicillin (26.5%), azithromycin, and metronidazole (25.3%) (Table 6). Similar results were observed previously in Sudan [14,16], where azithromycin (29.9%) and amoxicillin/clavulanic (26.8%) were found to be the most common antibiotics self-medicated by university students [17]. Multiple studies in Africa and the Middle-East concluded the extensive use of beta-lactam antibiotics especially amoxicillin and amoxicillin/clavulanic as SM [10,11]. It is however, worth mentioning that earlier studies in Sudan reported amoxicillin as the most common antibiotic used in comparison to the present study and a recent study in 2022 [12,16]. This shift can be explained by the fact that patients always seek the most effective antibiotics, or it might be due to extensive promotion applied by different companies to promote their antibiotics (amoxicillin/clavulanic).

Besides accelerating antimicrobial resistance, SMA can also be associated with ADR. One-fifth (21.8%) of study participants reported that they experienced ADR (Table 6). This is slightly lower than a previous study in Malaysia (28.3%) [5]. Alarmingly, a considerable amount of the participants either switched the antibiotics or continued the antibiotic with the rate of 20.8% and 11.3%, respectively. ADRs associated with antibiotics ranged from mild side effects such as GIT symptoms to life-threatening conditions such as anaphylactic shock which is associated with a large number of antibiotics impacting patients' health as well as cost [25,38].

The finding from the present study can be partially generalized to the overall Sudanese community owing to the large and diverse sample size. However, one of the limitations of this study was the recall bias since not all participants were able to exactly remember for instance the types of antibiotics. Further, the study was subjected to selection bias, since it was conducted during the daytime in public areas, it is for this reason most of the participants were aged below 39 years old. Additionally, the questionnaire used in the present study adopted close-ended limited options which made it difficult for some respondents to express their opinions.

4. Materials and Methods

4.1. Study Design and Setting

The study adopted a cross-sectional descriptive study design, conducted in all Sudan states (all 18 states) through the period between 1 June and 15 December 2021.

4.2. Study Population

All Sudanese adult aged above 18 years old and willing to participate in the study were considered eligible.

4.3. Sample Size and Sampling Technique

According to the last census, the total population of Sudan is around 46,000,000. Using the formula below:

$$n = Z^2 p (1-p)/w^2$$

where n: sample size, Z: the critical vale (using confidence interval of 99% (Z = 2.326)), p: proportion of the target population estimated to have a particular characteristic (since there were no previous nationwide study the frequency of occurrence was assumed to be, p = 50%), (1 − p): (frequency of not occurrence of an event), w: desired margin of error tolerated (degree of precision, w = 4%). Thus, the calculated sample size was 1041 participants. We collected data from 1492 accounting for missing data. A multistage stratified sampling technique was applied to the participants. Sudan was divided into 18 states. Each state was considered a stratum, and then within each stratum, participants were selected randomly using a convenience sampling technique. Samples were collected from public places such as markets, parks, and bus stations.

4.4. Operational Definitions and Study Variables

SMA (dependent variables) was defined as the selection and use of antibiotics by participants, within the last 12 months, to manage at least one self-recognized illness or symptom without professional prescription and supervision regarding indication, dosage, and duration of treatment. Independent variables (predictors of SMA) were carefully selected based on previous studies, including: participants' gender, age, monthly income, insurance status, and educational status (all were categorical variables).

4.5. Data Collection

The current study used semi-structured questionnaires for data collection (participants who found difficulties in writing were interviewed by the trained data collectors based on the questionnaire). A comprehensive search of the literature for potential studies reporting SMA was carried out through different databases to get guidance in designing the questionnaire [20,23,24,36]. The questionnaire consisted of 25 items (provided in Supplementary Materials Table S2), which can be broadly divided into two main sections; the first section gives information regarding the demographical characteristics of the study participants, which includes gender, age, economic status, insurance status, and levels of education, while the second section starts with a main question which seeks information about any previous use of antibiotics without prescription in the last 12 months through a closed-end format (yes/no). Participants whose answer is 'yes' in the previous question were further asked to explain the main reasons and major ailment that led participants to self-medicate (multiple choice questions). It also emphasizes the practice of the participants through enquiring about the sources, selection, and adherence to antibiotic regimens (closed and close multiple choice questions). Furthermore, commonly used antibiotics and adverse drug reaction histories were also reported (closed and close multiple choice questions). For the purpose of validation, two experts in pharmacy practice were asked to highlight the main weakness of the developed questionnaire, and their comments were considered in the final version. Additionally, a pilot study was distributed to 20 individuals to confirm the clarity of the questions, the questionnaire was further validated through Cronbach alpha ($\alpha = 0.78$). Responses from the pilot study were excluded from the study. To ensure the quality of the data; data was collected only through trained fifth-year pharmacy students who were taught courses in research methodology and given a comprehensive presentation on the research topics. Furthermore, data collectors were asked to check the completeness of each questionnaire.

4.6. Data Analysis

Data were entered into a Microsoft Excel spreadsheet, coded, and exported to the statistical software package SPSS (version 25.0). Both descriptive and inferential statistics were used to analyze the data. The main parts of the questionnaire were expressed in terms of frequency and percentage. A Chi-square test was employed to study the relationship between socio-demographic factors and other variables. A binary logistic regression model was used to assess the association between prevalence SM and explanatory variables. Regardless of their *p*-value in the unadjusted analysis, all variables were included in the final multiple regression model, and the model appropriateness was tested using Hosmer and Lemeshow test. Both crude odds ratio (COR) and adjusted odds ratios (AOR) were reported with a 95% confidence interval (95% CI). Finally, a *p*-value less than 0.05 was considered significant.

4.7. Ethical Consideration

Ethical approval was obtained from the ethical committee at the University of Khartoum, Faculty of Pharmacy (FPEC-26-2021). Before conducting the study, all participants signed written informed consent after a clear explanation of the research objectives, and each participant had the right to withdraw at any time from the study. To ensure confidentiality, all questionnaires were coded and personal identifiers remained anonymous throughout the study.

5. Conclusions

Two out of three individuals in Sudan SMA mainly to manage URT ailments, this mal-practice was explained by most of the participants by it is convenience and cost-saving. Amoxicillin/clavulanic were the most commonly used antibiotics. SMA was associated with participant's level of education and insurance status. The findings from the present study indicate the necessity of activating antimicrobial stewardship programs throughout the country, as well as implementing effective legislation to prohibit dispensing antibiotics without prescription.

Supplementary Materials: The following supporting information can be downloaded at: https://www.mdpi.com/article/10.3390/antibiotics12030612/s1, Table S1: Stratification of the sample based on states; Table S2: questionnaire for data collection.

Author Contributions: Data collection A.A.B., M.M.M. and E.A.M.; conceptualization, M.A.H.; methodology, M.A.H. and B.A.Y.; software, A.O.M.; validation, M.A.H., B.A.Y. and R.E.; formal analysis, A.O.M. and O.A.A.; writing—original draft preparation, A.O.M.; writing—review and editing, M.A.H. and B.A.Y.; supervision, M.A.H., B.A.Y., W.O. and R.A.M.; funding acquisition, R.A.M. All authors have read and agreed to the published version of the manuscript.

Funding: This research was funded by King Saud University, Riyadh, Saudi Arabia, Grant number (RSP2023R119).

Institutional Review Board Statement: The study was conducted in accordance with the Declaration of Helsinki, and approved by the Institutional Review Board (or Ethics Committee) of the ethical committee at University of Khartoum, Faculty of Pharmacy (FPEC-26-2021).

Informed Consent Statement: Informed consent was obtained from all subjects involved in the study.

Data Availability Statement: Most of the relevant data are available in the main text, further data are available from the corresponding author upon reasonable request.

Acknowledgments: The authors extend their appreciation to Researchers Supporting Project number (RSP2023R119), King Saud University, Riyadh, Saudi Arabia for funding this work.

Conflicts of Interest: The authors declare no conflict of interest.

References

1. Nusair, M.B.; Al-Azzam, S.; Alhamad, H.; Momani, M.Y. The prevalence and patterns of self-medication with antibiotics in Jordan: A community-based study. *Int. J. Clin. Pract.* **2020**, *75*, e13665. [CrossRef] [PubMed]
2. World Health Organization. *Guidelines for the Regulatory Assessment of Medicinal Products for Use in Self-Medication*; World Health Organization: Geneva, Switzerland, 2000.
3. Noone, J.; Blanchette, C.M. The value of self-medication: Summary of existing evidence. *J. Med. Econ.* **2017**, *21*, 201–211. [CrossRef] [PubMed]
4. Ruiz, M.E. Risks of Self-Medication Practices. *Curr. Drug Saf.* **2010**, *5*, 315–323. [CrossRef]
5. Dadgostar, P. Antimicrobial Resistance: Implications and Costs. *Infect. Drug Resist.* **2019**, *12*, 3903–3910. [CrossRef]
6. Yin, X.; Mu, K.; Yang, H.; Wang, J.; Chen, Z.; Jiang, N.; Yang, F.; Zhang, G.; Wu, J. Prevalence of self-medication with antibiotics and its related factors among Chinese residents: A cross-sectional study. *Antimicrob. Resist. Infect. Control* **2021**, *10*, 89. [CrossRef]
7. Irfan, M.; Almotiri, A.; AlZeyadi, Z.A. Antimicrobial Resistance and Its Drivers—A Review. *Antibiotics* **2022**, *11*, 1362. [CrossRef] [PubMed]

8. Torres, N.F.; Chibi, B.; Kuupiel, D.; Solomon, V.P.; Mashamba-Thompson, T.P.; Middleton, L.E. The use of non-prescribed antibiotics; prevalence estimates in low-and-middle-income countries. A systematic review and meta-analysis. *Arch. Public Health* **2021**, *79*, 1–15. [CrossRef] [PubMed]
9. World Health Organization. *Antimicrobial Resistance: Global Report on Surveillance*; World Health Organization: Geneva, Switzerland, 2014.
10. Alhomoud, F.; Aljamea, Z.; Almahasnah, R.; Alkhalifah, K.; Basalelah, L.; Alhomoud, F.K. Self-medication and self-prescription with antibiotics in the Middle East—Do they really happen? A systematic review of the prevalence, possible reasons, and outcomes. *Int. J. Infect. Dis.* **2017**, *57*, 3–12. [CrossRef]
11. Yeika, E.V.; Ingelbeen, B.; Kemah, B.L.; Wirsiy, F.S.; Fomengia, J.N.; Van der Sande, M.A. Comparative assessment of the prevalence, practices and factors associated with self-medication with antibiotics in Africa. *Trop. Med. Int. Health* **2021**, *26*, 862–881. [CrossRef] [PubMed]
12. Awad, A.I.; Eltayeb, I.B. Self-Medication Practices with Antibiotics and Antimalarials Among Sudanese Undergraduate University Students. *Ann. Pharmacother.* **2007**, *41*, 1249–1255. [CrossRef] [PubMed]
13. Awad, A.I.; Eltayeb, I.B.; Capps, P.A. Self-medication practices in Khartoum State, Sudan. *Eur. J. Clin. Pharmacol.* **2006**, *62*, 317–324. [CrossRef] [PubMed]
14. Elhada, A.; Eltayeb, I.B.; Mudawi, M.M. Pattern of self-medication with antibiotics in Khartoum State, Sudan. *World J. Pharm. Res.* **2014**, *3*, 678–692.
15. Abdelrahman Hussain, M.; Osman Mohamed, A.; Sandel Abkar, A.; Siddig Mohamed, F.; Khider Elzubair, H. Knowledge, Attitude and Practice of Community Pharmacists in Relation to Dispensing Antibiotics Without Prescription in Sudan: A Cross-sectional Study. *Integr. Pharm. Res. Pract.* **2022**, *11*, 107–116. [CrossRef]
16. Awad, A.; Eltayeb, I.; Matowe, L.; Thalib, L. Self-medication with antibiotics and antimalarials in the community of Khartoum State, Sudan. *J. Pharm. Pharm. Sci.* **2005**, *8*, 326–331. [PubMed]
17. Elmahi, O.K.O.; Musa, R.A.E.; Shareef, A.A.H.; Omer, M.E.A.; Elmahi, M.A.M.; Altamih, R.A.A.; Mohamed, R.I.H.; Alsadig, T.F.M. Perception and practice of self-medication with antibiotics among medical students in Sudanese universities: A cross-sectional study. *PLoS ONE* **2022**, *17*, e0263067. [CrossRef] [PubMed]
18. Ocan, M.; Bwanga, F.; Bbosa, G.S.; Bagenda, D.; Waako, P.; Ogwal-Okeng, J.; Obua, C. Patterns and Predictors of Self-Medication in Northern Uganda. *PLoS ONE* **2014**, *9*, e92323. [CrossRef]
19. Oleim, S.H.; Noor, S.K.; Bushara, S.O.; Ahmed, M.H.; Elmadhoun, W. The Irrational Use of Antibiotics Among Doctors, Pharmacists and the Public in River Nile State, Sudan. *Sudan J. Med. Sci.* **2019**, *14*, 276–288. [CrossRef]
20. Ateshim, Y.; Bereket, B.; Major, F.; Emun, Y.; Woldai, B.; Pasha, I.; Habte, E.; Russom, M. Prevalence of self-medication with antibiotics and associated factors in the community of Asmara, Eritrea: A descriptive cross sectional survey. *BMC Public Health* **2019**, *19*, 726. [CrossRef] [PubMed]
21. Horumpende, P.G.; Said, S.H.; Mazuguni, F.S.; Antony, M.L.; Kumburu, H.H.; Sonda, T.B.; Mwanziva, C.E.; Mshana, S.E.; Mmbaga, B.T.; Kajeguka, D.C.; et al. Prevalence, determinants and knowledge of antibacterial self-medication: A cross sectional study in North-eastern Tanzania. *PLoS ONE* **2018**, *13*, e0206623. [CrossRef] [PubMed]
22. Abduelkarem, A.R.; Othman, A.M.; Abuelkhair, Z.R.; Ghazal, M.M.; Alzouobi, S.B.; El Zowalaty, M. Prevalence Of Self-Medication With Antibiotics Among Residents In United Arab Emirates. *Infect. Drug Resist.* **2019**, *12*, 3445–3453. [CrossRef] [PubMed]
23. Rajendran, A.; Kulirankal, K.G.; Rakesh, P.; George, S. Prevalence and pattern of antibiotic self-medication practice in an urban population of Kerala, India: A cross-sectional study. *Indian J. Community Med.* **2019**, *44* (Suppl. S1), S42.
24. Haque, M.; Rahman, N.A.A.; McKimm, J.; Kibria, G.M.; Majumder, M.A.A.; Haque, S.Z.; Islam, M.Z.; Binti Abdullah, S.L.; Daher, A.M.; Zulkifli, Z.; et al. Self-medication of antibiotics: Investigating practice among university students at the Malaysian National Defence University. *Infect. Drug Resist.* **2019**, *12*, 1333. [CrossRef] [PubMed]
25. Ferreira, J.; Placido, A.I.; Afreixo, V.; Ribeiro-Vaz, I.; Roque, F.; Herdeiro, M.T. Descriptive Analysis of Adverse Drug Reactions Reports of the Most Consumed Antibiotics in Portugal, Prescribed for Upper Airway Infections. *Antibiotics* **2022**, *11*, 477. [CrossRef]
26. Mousnad, M.A.; Shafie, A.A.; Ibrahim, M.I.M. Determination of the main factors contributing to increases in medicine expenditures for the National Health Insurance Fund in Sudan. *J. Pharm. Health Serv. Res.* **2013**, *4*, 159–164. [CrossRef]
27. Babiker, M.; Habbani, K.; Kheir, S.; Awad, M. Pros and cons of national health insurance fund in Sudan: A critical review. *J. Qual. Healthc. Econ.* **2021**, *4*, 000241.
28. Salim, A.M.A.; Hamed, F.H.M. Exploring health insurance services in Sudan from the perspectives of insurers. *SAGE Open Med.* **2018**, *6*, 1–10. [CrossRef] [PubMed]
29. Aslam, A.; Zin, C.S.; Ab Rahman, N.S.; Gajdács, M.; Ahmed, S.I.; Jamshed, S. Self-Medication Practices with Antibiotics and Associated Factors among the Public of Malaysia: A Cross-Sectional Study. *Drug Health Patient Saf.* **2021**, *13*, 171–181. [CrossRef]
30. Jamhour, A.; El-Kheir, A.; Salameh, P.; Hanna, P.A.; Mansour, H. Antibiotic knowledge and self-medication practices in a developing country: A cross-sectional study. *Am. J. Infect. Control* **2017**, *45*, 384–388. [CrossRef] [PubMed]
31. Saha, A.; Marma, K.K.S.; Rashid, A.; Tarannum, N.; Das, S.; Chowdhury, T.; Afrin, N.; Chakraborty, P.; Emran, M.; Mehedi, H.M.H.; et al. Risk factors associated with self-medication among the indigenous communities of Chittagong Hill Tracts, Bangladesh. *PLoS ONE* **2022**, *17*, e0269622. [CrossRef]

32. Mohamed, S.S.; Mahmoud, A.A.; Ali, A.A. The role of Sudanese community pharmacists in patients' self-care. *Pharm. Weekbl.* **2014**, *36*, 412–419. [CrossRef] [PubMed]
33. Ibrahim, A.; Scott, J. Community pharmacists in Khartoum State, Sudan: Their current roles and perspectives on pharmaceutical care implementation. *Int. J. Clin. Pharm.* **2013**, *35*, 236–243. [CrossRef] [PubMed]
34. Elden, N.M.K.; Nasser, H.A.; Alli, A.; Mahmoud, N.; Shawky, M.A.; Ibrahim, A.A.E.A.; Fahmy, A.K. Risk Factors of Antibiotics Self-medication Practices among University Students in Cairo, Egypt. *Open Access Maced. J. Med. Sci.* **2020**, *8*, 7–12. [CrossRef]
35. Roien, R.; Bhandari, D.; Hosseini, S.M.R.; Mosawi, S.H.; Ataie, M.A.; Ozaki, A.; Martellucci, C.A.; Kotera, Y.; Delshad, M.H.; Sawano, T.; et al. Prevalence and determinants of self-medication with antibiotics among general population in Afghanistan. *Expert Rev. Anti-Infect. Ther.* **2021**, *20*, 315–321. [CrossRef] [PubMed]
36. Moglad, E.H. Antibiotics Profile, Prevalence of Extended-Spectrum Beta-Lactamase (ESBL), and Multidrug-Resistant Enterobacteriaceae from Different Clinical Samples in Khartoum State, Sudan. *Int. J. Microbiol.* **2020**, *2020*, 8898430. [CrossRef]
37. Ibrahim, M.E.; Bilal, N.E.; Hamid, M. Increased multi-drug resistant Escherichia coli from hospitals in Khartoum state, Sudan. *Afr. Health Sci.* **2013**, *12*, 368–375. [CrossRef] [PubMed]
38. Roger, J.Y.; Krantz, M.S.; Phillips, E.J.; Stone, C.A., Jr. Emerging causes of drug-induced anaphylaxis: A review of anaphylaxis-associated reports in the FDA Adverse Event Reporting System (FAERS). *J. Allergy Clin. Immunol. Pract.* **2021**, *9*, 819–829.e2.

Disclaimer/Publisher's Note: The statements, opinions and data contained in all publications are solely those of the individual author(s) and contributor(s) and not of MDPI and/or the editor(s). MDPI and/or the editor(s) disclaim responsibility for any injury to people or property resulting from any ideas, methods, instructions or products referred to in the content.

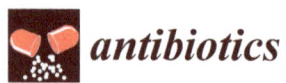

Article

Effects of a Primary Care Antimicrobial Stewardship Program on Meticillin-Resistant *Staphylococcus aureus* Strains across a Region of Catalunya (Spain) over 5 Years

Alfredo Jover-Sáenz [1,*], María Ramírez-Hidalgo [1], Alba Bellés Bellés [2], Esther Ribes Murillo [3], Meritxell Batlle Bosch [4], Anna Ribé Miró [4], Alba Mari López [5], José Cayado Cabanillas [5], Neus Piqué Palacín [5], Sònia Garrido-Calvo [6], Mireia Ortiz Valls [6], María Isabel Gracia Vilas [7], Laura Gros Navés [8], María Jesús Javierre Caudevilla [9], Lidia Montull Navarro [10], Cecilia Bañeres Argiles [10], Pilar Vaqué Castilla [11], José Javier Ichart Tomás [12], Mireia Saura Codina [12], Ester Andreu Mayor [13], Roser Martorell Solé [14], Ana Vena Martínez [15], José Manuel Albalad Samper [16], Susana Cano Marrón [17], Cristina Soler Elcacho [17], Andrés Rodríguez Garrocho [17], Gemma Terrer Manrique [17], Antoni Solé Curcó [18], David de la Rica Escuin [19], María José Estadella Servalls [20], Ana M. Figueres Farreny [21], Luís Miguel Montaña Esteban [22], Lidia Sanz Borrell [22], Arancha Morales Valle [23], Mercè Pallerola Planes [24], Aly Hamadi [24], Francesc Pujol Aymerich [25], Francisca Toribio Redondo [26], María Cruz Urgelés Castillón [27], Juan Valgañon Palacios [28], Marc Olivart Parejo [29], Joan Torres-Puig-gros [30], the P-ILEHRDA Group [†] and on behalf of Clinical Microbiology and Antibiotic Resistance Group -IRBLleida- [†]

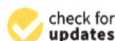

Citation: Jover-Sáenz, A.; Ramírez-Hidalgo, M.; Bellés Bellés, A.B.; Ribes Murillo, E.; Batlle Bosch, M.; Ribé Miró, A.; Mari López, A.; Cayado Cabanillas, J.; Piqué Palacín, N.; Garrido-Calvo, S.; et al. Effects of a Primary Care Antimicrobial Stewardship Program on Meticillin-Resistant *Staphylococcus aureus* Strains across a Region of Catalunya (Spain) over 5 Years. *Antibiotics* **2024**, *13*, 92. https://doi.org/10.3390/antibiotics13010092

Academic Editors: Juan Manuel Vázquez-Lago, Ana Estany-Gestal and Angel Salgado-Barreira

Received: 20 December 2023
Revised: 8 January 2024
Accepted: 15 January 2024
Published: 18 January 2024

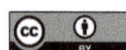

Copyright: © 2024 by the authors. Licensee MDPI, Basel, Switzerland. This article is an open access article distributed under the terms and conditions of the Creative Commons Attribution (CC BY) license (https://creativecommons.org/licenses/by/4.0/).

[1] Unidad Territorial Infección Nosocomial (UTIN), Hospital Universitari Arnau de Vilanova de Lleida (HUAV), 25198 Lleida, Spain; mframirez.lleida.ics@gencat.cat
[2] Sección de Microbiología, Hospital Universitari Arnau de Vilanova de Lleida (HUAV), 25198 Lleida, Spain; abelles.lleida.ics@gencat.cat
[3] Unidad de Farmacia de Atención Primaria, Institut Català de la Salut (ICS), 25007 Lleida, Spain; eribes.lleida.ics@gencat.cat
[4] Equipo de Atención Priamaria (EAP) Les Borges Blanques, 25400 Lleida, Spain; mbatlle.lleida.ics@gencat.cat (M.B.B.); aribem.lleida.ics@gencat.cat (A.R.M.)
[5] EAP Pla d'Urgell, 25001 Lleida, Spain; amari.lleida.ics@gencat.cat (A.M.L.); jcayado.lleida.ics@gencat.cat (J.C.C.); npique.lleida.ics@gencat.cat (N.P.P.)
[6] EAP Balàfia-Pardinyes, 25005 Lleida, Spain; sgarrido.lleida.ics@gencat.cat (S.G.-C.); mortiz.lleida.ics@gencat.cat (M.O.V.)
[7] EAP Rambla de Ferran, 25007 Lleida, Spain; mgracia.lleida.ics@gencat.cat
[8] EAP Lleida Rural Nord, 25110 Lleida, Spain; lgros@gss.cat
[9] Centre Penitenciari de Ponent, 25199 Lleida, Spain; jjavierrec@gencat.cat
[10] EAP Eixample, 25006 Lleida, Spain; lmontull.lleida.ics@gencat.cat (L.M.N.); cbaneres.lleida.ics@gencat.cat (C.B.A.)
[11] EAP Primer de Maig, 25002 Lleida, Spain; pvaque.lleida.ics@gencat.cat
[12] Servicio de Urgencias, Hospital Universitari Arnau de Vilanova de Lleida (HUAV), 25198 Lleida, Spain; jxichart.lleida.ics@gencat.cat (J.J.I.T.); msaura.lleida.ics@gencat.cat (M.S.C.)
[13] Col·legi Oficial de Podòlegs, 25001 Lleida, Spain; eandreu.lleida.ics@gencat.cat
[14] EAP Cervera, 25200 Lleida, Spain; rmartorell.lleida.ics@gencat.cat
[15] Servei de Geriatria, Hospital Universitari Santa Maria, 25198 Lleida, Spain; anav@gss.cat
[16] EAP Ponts, 25740 Lleida, Spain; jalbalad.lleida.ics@gencat.cat
[17] EAP Onze de Setembre, 25005 Lleida, Spain; scano.lleida.ics@gencat.cat (S.C.M.); csoler.lleida.ics@gencat.cat (C.S.E.); arodriguezg.lleida.ics@gencat.cat (A.R.G.); gterrer.lleida.ics@gencat.cat (G.T.M.)
[18] EAP Bellpuig, 25250 Lleida, Spain; ajsole.lleida.ics@gencat.cat
[19] EAP Artesa de Segre, 25730 Lleida, Spain; drica.lleida.ics@gencat.cat
[20] EAP Cappont, 25001 Lleida, Spain; mjestadella.lleida.ics@gencat.cat
[21] EAP Almacelles, 25100 Lleida, Spain; afigueres.lleida.ics@gencat.cat
[22] EAP Seròs, 25183 Lleida, Spain; lmontana.lleida.ics@gencat.cat (L.M.M.E.); lsanz.lleida.ics@gencat.cat (L.S.B.)
[23] EAP Lleida Rural Sud, 25171 Lleida, Spain; amorales.lleida.ics@gencat.cat
[24] EAP Balaguer, 25600 Lleida, Spain; mpallerola.lleida.ics@gencat.cat (M.P.P.); ahamadi.lleida.ics@gencat.cat (A.H.)
[25] EAP Alcarràs, 25180 Lleida, Spain; fpujol.lleida.ics@gencat.cat
[26] EAP Alfarràs-Almenar, 25120 Lleida, Spain; ftoribio.lleida.ics@gencat.cat
[27] EAP Bordeta-Magraners, 25001 Lleida, Spain; curgeles.lleida.ics@gencat.cat

[28] EAP La Granadella, 25177 Lleida, Spain; jvalganon.lleida.ics@gencat.cat
[29] EAP Tàrrega, 25300 Lleida, Spain; molivart.lleida.ics@gencat.cat
[30] Departament de Salut Pública, Universitat de Lleida (UdL), 25006 Lleida, Spain; joan.torres1958@gmail.com
* Correspondence: ajover.lleida.ics@gencat.cat; Tel.: +34-647-488-911; Fax: +34-973-248-154
† P-ILEHRDA and Clinical Microbiology and Antibiotic Resistance Groups are listed in the Acknowledgment section.

Abstract: Primary care antimicrobial stewardship program (ASP) interventions can reduce the overprescription of unnecessary antibiotics, but the impact on the reduction in bacterial resistance is less known, and there is a lack of available data. We implemented a prolonged educational counseling ASP in a large regional outpatient setting to assess its feasibility and effectiveness. Over a 5-year post-implementation period, which was compared to a pre-intervention period, a significant reduction in antibiotic prescriptions occurred, particularly those associated with greater harmful effects and resistance selection. There was also a decrease in methicillin-resistant *Staphylococcus aureus* (MRSA) strains and in their co-resistance to other antibiotics, particularly those with an ecological impact.

Keywords: antimicrobial stewardship; use antimicrobials; multidrug-resistant microorganisms; community-onset; epidemiology; MRSA

1. Introduction

Staphylococcus aureus is a microorganism recognized for being both a commensal and an opportunistic pathogen in humans and animals [1]. The methicillin-resistant *Staphylococcus aureus* (MRSA) strain has become a relevant lineage, with a continuously increasing prevalence in hospitals, communities, and livestock environments that poses a threat to public health. Moreover, the high pathogenicity of MRSA, which is attributable to various virulence factors, such as SCCmec acquired through genetic transfer from the mecA gene, as well as antibiotic resistance, compromises host immunity, making it responsible for causing severe infections in both humans and animals [2].

Traditionally, MRSA has been considered one of the primary multidrug-resistant pathogens causing healthcare-associated infections (HA-MRSA), and it has reached endemic proportions in many countries. It has become a leading cause and potentially fatal agent of invasive infections, skin and soft tissue infections, and pneumonia [3]. In the United States, the estimated annual cost of these infections is around USD 2.7 million, with a significant loss of lives that amounts to 20,000 deaths per year [4,5]. Alarmingly, its aggressive nature has extended to the community setting in the last two decades, where it is known as community-acquired MRSA (CA-MRSA), with greater pathogenicity and transmissibility affecting both young and healthy individuals [6]. In this context, the level of colonization in the general population can increase in environments with a high presence of livestock animals, as observed in Catalonia, Spain, where 75.6% of pig industry workers are colonized by MRSA, particularly with the ST398 strain [7].

Strategies to prevent acquisition rely not only on controlling the spread of clones and horizontal gene transfer, but also on reducing antibiotic pressure in the environment. There is a clear association between the volume of antibiotic prescriptions and the presence of multidrug-resistant microorganisms (MDR) [8,9]. This prevalence may be even higher when broad-spectrum antibiotics are used. Recent epidemiological studies conducted in our country showed a consistently high prevalence of MRSA in the community, exceeding 10% over the last decade [10]. Unfortunately, despite this, it is not only the antibiotic prescription rates in Spanish primary care that are high; the level of use of broad-spectrum antimicrobials remains two to three times higher than that observed in most European countries [11].

Several meta-analyses have demonstrated a direct relationship between exposure to certain antimicrobial classes and microbiological resistance [12]. Cephalosporins and beta-lactams combined with beta-lactamase inhibitors are potential selectors of resistant strains, but fluoroquinolones (FQ) are the most concerning and dangerous antibiotics [13,14]. Recent guidelines from the Infectious Diseases Society of America (IDSA) recommend reserving their use to protect the ecosystem from MDR and harm [15].

Antimicrobial Stewardship Programs (ASPs) play a crucial role in reducing emergencies and the transmission of resistant pathogens through the advice they provide in prescription practices. The implementation of ASP actions and the data of long-term outcomes in the community are limited [16–18]. Previous work by our group from 2017 to 2021 showed a pronounced decrease in the incidence densities (ID) of multidrug-resistant enterobacteriaceae, such as *Escherichia coli* ESBL-producing strains, after a period of ASP intervention [19]. During this intervention, there was a marked reduction in antimicrobial consumption. The program followed a non-mandatory educational advisory model, focusing on the overall reduction in third-generation cephalosporins, amoxicillin-clavulanic acid (co-amoxclav), azithromycin, and clindamycin use, with a specific emphasis on FQ. This prompted us to investigate whether a similar trend existed for MRSA and *Clostridioides difficile*, which also indicated prescription quality.

In this study, we evaluate our hypothesis regarding the change in community-associated MRSA incidence by following the prescriptive modification of these antimicrobials through an ASP in primary care over a 5-year period.

2. Materials and Methods

2.1. Design, Setting, and Study Periods

This quasi-experimental before-and-after comparison study was conducted in the Lleida region, which is part of the public healthcare network of Catalonia (CatSalut), Spain, during the period from January 2014 to December 2021, with an interventionist approach starting in January 2017 (5 years). The general practitioners and pediatricians in the region served a reference population of 340,000 inhabitants across 23 primary care centers in direct coordination with a regional microbiology laboratory and a level III referral hospital.

In 2016, the Infection and Antibiotic Policy Territorial Commission, consisting of professionals from various specialties, groups, and administrations, launched a specific ASP for the community [20], as part of a larger regional translational program (P-ILEHRDA) that already encompassed other settings such as acute hospitals, long-term care facilities, and geriatric residences. The program design was based on the consensus document on ASPs published by the Spanish Society of Infectious Diseases and Clinical Microbiology (SEIMC), adapted to the territorial characteristics [21]. Administrative recognition from the management was obtained for its implementation.

The ASP implementation relied on interdisciplinary and multidisciplinary actions from professionals, including operational teams in each primary care center composed of at least a general practitioner, a nurse, and a pediatrician. Additionally, a coordinating technical team included general practitioners, hospital infectious disease specialists, pediatricians, microbiologists, primary care pharmacists, community pharmacists, geriatricians, emergency physicians, podiatrists, and dentists. The clinical references were selected based on their interest, knowledge, experience, analytical skills, relationship with the teams, and proficiency in providing training.

The program encompassed the following educational and training actions: (1) Periodic development and updating of regional diagnostic and antibiotic treatment protocols for the most prevalent infections (urinary tract, respiratory, skin and soft tissue, and odontogenic infections), based on scientific evidence; (2) the creation of a free-download APP (ProAPP Lleida) for access to this documentation, which was also available on the institution's intranet; (3) regular general and specific structured training, both in-person and online, for professionals through the courses, sessions, workshops, or seminars; (4) daily review by operational teams of all the positive microbiological results from the centers and weekly review of prescriptions for the study's specific antibiotics, except on weekends and holidays; (5) daily non-mandatory virtual written educational advice on computerized SAP "Systems, Applications, Products in Data Processing" or E-cap "Primary Care Clinical Station" and direct personalized advice, in-person or by telephone, to prescribing medical professionals. The advice emphasized the appropriateness of empirical treatments, treatments tailored to microbiological results, dose adjustments, therapeutic de-escalation, shortened duration of treatment, presence of toxicity, or interactions; (6) preparation of monitoring reports on consumption, incidence density of multidrug-resistant microorganisms, and local microbiological sensitivity for annual comparative evaluation between the centers and feedback to the teams. The actions were not contingent on extra remuneration for professionals. The work and action diagram has been described in previous publications [19].

No restrictive prescription measures were implemented in any of the study periods. The typology of recommendations was prospectively collected to assess the incidence over time. The advisories were only discontinued in 2020 due to the onset of the SARS-CoV-2 pandemic.

2.2. Sources of Information

The information on community prescription and microbiological resistance was obtained from the regional dispensing data and the databases of an integrated departmental management program, respectively. For the temporal analysis, the updated semiannual number of inhabitants with a health card was collected.

2.3. Measurement of Consumption and Microbiological Impact Outcomes

The primary outcome of the study was the change in the overall consumption of antimicrobials in the community, specifically non-recommended antimicrobials (NRA), due to a higher risk of resistance or a high spectrum index (HSI). These included FQ, cephalosporins, co-amoxiclav, clindamycin, and azithromycin, which were analyzed every semester during the intervention period from 2017 to 2021 and compared to a previous reference period.

The secondary outcome focused on the trend in the evolution of *S. aureus*, both methicillin-sensitive (MSSA) and methicillin-resistant (MRSA), and their resistance to levofloxacin, clindamycin, and erythromycin.

A third input considered in the study was the presence of cases of pathological diarrhea caused by *C. difficile* in the community, whether requiring hospital admission or not; this was attributed to the outcomes of the ASP.

2.4. Evaluation Methods

The calculation of antimicrobial pharmaceutical consumption utilized the methodology of the Anatomical Therapeutic Chemical Classification System and Defined Daily Doses (ATC/DDDs) established by the World Health Organization (WHO), which was revised in 2023 (http://www.whocc.no/atc_ddd_index/) (accessed on 26 September 2023). The consumption was expressed as the number per 1000 inhabitants per day over the study population with a health card (DID). Defined Daily Doses (DDDs) represent the average maintenance doses per day for the antibiotic used in its first indication.

The evolutionary impact on resistances was assessed by calculating the ID per 1000 inhabitants per day for the mentioned microorganisms, semiannually; this assessment was similar to that for the antimicrobial consumption. Only one culture per person and semester was considered for the calculation. It was assumed that there would be a 6-month delay between the intervention, implementation, and any associated changes in resistance, as suggested in some articles [22]. Therefore, the temporal analysis of resistances extended for an additional 6 months beyond the study period. The resistance percentage was identified as resistant samples among the total antibiograms performed. The standard international criteria proposed by Magiorakos et al. [23] were used for defining bacterial multidrug resistance. The identification of new cases, based on a single clinical sample, was provided by the Regional Microbiology Section, which determined antibiotic resistance by following the recommendations of the European Committee on Antimicrobial Susceptibility Testing (EUCAST) [24].

While *C. difficile* is not considered an MDR, it is included in national and European surveillance due to its clinical–epidemiological significance. The definitions recently issued by the European Society of Clinical Microbiology and Infectious Diseases [25] were used for the calculations and case identification.

2.5. Statistical Analysis

The continuous quantitative variables were expressed as mean ± standard deviation (SD), while the categorical quantitative variables were presented as frequencies and percentages (%). The graphical representations of the antibiotic consumption and resistance evolution were created using line histograms, highlighting the cut-off point between the pre- and post-intervention periods. The main measure of association used was the relative risk (RR) or relative change between incidence densities. For the resistance measured in the rates, the odds ratio (OR) was employed. To assess the impact in absolute terms (in ID), attributable risk (absolute effect) was used, and in relative terms, the preventable fraction (relative effect) in the intervention was used and was expressed as a percentage. The analysis of the attributable effects of intervention was calculated by comparing the pre- and post-intervention periods at three cut-off points: the beginning, the middle, and the end of the intervention period. The temporal trend in each period, pre- and post-intervention, was analyzed using the chi-square test. Changes in quantitative variables such as ID were analyzed using the Student–Fisher *t*-test and one-way ANOVA. All the estimates were accompanied by the corresponding 95% confidence interval (CI). The accepted confidence level was $p < 0.05$, and the statistical package used was EPIDAT (version 3.1) from the Pan American Health Organization.

3. Results

During the study period (2014 to 2021), a total of 11,814,508 DDDs of oral antimicrobials were dispensed; they were prescribed by 349 primary care consultants (312 general practitioners and 37 pediatricians) in the Lleida health region. The average semiannual post-intervention population consisted of 342,086 inhabitants, compared to 335,046 inhabitants in the pre-intervention period (2014 to 2016).

Between 2017 and 2021, a total of 6856 interventions were conducted, including 1636 (23.9%) educational advisories related to positive microbiological samples for *S. aureus*; these were primarily cutaneous. There was an average annual trend of 36.6% growth in interventions, interrupted only in 2020 due to the SARS-CoV-2 pandemic. Antibiotic modification or suspension in advisory sessions was present in 1059 cases (64.7%).

3.1. Impact on Antibiotic Consumption

Throughout the entire study period, penicillin was the most prescribed antibiotic, accounting for 66.0% of the prescriptions. The studied NRA (co-amoxiclav, cephalosporins, FQ, azithromycin, and clindamycin) constituted 46.6% of the total antibiotics used. The temporal evolution in DID of the global prescription of any antimicrobial, including the NRA, in any period, is shown in Figure 1. The community's overall use of antibacterials in DID decreased by 33.7% between 2017 and 2021, with the average DID between the periods experiencing a drop of −0.095 (0.325), with a standard deviation (SD) ($p < 0.0001$). Similarly, the NRA group also exhibited a significant decrease of 37.6%, declining from 1.476 (0.131) in 2014–2016 to 1.047 (0.287) in 2017–2021 (mean difference −0.432, [95% CI −0.163 to −0.701], $p = 0.004$). The semester changes in the consumption of beta-lactamase inhibitors, FQ, and cephalosporins per DID, in the pre- and post-intervention periods in the health region, are described in Figure 2.

Table 1 shows the significant reductions in the specific antibiotics used for Gram-positive infections at three points (initial, middle, and final periods) and their final impact: FQ, cephalosporins, co-amoxiclav, azithromycin, and clindamycin. Before the intervention, a significant decreasing trend in the dispensing of FQ and co-amoxiclav was observed. However, this decrease persisted in the post-intervention period, but a statistically significant early and drastic reduction occurred from the third semester of ASP implementation. The average drops in DID per semester for these ANR were −0.064 (0.173) and, specifically, −0.023 (0.137) for co-amoxiclav, −0.023 (0.030) for FQ, and −0.004 (0.014) for cephalosporins ($p < 0.001$). A similar inflection point occurred in the sixth semester for azithromycin −0.017 (0.041) and clindamycin −0.001 (0.004) ($p < 0.001$), and this decline, along with other ANR, persisted until the end of the period.

Table 1. Changes in antimicrobial prescription (ATC codes J01 and specific antimicrobials) before and after ASP intervention at 3 points (initial, middle, and final periods) and overall impact.

Prescribed Antibiotic	DID Pre-Intervention Period	Relative Change First Semester 2017 (95% CI)	Relative Change First Semester 2019 (95% CI)	Relative Change Second Semester 2021 (95% CI)	Absolute Effect Post-Intervention Period	Relative Effect (%)
Total antibiotics (J01)	2.496	0.892 (0.890 to 0.894)	0.790 (0.787 to 0.781)	0.670 (0.668 to 0.672)	−0.688 (−0.691 to −0.685)	27.57 (27.65 to 27.49)
Total antibiotics not recommended (ANR)	1.476	0.989 (0.987 to 0.992)	0.796 (0.793 to 0.797)	0.581 (0.579 to 0.583)	−0.079 (−0.079 to −0.079)	37.57 (37.48 to 37.66)
Co-amoxclav (J01CR02)	0.704	0.940 (0.938 to 0.943)	0.821 (0.819 to 0.824)	0.659 (0.657 to 0.662)	−0.250 (−0.251 to −0.249)	35.59 (35.50 to 35.68)
Quinolones (J01M)	0.311	0.903 (0.897 to 0.908)	0.588 (0.584 to 0.593)	0.328 (0.325 to 0.331)	−0.294 (−0.295 to −0.294)	94.74 (94.72 to 94.75)
Ciprofloxacin (J01MA02)	0.114	0.779 (0.770 to 0.788)	0.556 (0.549 to 0.564)	0.439 (0.433 to 0.446)	−0.052 (−0.052 to −0.051)	45.39 (45.07 to 45.70)
Levofloxacin (J01MA12)	0.132	1.055 (1.046 to 1.065)	0.730 (0.722 to 0.738)	0.338 (0.332 to 0.344)	−0.065 (−0.065 to 0.064)	49.18 (48.93 to 49.44)
Cephalosporins (J01D)	0.111	1.115 (1.104 to 1.126)	0.785 (0.776 to 0.794)	0.807 (0.798 to 0.816)	−0.025 (−0.026 to −0.025)	22.99 (22.61 to 23.38)
Cefuroxime (J01DC02)	0.061	0.739 (0.726 to 0.751)	0.614 (0.603 to 0.625)	0.433 (0.424 to 0.442)	−0.025 (−0.025 to −0.025)	40.96 (40.50 to 41.41)
Third-generation cephalosporins (J01DD)	0.046	1.223 (1.204 to 1.242)	0.967 (0.971 to 1.004)	1.275 (1.256 to 1.294)	0.001 (0.001 to 0.001)	2.32 (1.57 to 3.07)
Azithromycin (J01FA10)	0.152	1.204 (1.194 to 1.213)	1.119 (1.110 to 1.128)	0.533 (0.527 to 0.539)	−0.042 (−0.043 to −0.041)	27.67 (27.36 to 27.98)
Clindamycin (J01FF01)	0.021	0.771 (0.750 to 0.793)	0.720 (0.699 to 0.741)	0.846 (0.824 to 0.869)	−0.004 (−0.005 to −0.004)	21.57 (20.61 to 22.51)
Total recommended antibiotics (RA)	0.969	1.032 (1.028 to 1.035)	1.146 (1.143 to 1.150)	0.748 (0.746 to 0.751)	−0.052 (−0.052 to −0.051)	21.29 (21.17 to 22.42)
Amoxicillin (J01CA04)	0.925	1.028 (1.027 to 1.029)	1.081 (1.081 to 1.082)	0.711 (0.709 to 0.712)	−0.218 (−0.218 to −0.217)	23.53 (23.48 to 23.59)
Cloxacillin (J01CF02)	0.018	1.018 (0.991 to 1.046)	1.032 (1.005 to 1.060)	0.722 (0.700 to 0.745)	−0.004 (−0.005 to −0.004)	25.17 (24.18 to 26.15)
Cefadroxil (J01DB05)	0.001	1.652 (1.418 to 1.924)	2.702 (2.380 to 3.066)	8.835 (8.066 to 9.678)	0.002 (0.002 to 0.002)	84.02 (82.80 to 85.14)
Cotrimoxazole (J01EE01)	0.027	1.158 (1.134 to 1.182)	1.416 (1.390 to 1.443)	1.956 (1.924 to 1.988)	0.014 (0.013 to 0.014)	33.89 (33.26 to 34.52)

ATC; Anatomical Therapeutic Chemical. DID; defined daily doses per 1000 inhabitants per day. NRA; non-recommended antibiotics (co-amoxiclav, quinolones, cephalosporins, azithromycin, and clindamycin). RA; recommended antibiotics (amoxicillin, cloxacillin, cefadroxil, and cotrimoxazole).

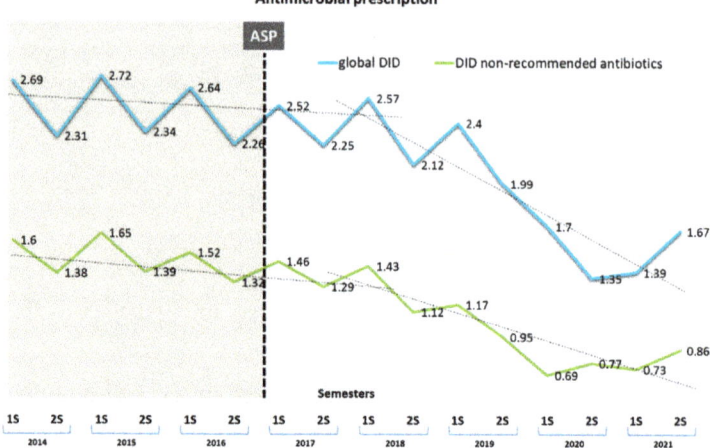

Figure 1. Semestral evolution of defined daily doses per 1000 inhabitants/day (DID). Global antimicrobial prescription (upper line) and non-recommended antimicrobials (NRA) (lower line). Shaded area represents the pre-antibiotic stewardship program (ASP) intervention period.

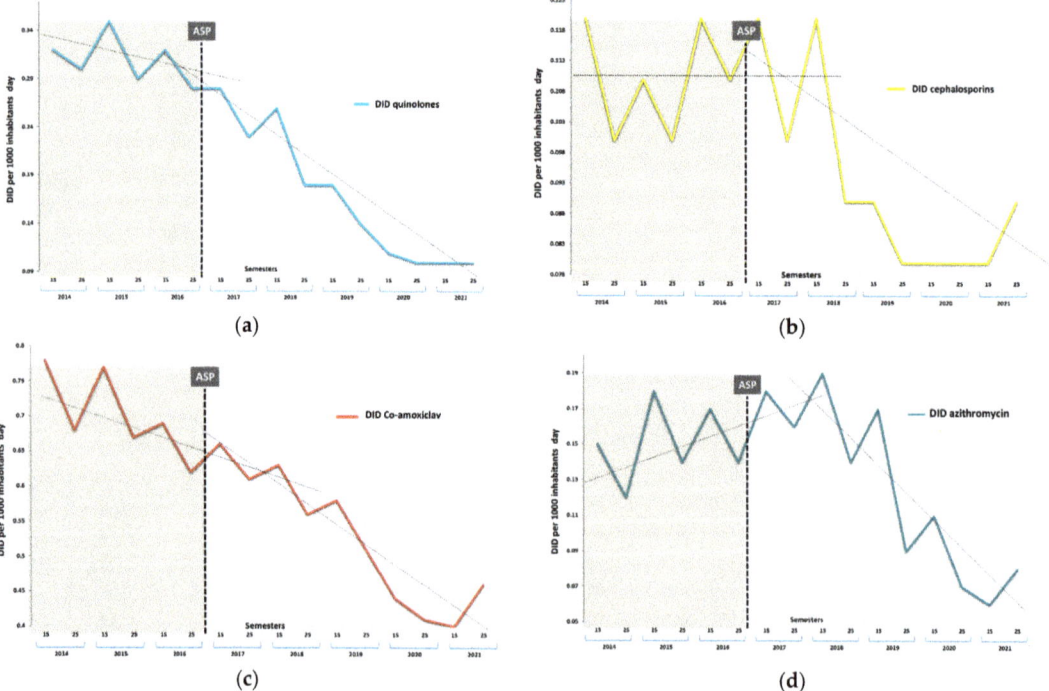

Figure 2. Cont.

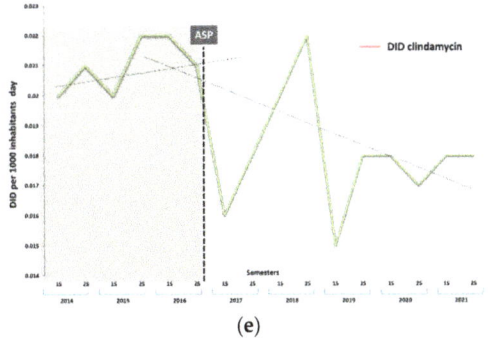
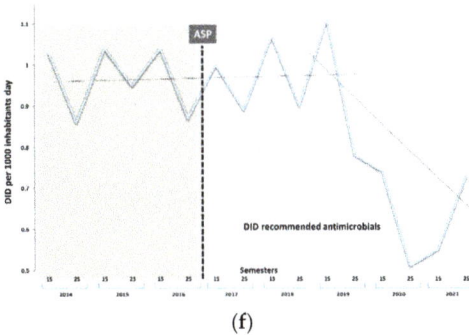

Figure 2. Antimicrobial prescription of other antimicrobials. Semestral evolution of defined daily doses per 1000 inhabitants/day (DID). (**a**) Quinolones, (**b**) cephalosporins, (**c**) co-amoxclav, (**d**) azithromycin, (**e**) clindamycin, (**f**) recommended antimicrobials—amoxicillin, cloxacillin, cefadroxil, cotrimoxazole. 1S; first semester, 2S; second semester.

Regarding the expected trends after those observed in the previous period, the intervention was also associated with significant changes in the post-intervention prescription, with additional significant decreases of −0.2 (95% CI −0.4 to −0.1), −0.4 (−0.5 to −0.3), −0.4 (−0.5 to −0.3), −0.3 (−0.4 to −0.1) ($p < 0.001$), and −0.1 (−0.2 to −0.05) ($p = 0.02$) in DID per semester for FQ, cephalosporins, co-amoxiclav, azithromycin, and clindamycin, respectively. In contrast, the recommended antibiotics (RA) (amoxicillin, cloxacillin, and cefadroxil) did not show a proportionally relevant inverse increase.

3.2. Impact on Antimicrobial Resistance

The antibiotic sensitivity was tested in 3586 clinical samples of *S. aureus* collected over 8.5 years, of which 948 (26.4%) were MRSA.

There were no statistically significant variations in the methicillin resistance rates between the two periods (26.4%) (948/3586). The overall resistance rates for clindamycin, levofloxacin, and erythromycin were 22.5% (807/3586), 33.1% (1187/3586), and 31.5% (1130/3586), respectively. The proportion of *S. aureus* resistant to levofloxacin significantly decreased between the two study periods by 15.1% (371/999 to 816/2587) (OR 0.68, [95% CI 0.58 to 0.79]) ($p < 0.001$). Conversely, the resistance increased in clindamycin and erythromycin, though only significantly in the first one, with a percentage of 53.4% (123/999 to 684/2587) (OR 2.29, [95% CI 1.86 to 2.31], $p < 0.001$). Table 2 presents the semestral comparison of microbiological resistance rates according to the *S. aureus* typology. It shows statistically significant drops in levofloxacin resistance rates, in both MSSA and MRSA, in the last two sections of the intervention period ($p = 0.035$). Resistance to the studied antibiotics increased significantly in the pre-intervention period in both bacteria ($p < 0.001$). After ASP initiation and throughout the post-intervention period, the resistance rates maintained a linear trend towards a general decrease in MRSA ($p < 0.005$), particularly to FQ (OR 0.74, [95% CI 0.64 to 0.86], $p < 0.001$).

Table 2. Rates of microbiological resistance of *S. aureus*.

	Antimicrobial Resistance	% (n/N) Pre-Intervention Resistance	Second S 2016 vs. Second S 2017				Second S 2016 vs. Second S 2019				Second S 2016 vs. First S 2022			
			% (n/N) Post-Intervention Resistance	OR CI 95%	p	Prevention Rate (%)	% (n/N) Pre-Intervention Resistance	% (n/N) Post-Intervention Resistance	OR CI 95%	p	Prevention Rate (%)	% (n/N) Pre-Intervention Resistance	% (n/N) Post-Intervention Resistance	OR CI 95%	p	Prevention Rate (%)
MSSA	Clindamycin	6.54 (48/734)	16.08 (23/143)	2.73 (1.60–4.67)	<0.001		6.53 (48/734)	17.89 (34/190)	3.11 (1.94–4.99)	<0.001	NA	6.53 (48/734)	19.10 (34/178)	3.37 (2.09–5.42)	<0.001	NA
	Levofloxacin	17.71 (130/734)	13.22 (19/143)	0.71 (0.42–1.19)	NS		17.71 (130/734)	6.84 (13/190)	0.34 (0.18–0.61)	<0.001	61.4 (33.2–77.6)	17.71 (130/734)	10.11 (18/178)	0.52 (0.30–0.88)	0.014	42.9 (9.10–64.1)
	Erythromycin	19.20 (141/734)	22.07 (33/143)	1.26 (0.82–1.93)	NS		19.20 (141/734)	21.57 (41/190)	1.15 (0.78–1.71)	NS	NA	19.20 (141/734)	22.47 (40/178)	1.21 (0.81–1.81)	NS	NA
MRSA	Clindamycin	28.30 (75/265)	38.35 (28/73)	1.57 (0.91–2.71)	NS		28.30 (75/265)	45.31 (29/64)	2.09 (1.19–3.67)	0.009	NA	28.30 (75/265)	51.11 (23/45)	2.64 (1.39–5.03)	0.002	NA
	Levofloxacin	90.94 (241/265)	93.15 (68/73)	1.35 (0.49–3.68)	NS		90.94 (241/265)	79.63 (50/64)	0.39 (0.18–0.81)	0.010	12.37 (0.27–23.01)	90.94 (241/265)	81.25 (39/45)	0.43 (0.18–0.99)	0.044	10.6 (−2.83–22.4)
	Erythromycin	42.64 (113/265)	56.62 (47/73)	1.75 (1.06–2.88)	0.026		42.64 (113/265)	46.87 (30/64)	1.18 (0.68–2.05)	NS	NA	42.64 (113/265)	51.11 (23/45)	1.40 (0.74–2.64)	NS	NA

(n/N); n: total positive antibiograms, N; total antibiograms, MSSA; methicillin-sensitive *staphylococcus aureus*. MRSA; methicillin-resistant *staphylococcus aureus*. NS; not significant. NA; not applicable; OR; qdds ratio.

Table 3 shows the resistance changes in the IDs at three points (initial, middle, and final periods), during the intervention and in terms of the overall impact. Comparatively, there were no decreases between periods in the IDs per 1000 inhabitants and per day of *S. aureus*. However, within the intervention period, both the IDs for MRSA and those according to the studied co-resistance typology to clindamycin, levofloxacin, and erythromycin significantly decreased during the intervention period ($p < 0.001$) (Figure 3). These IDs decreased by -0.109 cases (95% CI, -0.232 to -0.064) for methicillin; -0.091 cases (-0.105 to -0.063) for clindamycin; -0.128 (-0.230 to -0.097) for levofloxacin; and -0.112 (-0.116 to -0.084) for erythromycin, with a relative reduction of 62.1%, 58.0%, 55.4%, and 62.9% ($p < 0.001$) at the end of 5 years.

Table 3. Changes on incidence density before and after ASP intervention at 3 points (initial, middle, and final periods) and overall impact.

Antimicrobial Resistance	ID Pre-Intervention Period (95% CI)	Relative Change Second Semester 2017 (95% CI)	Relative Change Second Semester 2019 (95% CI)	Relative Change First Semester 2022 (95% CI)	Absolute Effect Post-Intervention Period	Relative Preventable Effect (%)
MSSA						
Clindamycin	0.024 (0.024 to 0.024)	2.860 (1.740 to 4.703)	4.170 (2.687 to 6.471)	4.071 (2.623 to 6.371)	0.065 (0.054 to 0.076)	73.11 (63.67 to 80.10)
Levofloxacin	0.065 (0.064 to 0.065)	0.872 (0.539 to 1.412)	0.588 (0.332 to 1.041)	0.795 (0.486 to 1.302)	−0.008 (−0.021 to 0.005)	12.33 (−8.65 to 29.25)
Erythromycin	0.071 (0.070 to 0.071)	1.397 (0.956 to 2.040)	1.712 (1.209 to 2.424)	1.630 (1.147 to 2.316)	0.041 (0.026 to 0.056)	39.92 (23.81 to 47.77)
MRSA						
Clindamycin	0.037 (0.037 to 0.038)	2.229 (1.444 to 3.440)	2.276 (1.483 to 3.494)	1.762 (1.104 to 2.812)	0.040 (0.028 to 0.052)	51.93 (38.18 to 62.62)
Levofloxacin	0.120 (0.119 to 0.120)	1.684 (1.287 to 2.204)	1.246 (0.921 to 1.685)	0.858 (0.604 to 1.218)	0.022 (0.003 to 0.041)	15.48 (1.80 to 27.26)
Erythromycin	0.056 (0.056 to 0.057)	2.483 (1.767 to 3.489)	1.563 (1.045 to 2.337)	1.169 (0.747 to 1.831)	0.045 (0.031 to 0.060)	44.73 (31.96 to 55.10)

ID; incidence density per 1000 inhabitants per day. MSSA; methicillin-sensitive *Staphylococcus aureus*. MRSA; methicillin-resistant *Staphylococcus aureus*.

The observed change in the inflection and decline occurred, with a significant linear trend, for both MRSA and its resistance phenotypes to the three studied antimicrobials, in the second semester of the intervention period ($p < 0.001$). From that moment, a modification of the slope of -0.011 cases (SD, 0.043) ($p < 0.001$) per 1000 inhabitants and day, per semester, was noted for MRSA, -0.004 cases (0.036) for clindamycin ($p = 0.005$), -0.015 cases (0.040) for levofloxacin ($p = 0.002$), and -0.010 cases (0.022) for erythromycin ($p < 0.001$).

Finally, there were 56 cases of community-acquired *C. difficile* infection. There were no instances of recurrence. The ID of the initial community-onset infection increased by 41.2% (0.004 to 0.009) during the intervention period (OR 1.24, [95% CI 0.71 to 2.18]), but this increase was not statistically significant (Figure 4).

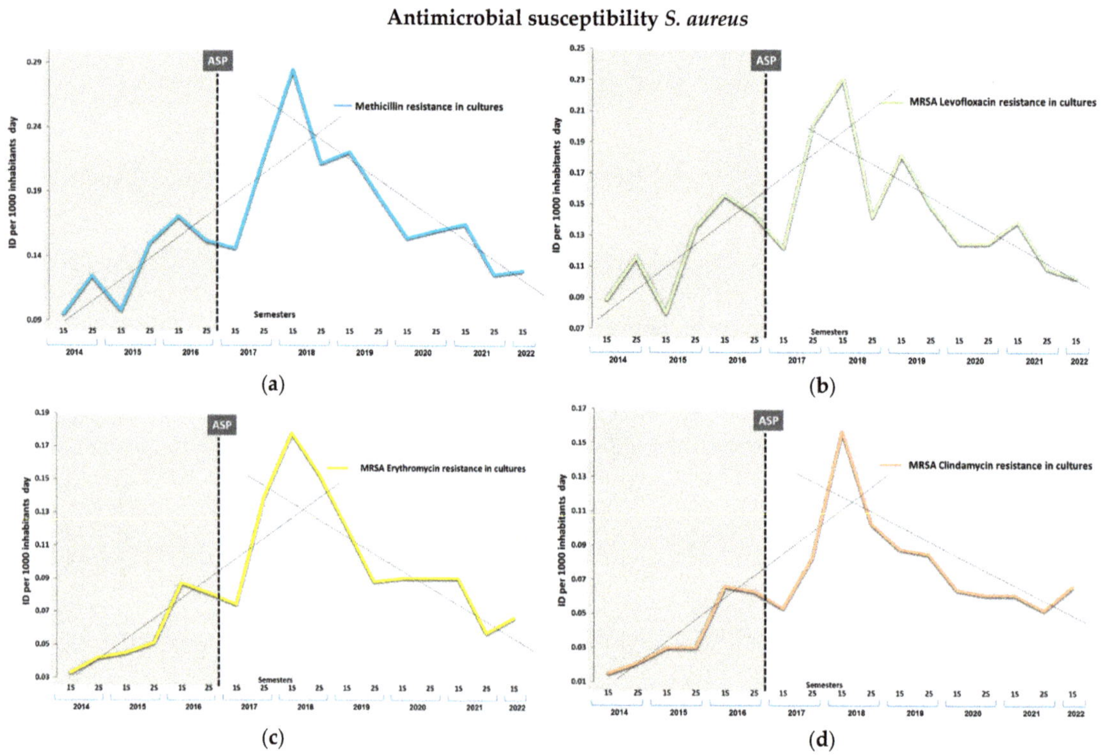

Antimicrobial susceptibility *S. aureus*

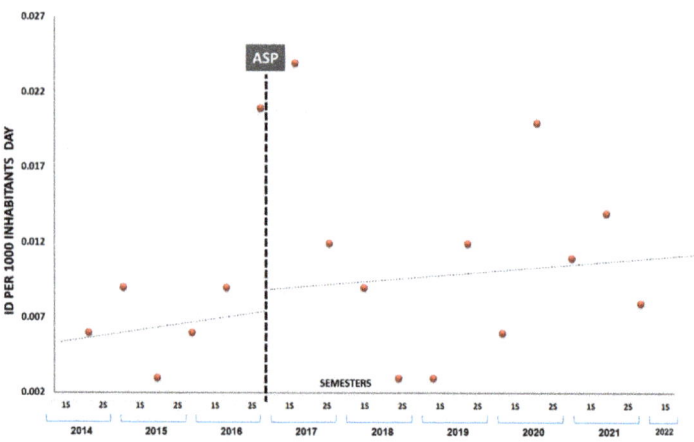

Figure 3. Semestral evolution MRSA (**a**) and antibiotic-resistant MRSA in general cultures per incidence density (ID) per 1000 inhabitants/day. (**b**) Levofloxacin resistance, (**c**) erythromycin resistance, (**d**) clindamycin resistance. 1S; first semester, 2S; second semester.

Figure 4. *C difficile* infection incidence density (ID) per 1000 inhabitants/day over study period.

4. Discussion

Our observational and quasi-experimental study suggests a long-term positive effect on community antimicrobial prescription following the implementation of an educational

ASP designed for primary care. It also indicates a linear trend and an association between antibiotic use and appropriateness and the incidence density of MRSA in the community.

In recent years, the attention to antimicrobial administration has been increasing [26]. In 2023, after several years of recommendations, the European Union (EU) urged all member states to implement real action plans against antimicrobial resistance and to promote the prudent use of antibiotics [27]. However, despite a significant reduction in the average consumption of community systemic treatments in the European Economic Area (EEA) during the period of 2012–2021 (19.3 DID vs. 15.0 DID), the weighted average proportion of the EU/EEA population in relation to the consumption of penicillins, cephalosporins, FQ, and broad-spectrum macrolides (except erythromycin) compared to the narrow-spectrum ones has shown a statistically significant increasing trend of 3.7 (range of countries: 0.1–20.7) in half of the countries, including Spain [28]. These data highlight the value of our intervention, which led to a behavioral change in prescription practices, with a significant reduction in the use of levofloxacin, clindamycin, azithromycin, and cephalosporins, resulting in an increase in the use of RA, specifically first-generation cephalosporins and cotrimoxazole. However, this observed increase was not inversely proportional to these antibiotics recommended by our P-ILEHRDA program, especially in the management of skin and soft tissue infections where Gram-positive microorganisms are present. We believe that improvements in microbiological sample collection techniques, with a focus on percutaneous aspiration rather than swabs, along with the avoidance of indiscriminate culturing of chronic ulcers, which are mostly colonized and are either diagnostic confusion elements or not amenable to antimicrobial treatment, may explain this finding [29–31].

Multimodal models with multifaceted interventions, like those in our study, are more effective than single interventions in changing antimicrobial prescription behavior [32,33]. The studies by Arnold et al. [34] demonstrated that continuous training and feedback of results to professionals improve clinical practice in a sustained and continuous manner, supporting our case when a lower level of counseling during the COVID-19 period did not interfere with the results. Furthermore, while most studies have focused exclusively on respiratory tract infections [35,36], our ASP was designed to address all prevalent types of infections, with a comprehensive approach that was in line with expert recommendations, societies, and previous studies [21,34,37]. Restrictive interventions were not included because, although they can have rapid effects on targeted antibiotic use, such measures are negatively viewed by professionals and do not help to adjust prescription behaviors [38,39].

Our study linked antibiotic dispensing data with around 4000 positive results for *S. aureus* in various samples, mainly skin-related and routinely collected; these results provided our study with sufficient power to detect the direct relationship between consumption and resistance.

The direct association between MRSA and the use of the studied ANR has been evidenced in various analyses, depending on the volume of the exposed population and the age group [40–42]. The relationship has also been established at both the host and the molecular and microbiological levels. A meta-analysis of associations between individual exposures to antibiotics and the risk of MRSA acquisition showed FQ, glycopeptides, cephalosporins, macrolides, and β-lactams to be the most notable [9]. In vitro studies have shown how exposure to most of these antibiotics causes a particular co-resistance in MRSA, as opposed to MSSA, especially to ciprofloxacin, erythromycin, and clindamycin; this is perhaps due to resistance transfer and competition between pathogens [42]. Several authors [13,43,44] have demonstrated how the selectivity and the reduction in the antibiotic pressure threshold on the population can determine the molecular epidemiology of MRSA and cause different phenotypes and shifts toward more susceptible sub-lineages within all clonal complexes. In this regard, our work, although we did not perform a molecular study, not only indicated a reduction in MRSA IDs but also a significant linear downward trend in the total of its co-resistances during the ASP period.

Eliminating the pressure from selected antibiotics such as FQ may not only favor a reduction in MRSA presence but also prompt a rapid decline in resistance. Previous reviews [12,22,45–47] have evaluated the temporal relationship between antibiotic consumption and resistance development in outpatient and primary care settings. Bell et al. [12] included 243 studies (case-control, cross-sectional, ecological, and experimental studies) on all antibiotics and bacteria. The time between consumption and resistance was 6 months or less in 53% and more than 6 months in 23%, and it was unclear in the remaining included studies [12]. The use of FQ has been associated with MRSA incidence shortly after exposure (between 1 and 5 months) [48–50] and with FQ resistance between 0 and 4 months [42,51]. Similarly, the use of lincosamides was associated with the incidence of MRSA and clindamycin resistance in the second month, and in the case of penicillin + β-lactamase inhibitors, this same relationship occurred with a delay of 1 to 5 months [40,42,48,52]. However, a reversal in the trend is feasible with the same temporal intensity if suspension occurs. Studies conducted in the United Kingdom [53,54] assessed the prevalence of ciprofloxacin resistance before, during, and after a national restriction on the use of FQ [22]. These works reported a reduction in resistance levels in less than 3 months. Our trend analysis showed changes in resistance with significant inflection points in MRSA ID, highlighting a steep decline in the early semesters after the start of our ASP, followed by a sustained, significant, and intense decline until the end of the study period. This ecological effect probably occurred because the outcomes were higher at the beginning of the program, when it was easier to improve, and then were maintained over time.

Implementing outpatient interventions to reduce inappropriate antibiotic use can substantially decrease the rates of community-acquired *C. difficile* infection [55,56]. Various studies [57] and a recent meta-analysis [58] that used data from eight studies in various regions of the world have shown that exposure to various categories of antibiotics, including clindamycin, FQ, cephalosporins, penicillins, macrolides, and cotrimoxazole, was associated with an increased risk of *C. difficile* in adults. Our study, despite a significant reduction in most of these antibiotics, did not observe a decrease in *C. difficile* infection. This aspect could be explained by two reasons: the first is the availability of improved protocols and the diagnostic suspicion regarding *C. difficile* as a cause of diarrhea. Alcalá et al. [59] demonstrated in our country that it was only suspected in 47.6% of the cases. The second was the implementation in our health area of new diagnostic techniques with higher sensitivity (PCR techniques in the diagnostic algorithm) at the end of 2016.

Finally, the results of our study have other strengths. First, measuring dispensed antibiotics rather than prescribed ones is considered to be a much stronger measure of exposure and consumption since it faithfully reflects the patients who, by picking up the medication at a pharmacy, have used it. Second, having a unique central microbiology laboratory avoids changes in study techniques and biased variability in the number of samples studied. On the other hand, our work has some limitations: first, the molecular recognition of *S. aureus* ribotypes and resistance genotypes, which could help to better identify interventions aimed at avoiding antibiotics that are considered to be a high risk, were not performed. Second, the synergistic role of standard universal strategies in preventing infection, such as decolonization or hand hygiene, has not been analyzed, with the understanding that the latter has increased during the SARS-CoV-2 pandemic. Third, only community data on overall and selected antibiotic consumption were collected, while antibiotics were also prescribed in hospitals, which, in our case, already had an ASP established with a similar action methodology, which could have magnified the results on the reduction in resistance.

5. Conclusions

The results of this study demonstrate that after five years, the implementation strategies of an educational community ASP, aimed at reducing antibiotic pressure, were associated with significant benefits in terms of both antimicrobial consumption and the local ecological impact of MRSA.

Author Contributions: Conceptualization, A.J.-S., M.R.-H., A.B.B., E.R.M., M.B.B., A.R.M., A.M.L., J.C.C., N.P.P., S.G.-C., M.O.V., M.I.G.V., L.G.N., M.J.J.C., L.M.N., C.B.A., P.V.C., J.J.I.T., M.S.C., E.A.M., R.M.S., A.V.M., J.M.A.S., S.C.M., C.S.E., A.R.G., G.T.M., A.S.C., D.d.l.R.E., M.J.E.S., A.M.F.F., L.M.M.E., L.S.B., A.M.V., M.P.P., A.H., F.P.A., F.T.R., M.C.U.C., J.V.P., M.O.P. and J.T.-P.-g.; methodology, A.J.-S., M.R.-H., A.B.B. and J.T.-P.-g.; formal analysis, J.T.-P.-g.; investigation, A.J.-S.; resources, A.J.-S.; writing—original draft, A.J.-S.; writing—review and editing, A.J.-S., M.R.-H., A.B.B. and E.R.M.; visualization, A.J.-S.; supervision, A.J.-S. and M.R.-H. All authors have read and agreed to the published version of the manuscript.

Funding: This research received no external funding.

Institutional Review Board Statement: Not applicable.

Informed Consent Statement: Not applicable.

Data Availability Statement: No new data were created or analyzed in this study. Data sharing is not applicable to this article.

Acknowledgments: To Montserrat Solanilla for the effort in carrying out the administrative work and Fernando Barcenilla for the critical review. We acknowledge the contribution of other P-ILEHRDA members: M. Mar Álvarez Ceballos (ABS Balàfia), Miracle Camarasa Barbosa (ABS Bellpuig), José Cardona Serra (ABS Almenar), M. Carme Farran Balcells (ABS Tàrrega), Xavier Farré Masip (ABS La Granadella), Carme Florensa Piro (ABS Les Borges Blanques), Asunción Garrido Díaz (ABS Cappont), Jaume Garriga Masana (ABS Artesa de Segre), Iñigo M. Lorente Doria (ABS Primer de maig), Cristina Puras Castells (ABS Primer de maig), Marina Domenjo Solsona (ABS Tàrrega), Antoni Plana Blanco (ABS Balàfia), Sara Porta Acosta (ABS Seròs), Jesús Pujol Salud (ABS Balaguer), M. Bernarda Rodríguez Calaveras (ABS Bordeta), Laia Sabaté Navarro (ABS Eixample), Eva Serra Llavall (ABS Ponts), Mercè Solà Amorós (ABS Almenar), Núria Tarraubella Balanyà (ABS Bordeta), Mireia Villalta Martí (ABS Agramunt), Marc Villanueva Navarro (ABS Pla d'Urgell), Alejandra Villuendas Tirado (ABS Rambla de Ferran), Núria Arco Huguet (ABS Balaguer), Viktoriya Atroshchenko Shushko (ABS Cervera), Daniel Gros Esteban (ABS Eixample), Sara Martí (ABS Rural nord), Raquel Plasencia Atienza (ABS Rural sud), Victoria San José Inés (ABS Alcarràs), Mihaela Cozar (ABS Rambla de Ferran). Finally, our most sincere thanks to the medical specialists and nursing of primary care for their support in accepting and applying the recommendations. Part of this work was presented at the XXIX CAMFIC Congress, Lleida, Spain (oral communication 8435). All individuals included in this section have consented to the acknowledgement.

Conflicts of Interest: The authors declare no conflicts of interest.

References

1. Stefani, S.; Chung, D.R.; Lindsay, J.A.; Friedrich, A.W.; Kearns, A.M.; Westh, H.; MacKenzie, F.M. Meticillin-resistant *Staphylococcus aureus* (MRSA): Global epidemiology and harmonisation of typing methods. *Int. J. Antimicrob. Agents* **2012**, *39*, 273–282. [CrossRef] [PubMed]
2. Shoaib, M.; Aqib, A.I.; Muzammil, I.; Majeed, N.; Bhutta, Z.A.; Kulyar, M.F.; Fatima, M.; Zaheer, C.-N.F.; Muneer, A.; Murtaza, M.; et al. MRSA compendium of epidemiology, transmission, pathophysiology, treatment, and prevention within one health framework. *Front. Microbiol.* **2023**, *13*, 1067284. [CrossRef] [PubMed]
3. Diekema, D.J.; Pfaller, M.A.; Shortridge, D.; Zervos, M.; Jones, R.N. Twenty-year trends in antimicrobial susceptibilities among *Staphylococcus aureus* from the SENTRY antimicrobial surveillance program. *Open Forum Infect. Dis.* **2019**, *6* (Suppl. S1), S47–S53. [CrossRef] [PubMed]
4. Kourtis, A.; Hatfield, K.; Baggs, J.; Mu, Y.; See, I.; Epson, E.; Nadle, J.; Kainer, M.A.; Dumyati, G.; Petit, S.; et al. Vital signs: Epidemiology and recent trends in methicillin-resistant and in methicillin-susceptible *Staphylococcus aureus* bloodstream infections—United States. *MMWR Morb. Mortal. Wkly. Rep.* **2019**, *68*, 214–219. [CrossRef] [PubMed]
5. Garcia Reeves, A.B.; Trogdon, J.G.; Stearns, S.C.; Lewis, J.W.; Weber, D.J.; Weinberger, M. Are rates of methicillin-resistant Staphylococcus aureus and Clostridioides difficile associated with quality and clinical outcomes in US acute care hospitals? *Am. J. Med. Qual.* **2021**, *36*, 90–98. [CrossRef] [PubMed]
6. DeLeo, F.R.; Otto, M.; Kreiswirth, B.N.; Chambers, H.F. Community-associated meticillin-resistant *Staphylococcus aureus*. *Lancet* **2010**, *375*, 1557–1568. [CrossRef] [PubMed]
7. Quero, S.; Serras-Pujol, M.; Párraga-Niño, N.; Torres, C.; Navarro, M.; Vilamala, A.; Puigoriol, E.; Ríos, J.D.d.L.; Arqué, E.; Serra-Pladevall, J.; et al. Methicillin-resistant and methicillin-sensitive *Staphylococcus aureus* in pork industry workers, Catalonia, Spain. *One Health* **2023**, *16*, 100538. [CrossRef]

8. Aldeyab, M.A.; Bond, S.E.; Conway, B.R.; Lee-Milner, J.; Sarma, J.B.; Lattyak, W.J. A threshold logistic modelling approach for identifying thresholds between antibiotic use and methicillin-resistant *Staphylococcus aureus* incidence rates in hospitals. *Antibiotics* **2022**, *11*, 1250. [CrossRef]
9. Tacconelli, E.; De Angelis, G.; Cataldo, M.A.; Pozzi, E.; Cauda, R. Does antibiotic exposure increase the risk of methicillin-resistant *Staphylococcus aureus* (MRSA) isolation? A systematic review and meta-analysis. *J. Antimicrob. Chemother.* **2008**, *61*, 26–38. [CrossRef]
10. Vázquez-Sánchez, D.A.; Grillo, S.; Carrera-Salinas, A.; González-Díaz, A.; Cuervo, G.; Grau, I.; Camoez, M.; Martí, S.; Berbel, D.; Tubau, F.; et al. Molecular epidemiology, antimicrobial susceptibility, and clinical features of methicillin-resistant *Staphylococcus aureus* bloodstream infections over 30 Years in Barcelona, Spain (1990–2019). *Microorganisms* **2022**, *10*, 2401. [CrossRef]
11. Bruyndonckx, R.; Hoxha, A.; Quinten, C.; Ayele, G.M.; Coenen, S.; Versporten, A.; ESAC-Net Study Group. Change-points in antibiotic consumption in the community, European Union/European Economic Area, 1997–2017. *J. Antimicrob. Chemother.* **2021**, *76* (Suppl. S2), ii68–ii78. [CrossRef] [PubMed]
12. Bell, B.G.; Schellevis, F.; Stobberingh, E.; Goossens, H.; Pringle, M. A systematic review and meta-analysis of the effects of antibiotic consumption on antibiotic resistance. *BMC Infect. Dis.* **2014**, *14*, 13. [CrossRef] [PubMed]
13. Lawes, T.; Lopez-Lozano, J.M.; Nebot, C.A.; Macartney, G.; Subbarao-Sharma, R.; Dare, C.R.; Wares, K.D.; Gould, I.M. Effects of national antibiotic stewardship and infection control strategies on hospital-associated and communityassociated meticillin-resistant Staphylococcus aureus infections across a region of Scotland: A non-linear time-series study. *Lancet Infect. Dis.* **2015**, *15*, 1438–1449. [CrossRef] [PubMed]
14. Kurotschka, P.K.; Fulgenzio, C.; Da Cas, R.; Traversa, G.; Ferrante, G.; Massidda, O.; Gágyor, I.; Aschbacher, R.; Moser, V.; Pagani, E.; et al. Effect of fluoroquinolone use in primary care on the development and gradual decay of Escherichia coli resistance to fluoroquinolones: A matched case-control study. *Antibiotics* **2022**, *11*, 822. [CrossRef] [PubMed]
15. Gupta, K.; Hooton, T.M.; Naber, K.G.; Wullt, B.; Colgan, R.; Miller, L.G.; Moran, G.J.; Nicolle, L.E.; Raz, R.; Schaeffer, A.J.; et al. Infectious Diseases Society of America; European Society for Microbiology and Infectious Diseases. International clinical practice guidelines for the treatment of acute uncomplicated cystitis and pyelonephritis in women: A 2010 update by the Infectious Diseases Society of America and the European Society for Microbiology and Infectious Diseases. *Clin. Infect Dis.* **2011**, *52*, e103–e120. [CrossRef] [PubMed]
16. Hammond, A.; Stuijfzand, B.; Avison, M.B.; Hay, A.D. Antimicrobial resistance associations with national primary care antibiotic stewardship policy: Primary care-based, multilevel analytic study. *PLoS ONE* **2020**, *15*, e0232903. [CrossRef]
17. Gágyor, I.; Hay, A.D. Outcome selection in primary care antimicrobial stewardship research. *J. Antimicrob. Chemother.* **2021**, *77*, 7–12. [CrossRef]
18. Avent, M.L.; Cosgrove, S.E.; Price-Haywood, E.G.; van Driel, M.L. Antimicrobial stewardship in the primary care setting: From dream to reality? *BMC Fam. Pract.* **2020**, *21*, 134. [CrossRef]
19. Jover-Sáenz, A.; Ramírez-Hidalgo, M.; Bellés Bellés, A.; Ribes Murillo, E.; Batlle Bosch, M.; Cayado Cabanillas, J.; Garrido-Calvo, S.; Vilas, M.I.G.; Navés, L.G.; Caudevilla, M.J.J.; et al. Impact of a Primary Care Antimicrobial Stewardship Program on Bacterial Resistance Control and Ecological Imprint in Urinary Tract Infections. *Antibiotics* **2022**, *11*, 1776. [CrossRef]
20. Jover-Sáenz, A.; Grup d'estudi i equip PROAP. P-ILERDA -Programa integrat local extrahospitalari de racionalització, millora i desprescripció antibiòtica a Lleida-. Primers resultats d'un programa d'optimització d'ús d'antimicrobians (PROA) en atenció primària. *Annals Medicina* **2018**, *4*, 160–166. (In Catalan)
21. Rodríguez-Baño, J.; Paño-Pardo, J.R.; Alvarez-Rocha, L.; Asensio, Á.; Calbo, E.; Cercenado, E.; Cisneros, J.M.; Cobo, J.; Delgado, O.; Garnacho-Montero, J.; et al. Programs for optimizing the use of antibiotics (PROA) in Spanish hospitals: GEIH-SEIMC, SEFH and SEMPSPH consensus document. *Enferm. Infecc. Microbiol. Clin.* **2012**, *30*, 22.e1–22.e23. [CrossRef]
22. Bakhit, M.; Hoffmann, T.; Scott, A.M.; Beller, E.; Rathbone, J.; Del Mar, C. Resistance decay in individuals after antibiotic exposure in primary care: A systematic review and meta-analysis. *BMC Med.* **2018**, *16*, 126. [CrossRef]
23. Magiorakos, A.P.; Srinivasan, A.; Carey, R.B.; Carmeli, Y.; Falagas, M.E.; Giske, C.G.; Harbarth, S.; Hindler, J.F.; Kahlmeter, G.; Olsson-Liljequist, B.; et al. Multidrug-resistant, extensively drug-resistant and pandrug-resistant bacteria: An international expert proposal for interim standard definitions for acquired resistance. *Clin. Microbiol. Infect.* **2012**, *18*, 268–281. [CrossRef]
24. The European Committee on Antimicrobial Susceptibility Testing. Breakpoint Tables for Interpretation of MICs and Zone Diameters, Version 8.0. 2018. Available online: http://www.eucast.org/clinical_breakpoints/ (accessed on 5 December 2023).
25. van Prehn, J.; Reigadas, E.; Vogelzang, E.H.; Bouza, E.; Hristea, A.; Guery, B.; Krutova, M.; Norén, T.; Allerberger, F.; Coia, J.E.; et al. Guideline Committee of the European Study Group on *Clostridioides difficile*. European Society of Clinical Microbiology and Infectious Diseases: 2021 update on the treatment guidance document for *Clostridioides difficile* infection in adults. *Clin. Microbiol. Infect.* **2021**, *27* (Suppl. S2), S1–S21. [CrossRef]
26. Antimicrobial Resistance Collaborators. Global burden of bacterial antimicrobial resistance in 2019: A systematic analysis. *Lancet* **2022**, *399*, 629–655. [CrossRef] [PubMed]
27. Consejo de la Unión Europea. Recomendación del Consejo sobre la intensificación de las medidas de la UE para luchar contra la resistencia a los antimicrobianos de acuerdo con el concepto «Una sola salud». *D. Of. De La Unión Eur.* **2023**, *220*, 1–20.
28. European Centre for Disease Prevention and Control. Antimicrobial Consumption in the EU/EEA (ESAC-Net) AER for 2021 (europa.eu). Available online: https://www.ecdc.europa.eu/en/publications-data/surveillance-antimicrobial-consumption-europe-2021 (accessed on 4 October 2023).

29. Lee, P.C.; Turnidge, J.; McDonald, P.J. Fine-needle aspiration biopsy in diagnosis of soft tissue infections. *J. Clin. Microbiol.* **1985**, *22*, 80–83. [CrossRef]
30. Miller, J.M.; Binnicker, M.J.; Campbell, S.; Carroll, K.C.; Chapin, K.C.; Gilligan, P.H.; Gonzalez, M.D.; Jerris, R.C.; Kehl, S.C.; Patel, R.; et al. A guide to utilization of the microbiology laboratory for diagnosis of infectious diseases: 2018 update by the Infectious Diseases Society of America and the American Society for Microbiology. *Clin. Infect. Dis.* **2018**, *67*, e1–e94. [CrossRef] [PubMed]
31. Ezemma, O.; Korman, A.M.; Wang, H.E.; Kaffenberger, B. Diagnostic methods for the confirmation of non-purulent cellulitis: A review. *Arch. Dermatol. Res.* **2023**, *315*, 2519–2527. [CrossRef] [PubMed]
32. Figueiras, A.; López-Vázquez, P.; Gonzalez-Gonzalez, C.; Vázquez-Lago, J.M.; Piñeiro-Lamas, M.; López-Durán, A.; Sánchez, C.; Herdeiro, M.T.; GREPHEPI Group. Impact of a multifaceted intervention to improve antibiotic prescribing: A pragmatic cluster-randomised controlled trial. *Antimicrob. Resist. Infect. Control.* **2020**, *9*, 195. [CrossRef]
33. Rocha, V.; Estrela, M.; Neto, V.; Roque, F.; Figueiras, A.; Herdeiro, M.T. Educational interventions to reduce prescription and dispensing of antibiotics in primary care: A systematic review of economic impact. *Antibiotics* **2022**, *11*, 1186. [CrossRef]
34. Arnold, S.R.; Straus, S.E. Interventions to improve antibiotic prescribing practices in ambulatory care. *Evid. Based Child. Health* **2006**, *1*, 623–690. [CrossRef]
35. Drekonja, D.M.; Filice, G.A.; Greer, N.; Olson, A.; MacDonald, R.; Rutks, I.; Wilt, T.J. Antimicrobial stewardship in outpatient settings: A systematic review. *Infect. Control Hosp. Epidemiol.* **2015**, *36*, 142–152. [CrossRef]
36. Dyar, O.J.; Beović, B.; Vlahović-Palčevski, V.; Verheij, T.; Pulcini, C. How can we improve antibiotic prescribing in primary care? *Expert. Rev. Anti-Infect. Ther.* **2016**, *14*, 403–413. [CrossRef] [PubMed]
37. McNulty, C.; Hawking, M.; Lecky, D.; Jones, L.; Owens, R.; Charlett, A.; Butler, C.; Moore, P.; Francis, N. Effects of primary care antimicrobial stewardship outreach on antibiotic use by general practice staff: Pragmatic randomized controlled trial of the TARGET antibiotics work-shop. *J. Antimicrob. Chemother.* **2018**, *73*, 1423–1432. [CrossRef]
38. Rice, L.B. Antimicrobial stewardship and antimicrobial resistance. *Med. Clin. North. Am.* **2018**, *102*, 805–818. [CrossRef]
39. Chin, J.; Green, S.B.; McKamey, L.J.; Gooch, M.D.; Chapin, R.W.; Gould, A.P.; Milliken, S.F.; Blanchette, L.M. Restriction-free antimicrobial stewardship initiative targeting fluoroquinolone reduction across a regional health-system. *Infect. Prev. Pract.* **2019**, *1*, 100019. [CrossRef]
40. López-Lozano, J.M.; Lawes, T.; Nebot, C.; Beyaert, A.; Bertrand, X.; Hocquet, D.; Aldeyab, M.; Scott, M.; Conlon-Bingham, G.; Farren, D.; et al. A nonlinear time-series analysis approach to identify thresholds in associations between population antibiotic use and rates of resistance. *Nat. Microbiol.* **2019**, *4*, 1160–1172. [CrossRef] [PubMed]
41. Schneider-Lindner, V.; Quach, C.; Hanley, J.A.; Suissa, S. Antibacterial drugs and the risk of community-associated methicillin-resistant *Staphylococcus aureus* in children. *Arch. Pediatr. Adolesc. Med.* **2011**, *165*, 1107–1114. [CrossRef] [PubMed]
42. Lawes, T.; López-Lozano, J.M.; Nebot, C.; Macartney, G.; Subbarao-Sharma, R.; Dare, C.R.; Edwards, G.F.S.; Gould, I.M. Turning the tide or riding the waves? Impacts of antibiotic stewardship and infection control on MRSA strain dynamics in a Scottish region over 16 years: Non-linear time series analysis. *BMJ Open* **2015**, *5*, e006596. [CrossRef] [PubMed]
43. El Mammery, A.; Ramírez de Arellano, E.; Cañada-García, J.E.; Cercenado, E.; Villar-Gómara, L.; Casquero-García, V.; García-Cobos, S.; Lepe, J.A.; Bordes, E.R.d.G.; Calvo-Montes, J.; et al. An increase in erythromycin resistance in methicillin-susceptible *Staphylococcus aureus* from blood correlates with the use of macrolide/lincosamide/streptogramin antibiotics. EARS-Net Spain (2004–2020). *Front. Microbiol.* **2023**, *14*, 1220286. [CrossRef]
44. Oteo, J.; Aracil, M.B. Caracterización de mecanismos de resistencia por biología molecular: *Staphylococcus aureus* resistente a meticilina, β-lactamasas de espectro extendido y carbapenemasas. *Enferm. Infecc. Microbiol. Clin.* **2015**, *33* (Suppl. S2), 27–33. [CrossRef] [PubMed]
45. Poku, E.; Cooper, K.; Cantrell, A.; Harnan, S.; Sin, M.A.; Zanuzdana, A.; Hoffmann, A. Systematic review of time lag between antibiotic use and rise of resistant pathogens among hospitalized adults in Europe. *JAC Antimicrob. Resist.* **2023**, *5*, dlad001. [CrossRef] [PubMed]
46. Costelloe, C.; Metcalfe, C.; Lovering, A.; Mant, D.; Hay, A.D. Effect of antibiotic prescribing in primary care on antimicrobial resistance in individual patients: Systematic review and meta-analysis. *BMJ* **2010**, *340*, c2096. [CrossRef] [PubMed]
47. Bakhit, M.; Del Mar, C.; Scott, A.M.; Hoffmann, T. An analysis of reporting quality of prospective studies examining community antibiotic use and resistance. *Trials* **2018**, *19*, 656. [CrossRef] [PubMed]
48. Aldeyab, M.A.; Monnet, D.L.; Lopez-Lozano, J.M.; Hughes, C.M.; Scott, M.G.; Kearney, M.P.; Magee, F.A.; McElnay, J.C. Modelling the impact of antibiotic use and infection control practices on the incidence of hospital-acquired methicillin-resistant *Staphylococcus aureus*: A time-series analysis. *J. Antimicrob. Chemother.* **2008**, *62*, 593–600. [CrossRef]
49. Kaier, K.; Hagist, C.; Frank, U.; Conrad, A.; Meyer, E. Two time-series analyses of the impact of antibiotic consumption and alcohol-based hand disinfection on the incidences of nosocomial methicillin-resistant *Staphylococcus aureus* infection and *Clostridium difficile* infection. *Infect. Control Hosp. Epidemiol.* **2009**, *30*, 346–353. [CrossRef]
50. Mahamat, A.; MacKenzie, F.M.; Brooker, K.; Monnet, D.L.; Daures, J.P.; Gould, I.M. Impact of infection control interventions and antibiotic use on hospital MRSA: A multivariate interrupted time-series analysis. *Int. J. Antimicrob. Agents.* **2007**, *30*, 169–176. [CrossRef]
51. Berger, P.; Pascal, L.; Sartor, C.; Delorme, J.; Monge, P.; Ragon, C.P.; Charbit, M.; Sambuc, R.; Drancourt, M. Generalized additive model demonstrates fluoroquinolone use/resistance relationships for *Staphylococcus aureus*. *Eur. J. Epidemiol.* **2004**, *19*, 453–460. [CrossRef]

52. Vernaz, N.; Sax, H.; Pittet, D.; Bonnabry, P.; Schrenzel, J.; Harbarth, S. Temporal effects of antibiotic use and hand rub consumption on the incidence of MRSA and *Clostridium difficile*. *J. Antimicrob. Chemother.* **2008**, *62*, 601–607. [CrossRef] [PubMed]
53. Aldeyab, M.A.; Scott, M.G.; Kearney, M.P.; Alahmadi, Y.M.; Magee, F.A.; Conlon, G.; McELNAY, J.C. Impact of an enhanced antibiotic stewardship on reducing methicillin-resistant *Staphylococcus aureus* in primary and secondary healthcare settings. *Epidemiol. Infect.* **2014**, *142*, 494–500. [CrossRef] [PubMed]
54. Parienti, J.J.; Cattoir, V.; Thibon, P.; Lebouvier, G.; Verdon, R.; Daubin, C.; du Cheyron, D.; Leclercq, R.; Charbonneau, P. Hospital-wide modification of fluoroquinolone policy and meticillin-resistant *Staphylococcus aureus* rates: A 10-year interrupted time-series analysis. *J. Hosp. Infect.* **2011**, *78*, 118–122. [CrossRef] [PubMed]
55. Dantes, R.; Mu, Y.; Hicks, L.A.; Cohen, J.; Bamberg, W.; Beldavs, Z.G.; Dumyati, G.; Farley, M.M.; Holzbauer, S.; Meek, J.; et al. Association between outpatient antibiotic prescribing practices and community-associated *Clostridium difficile* infection. *Open Forum Infect. Dis.* **2015**, *2*, ofv113. [CrossRef] [PubMed]
56. Rhea, S.; Jones, K.; Endres-Dighe, S.; Munoz, B.; Weber, D.J.; Hilscher, R.; MacFarquhar, J.; Sickbert-Bennett, E.; DiBiase, L.; Marx, A.; et al. Modeling inpatient and outpatient antibiotic stewardship interventions to reduce the burden of *Clostridioides difficile* infection in a regional healthcare network. *PLoS ONE* **2020**, *15*, e0234031. [CrossRef]
57. Miller, A.C.; Arakkal, A.T.; Sewell, D.K.; Segre, A.M.; Tholany, J.; Polgreen, P.M.; CDC MInD-Healthcare Group. Comparison of different antibiotics and the risk for community-associated *Clostridioides difficile* infection: A Case-Control Study. *Open Forum Infect. Dis.* **2023**, *10*, ofad413. [CrossRef] [PubMed]
58. Deshpande, A.; Pasupuleti, V.; Thota, P.; Pant, C.; Rolston, D.D.; Sferra, T.J.; Hernandez, A.V.; Donskey, C.J. Community-associated *Clostridium difficile* infection and antibiotics: A meta-analysis. *J. Antimicrob. Chemother.* **2013**, *68*, 1951–1961. [CrossRef]
59. Alcalá, L.; Martín, A.; Marín, M.; Sánchez-Somolinos, M.; Catalán, P.; Peláez, T.; Bouza, E.; Spanish *Clostridium difficile* Study Group. The undiagnosed cases of *Clostridium difficile* infection in a whole nation: Where is the problem? *Clin. Microbiol. Infect.* **2012**, *18*, E204–E213. [CrossRef] [PubMed]

Disclaimer/Publisher's Note: The statements, opinions and data contained in all publications are solely those of the individual author(s) and contributor(s) and not of MDPI and/or the editor(s). MDPI and/or the editor(s) disclaim responsibility for any injury to people or property resulting from any ideas, methods, instructions or products referred to in the content.

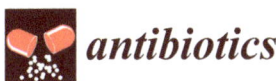

Article

Acculturation and Subjective Norms Impact Non-Prescription Antibiotic Use among Hispanic Patients in the United States

Lindsey A. Laytner [1,2,*], Kiara Olmeda [1], Juanita Salinas [1], Osvaldo Alquicira [3], Susan Nash [1], Roger Zoorob [1], Michael K. Paasche-Orlow [4], Barbara W. Trautner [2,5,6] and Larissa Grigoryan [1,2]

1. Department of Family and Community Medicine, Baylor College of Medicine, Houston, TX 77098, USA
2. Center for Innovations in Quality, Effectiveness and Safety (IQuESt), Houston, TX 77021, USA
3. Tilman J. Fertitta Family College of Medicine, Houston, TX 77021, USA
4. Department of Medicine, Tufts Medical Center, Boston, MA 02111, USA
5. Michael E. DeBakey Veterans Affairs Medical Center, Houston, TX 77030, USA
6. Department of Medicine, Section of Health Services Research, Baylor College of Medicine, Houston, TX 77030, USA
* Correspondence: lindsey.laytner@bcm.edu

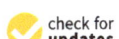

Citation: Laytner, L.A.; Olmeda, K.; Salinas, J.; Alquicira, O.; Nash, S.; Zoorob, R.; Paasche-Orlow, M.K.; Trautner, B.W.; Grigoryan, L. Acculturation and Subjective Norms Impact Non-Prescription Antibiotic Use among Hispanic Patients in the United States. *Antibiotics* **2023**, *12*, 1419. https://doi.org/10.3390/antibiotics12091419

Academic Editors: Juan Manuel Vázquez-Lago, Ana Estany-Gestal and Angel Salgado-Barreira

Received: 28 July 2023
Revised: 31 August 2023
Accepted: 2 September 2023
Published: 8 September 2023

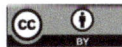

Copyright: © 2023 by the authors. Licensee MDPI, Basel, Switzerland. This article is an open access article distributed under the terms and conditions of the Creative Commons Attribution (CC BY) license (https:// creativecommons.org/licenses/by/ 4.0/).

Abstract: Using antibiotics without medical guidance (non-prescription antibiotic use) may contribute to antimicrobial resistance. Hispanic individuals are a growing demographic group in the United States (US) with a high prevalence of non-prescription antibiotic use. We investigated the effects of acculturation and subjective norms on Hispanic individuals' intentions to use antibiotics without a prescription from the following sources: (1) markets in the United States (not legal), (2) other countries (abroad), (3) leftovers from previous prescriptions, and (4) friends/relatives. We surveyed self-identified Hispanic outpatients in eight clinics from January 2020 to June 2021 using the previously validated Short Acculturation Scale for Hispanics (SASH). Of the 263 patients surveyed, 47% reported previous non-prescription use, and 54% expressed intention to use non-prescription antibiotics if feeling sick. Individuals with lower acculturation (Spanish-speaking preferences) expressed greater intentions to use antibiotics from abroad and from any source. Individuals with more friends/relatives who obtain antibiotics abroad were over 2.5 times more likely to intend to use non-prescription antibiotics from friends/relatives ($p = 0.034$). Other predictors of intention to use non-prescription antibiotics included high costs of doctor visits and perceived language barriers in the clinic. Antibiotic stewardship interventions in Hispanic communities in the United States should consider the sociocultural and healthcare barriers influencing non-prescription use and promote language-concordant healthcare.

Keywords: acculturation; subjective norms; socio-cultural factors; antibiotic resistance; non-prescription antibiotic use; antibiotic stewardship

1. Introduction

Using antibiotics without a prescription (non-prescription antibiotic use) is a common practice worldwide and is a safety threat to individuals and the public health [1–3]. Non-prescription antibiotic use can potentially increase the risks of adverse drug reactions or interactions, superinfection, gut dysbiosis, and the development of antimicrobial resistance [4–6].

Recent studies have documented the determinants of non-prescription antibiotic use across low-, middle-, and high-income countries and found that patient-level (sociocultural and sociodemographic) factors and healthcare system barriers contribute to non-prescription antibiotic use [7–9]. In the United States (US), Hispanic communities have one of the highest reported prevalence rates of non-prescription antibiotic use, with the prevalence ranging from 19 to 66% [9]. Prior studies have identified that these Hispanic communities use non-prescribed antibiotics from a variety of sources, including leftover prescriptions (e.g., from self, friends, or family); purchasing illegally under-the-counter through informal sources in the US (e.g., flea markets and ethnic or herbalist shops); or outside the US without a prescription (e.g., across the border in another country, including Mexico) [3,9–12].

Sociocultural factors include an individual's level of acculturation and their subjective norms. Acculturation and subjective norms can impact health behaviors in Hispanic communities [10–12]. Acculturation is "the process by which individuals adopt the attitudes, values, customs, beliefs, and behaviors of another culture" [13,14]. For example, less-acculturated individuals may continue certain health practices (e.g., non-prescription antibiotic use) that they had in their home countries. Subjective norms are often classified as the "expectations set by groups of important people (such as family, relatives, and friends) in terms of whether an individual should or should not engage in a behavior" [15]. For instance, individuals may engage in non-prescription antibiotic use because their friends and family also routinely engage in that behavior.

A recent study of a Hispanic community along the Texas border found that a higher generation score, a proxy measure of acculturation, was associated with lower cross-border purchases of antibiotics [11]. Another qualitative study of Hispanic primary care patients in Houston found that patients' subjective norms (e.g., friends and family frequently purchase non-prescription antibiotics) and social networks (e.g., friends, family, or other "trusted" persons) influenced their decisions to use non-prescription antibiotics [12]. However, these studies included medically underserved, impoverished Hispanic individuals and did not study the independent effects of sociocultural and healthcare system factors on non-prescription antibiotic use in sociodemographically diverse Hispanic communities.

2. Materials and Methods

We investigated the effects of Hispanic patients' sociocultural factors (acculturation and subjective norms) and the barriers to healthcare on the intention to use non-prescription antibiotics from four sources: (1) markets in the United States (under the counter, not legal), (2) other countries, (3) leftovers from previous prescriptions, and (4) friends/relatives.

2.1. Design and Recruitment

We conducted a large, cross-sectional survey to assess non-prescription antibiotic use in sociodemographically diverse outpatients. Data collection occurred between January 2020 and June 2021 in eight outpatient clinic waiting rooms (six public primary care and two private emergency departments) in Harris County, Texas [3]. Clinic staff gave flyers to patients who checked in for primary care visits. The flyer summarized the study, and interested patients volunteered to participate. Surveys were conducted anonymously in person when permitted during the pandemic or remotely via teleconferencing in patients' preferred language (English or Spanish). Each respondent was given a list of brand name and generic antibiotics that were accompanied by images of the most commonly used antibiotics in the US and Latin American countries.

Individuals who self-identified as Hispanic or Latino in the larger survey were included for analysis in this study [3]. This study was approved by the Institutional Review Board for Baylor College of Medicine and Affiliated Hospitals (protocol H-45709). Additional details on recruitment, survey design information, sample size calculations, response rate, and additional information were published elsewhere [3].

2.2. Survey Instrument

The survey instrument is available in Appendix A. Non-prescription antibiotic use was defined as the consumption of antibiotics not prescribed to that individual for his or her current health condition [3]. Intended use was defined as a professed intention for future non-prescription antibiotic use [9,16]. Individuals classified as non-prescription antibiotic users reported having "ever taken" oral antibiotics without a prescription. Individuals classified as intended users endorsed using antibiotics from one of four sources presented via the question "If you were feeling sick, would you take antibiotics in the following situations without contacting a doctor/nurse/dentist/clinic?" The sources presented to the patients were: (1) you can buy antibiotics without a prescription in the United States, (2) you can buy antibiotics without a prescription in another country, (3) friends or relatives give you antibiotics, and (4) you have leftover antibiotics from a previous prescription.

Survey questions were mapped to factors in the Kilbourne Framework for Advancing Health Disparities Research, including the patient, healthcare system, and clinical encounter factors [17]. Subjective norms and acculturation are patient factors that may contribute to non-prescription antibiotic use in Hispanic populations. Healthcare system barriers included lacking transportation to the doctor visits, long clinic waits, not having a regular doctor, and the high cost of doctor visits. Clinical encounter factors included language barriers at the clinic and during doctor visits.

2.3. Patient Factors

2.3.1. Sociodemographic Factors

Sociodemographic characteristics included age, gender, race/ethnicity, education, yearly household income, health insurance status, country of birth, and health literacy (Table 1). Individuals' insurance status was categorized into three groups: (1) private insurance or Medicare, (2) Medicaid (i.e., public health insurance for low-income children, families, seniors, and people with disabilities) or county financial assistance program (CFAP) (provides healthcare coverage/access to publicly funded clinics at very low or no cost to patients), or (3) self-pay (no insurance or CFAP). For health literacy, we used the Brief Health Literacy Screen measure validated in primary care settings [18,19]. Inadequate health literacy was defined as an answer to any of three screening questions that endorsed having problems associated with health literacy some or all of the time.

Table 1. Patient sociodemographic characteristics.

Characteristic	Total (N = 263)
Median age (y) (range)	51 (20–80)
No. (%) of female respondents	194 (73.8)
No. (%) of respondents with education level	
Less than high school	84 (31.9)
High school or GED	104 (39.5)
Some college and above	75 (28.5)
No. (%) of respondents with insurance status	
Private or Medicare	74 (28.1)
Medicaid or county financial assistance program *	173 (60.8)
Self-pay	16 (6.1)
No. (%) of patients attending Healthcare system	
Private	41 (15.6)
Public	222 (84.4)
No. (%) of patients attending clinic type	
Continuity clinic	102 (38.8)
Emergency Department	41 (15.6)
Walk in Clinic	120 (45.6)
No. of respondents with income/total no. of respondents (%)	
<$20,000	127 (48.3)
≥$20,000 but <$40,000	58 (22.1)
≥$40,000 but <$60,000	11 (4.2)
≥$60,000 but <$100,000	8 (3.0)
≥$100,000	6 (2.3)
Don't know/prefer not to say	53 (20.2)

Table 1. *Cont.*

Characteristic	Total (N = 263)
No. (%) of questionnaires completed in Spanish	155 (58.9)
No. (%) of respondents born in the United States/Other	
United States	81 (30.8)
Other [†]	182 (69.2)
Median years lived in the United States for the respondents born in other countries (y) (range) (n = 182)	23 (0–58)
No. (%) of respondents reporting non-prescription antibiotic use	
Reported prior non-prescription use	123 (46.8)
No. (%) Health Literacy [§]	
Adequate Health Literacy	198 (75.3)
Inadequate Health Literacy	65 (24.7)

* County financial assistance program includes those who have benefits from the county allowing access to public clinic providers at either very low cost or no cost. [†] Includes 1 Columbia, 1 Costa Rica, 6 Cuba, 1 Dominican Republic, 14 El Salvador, 6 Guatemala, 15 Honduras, 131 Mexico, 2 Nicaragua, 1 Panama, 1 Peru, and 3 Venezuela (countries are listed in alphabetical order). [§] Calculated using the three questions from the Brief Health literacy Screen measure [18,19].

2.3.2. Acculturation

Acculturation was assessed using the Short Acculturation Scale for Hispanics (SASH) developed and validated by Marin et al. and included the Language Use, Television and Media, and Social and Ethnic Relations subscale scores [20]. The SASH questionnaire contains 12 questions of equal weight: 5 assessing language preferences, 3 assessing media preferences, and 4 assessing social and ethnic preferences (Appendix A. Survey Instrument).

Each question was scored on Likert-type scales, ranging from 1 (Only Spanish/all Hispanic individuals) to 5 (Only English/all non-Hispanic individuals). Subscores with lower values (closer to 1) reflect preferences for Spanish-speaking interactions or Hispanic social interactions or entertainment. Higher scores (closer to 5) reflect a preference for English-speaking interactions or entertainment. The total points per subscale were averaged over the number of questions answered to generate the numerical score for that subscale. Cronbach's alpha was computed to determine the internal consistency of the set of questions representing each construct; one question was excluded from the ethnic and social relations subscale (Appendix B. SASH Reliability Statistics). The overall acculturation score was calculated using the sum of the language, television and media use, and ethnic and social relations subscores (Table 2).

Table 2. Acculturation by subscale means, interquartile range, and internal consistency [†].

Acculturation Subscales	Intended Use from Any Source		Cronbach's Alpha
	Yes (n = 95) Median (IQR *)	No (n = 167) Median (IQR *)	
Language Use Subscale Score	2.0 (1.2–3.4)	2.0 (1.4–3.2)	0.939
Media Subscale Score	3.0 (1.7–4.0)	3.0 (1.0–4.0)	0.969
Ethnic Social Relations Subscale Score	2.3 (2.0–2.7)	2.3 (2.0–3.0)	0.817
Total Acculturation (Overall, Aggregate Score)	2.5 (1.6–3.4)	2.4 (1.7–3.3)	0.939

* Interquartile Range. [†] The Short Acculturation Scale for Hispanics is comprised of three subscales (Language Use, Media, and Ethnic Social Relations). Scores range from 1 (all Latinos/Hispanics) to 5 (all non-Latinos/Hispanics). Higher score indicates higher levels of acculturation [20].

2.3.3. Subjective Norms

Subjective norms were identified by the following proxy questions: (1) "How many of your friends or relatives use antibiotics without contacting a doctor?" and (2) "How many of your friends or relatives get antibiotics from another country?" Each question was scored using Likert-type scales ranging from 1 (none/don't remember/don't know) to 4 (all/most/about half) (Table 3).

Table 3. Subjective norms (N = 263).

	Total No. (%)
How many of your friends or relatives use antibiotics without contacting a doctor?	
None/Don't Remember/Don't Know	105 (39.9)
Some	98 (37.3)
About Half	15 (5.7)
Most	33 (12.5)
All	12 (4.6)
How many of your friends or relatives get antibiotics from another country?	
None/Don't Remember/Don't Know	123 (46.8)
Some	97 (36.9)
About Half	15 (5.7)
Most	28 (10.6)

2.4. Healthcare System and Clinical Encounter Factors

Healthcare barriers were assessed using five questions relevant to our safety net patient population, including transportation, language barriers, long clinic waits, not having a regular doctor, and the high cost of doctor visits. Each question was scored dichotomously as "not a problem" or "a problem" (i.e., included answering that the barrier was a minor or major problem) (Appendix C).

2.5. Statistical Analysis

Descriptive statistics were performed on all study variables using SPSS version 28 (Chicago, IL, USA) [21]. Cronbach's alpha was computed to analyze the internal consistency of the set of questions representing the acculturation scale. We used univariate logistic regression to assess the patient and healthcare system factors associated with patients' intention to use non-prescription antibiotics from each source. Predictor variables that showed a univariate relationship ($p < 0.2$) with each source of intended non-prescription antibiotic use were considered for the multivariate analyses (Appendix D. Univariate Regression Results).

Multivariate logistic regression assessed the effects of patients' acculturation and subjective norms on their intention to use antibiotics without a prescription from one of the following sources: (1) stores or markets in the US, (2) another country, (3) friends/relatives, (4) a leftover prescription, and (5) any of these four sources (Tables 4–8).

3. Results

3.1. Patient Factors

3.1.1. Sociodemographic Characteristics

Table 1 shows the sociodemographic characteristics of the 263 patients surveyed. Most respondents were female (74%) and educated at the high school level (40%) or some college and above (29%). Approximately 61% of the patients had healthcare coverage through Medicaid or county financial assistance, followed by private insurance or Medicare (28%) and self-pay (6%). Most patients who reported their income had household incomes below 40,000 USD/year (70%). Approximately 59% of all patients preferred being surveyed in Spanish. More patients were born outside the US (69%) in Mexico (n = 131), followed by Honduras (n = 15) and El Salvador (n = 14). Foreign-born patients lived in the US for a median of 23.5 years. Nearly half (47%) of the participants reported prior non-prescription antibiotic use, and over 75% of patients were classified as having "adequate" health literacy levels (Table 1). Overall, 54% professed an intention to use/obtain non-prescription antibiotics if feeling sick from at least one source (Figure 1).

  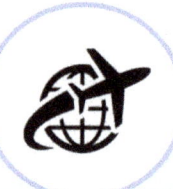 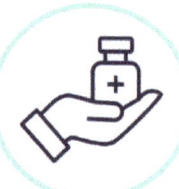 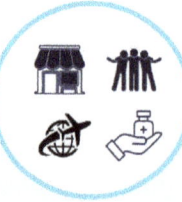

23% of patients intended to use non-prescription antibiotics from stores or markets in the US

25% of patients intended to use non-prescription antibiotics from friends and relatives

27% of patients intended to use non-prescription antibiotics purchased from abroad

47% of patients intended to use non-prescription antibiotics from leftover prescribed course(s)

54% of patients intended to use non-prescription antibiotics from any of these four sources

Figure 1. Prevalence of the intention to use non-prescription antibiotics in Hispanic patients surveyed (N = 263).

3.1.2. Acculturation

Table 2 includes the mean acculturation subscale and Cronbach's alpha scores for language use, TV and media, ethnic and social relations, and the total acculturation (overall, aggregate score). The median total acculturation score for respondents who professed intention for future non-prescription antibiotic use was 2.5/5.0 (IQR 1.6–3.4), and the Cronbach's alpha for the total acculturation was 0.939 (Table 2).

3.1.3. Subjective Norms

Table 3 lists the proportion of patients (N = 263) that reported friends/relatives that used non-prescribed antibiotics or purchased antibiotics from other countries (outside the US). Over 60% of patients reported that some to all of their friends or relatives had used antibiotics without contacting a doctor. About 53% reported that some to most of their friends or relatives have used or purchased non-prescribed antibiotics from another country (Table 3).

3.2. Healthcare System Factors

Appendix C displays the patient-reported barriers to healthcare in the last 12 months. Of the barriers to access, patients frequently expressed that long waiting times (26%), transportation (16%), and the high cost of doctor visits (16%) were problematic, followed by language barriers (8%) and not having a regular doctor (5%) (Appendix C).

3.3. Multivariate Results

Tables 4–8 display the multivariate logistic regression results of patient intentions to use non-prescription antibiotics from each of the four sources and overall.

Table 4. Multivariate results of the intended use of antibiotics from stores or markets in the US.

Intended Use of Antibiotics from Stores or Markets in the United States		
Predictors §	OR (95% CI)	p-Value
Prior Non-prescription Use		
No Prior Use	1 (reference)	1 (reference)
Prior Use	6.26 (3.13–12.51)	<0.001
Barriers To Healthcare Access		
For your medical appointments in the last 12 months, how much of a problem are:		
High cost of doctor visits		
Not a problem	1 (reference)	1 (reference)
A problem	3.1 (1.43–6.69)	0.004

§ The following predictors were not significant in the multivariate model: Acculturation (Language Use Subscale, Media Subscale, and Ethnic Social Relations Subscale); Subjective Norms (How many of your friends or relatives get antibiotics without contacting a doctor? How many of your friends or relatives get antibiotics from another country?); Sociodemographics (Age, Healthcare System, Insurance, Language, Education, and Country of Birth); and Barriers to Healthcare Access (For your medical appointments in the last 12 months, how much of a problem is not having a regular doctor?).

Table 5. Multivariate results of the intended use of antibiotics bought without a prescription from another country.

Intended Use of Antibiotics Bought without a Prescription from Another Country		
Predictors §	OR (95% CI)	p-Value
Acculturation ¶		
Ethnic Social Relations Subscale	0.54 (0.33–0.86)	0.009
Prior Non-prescription Use		
No Prior Use	1 (reference)	1 (reference)
Prior Use	10.49 (5.13–21.46)	<0.001

¶ The Short Acculturation Scale for Hispanics is comprised of three subscales (Language Use, Media, and Ethnic Social Relations). Scores range from 1 (all Latinos/Hispanics) to 5 (all non-Latinos/Hispanics). Higher score indicates higher levels of acculturation [20]. § The following predictors were not significant in the multivariate model: Acculturation (Language Use Subscale and Media Subscale); Subjective Norms (How many of your friends or relatives get antibiotics without contacting a doctor? How many of your friends or relatives get antibiotics from another country?); Sociodemographics (Age, Years lived in the US, and Education); and Barriers to Healthcare Access (For your medical appointments in the last 12 months, how much of a problem are high cost of doctor visits, a language barrier, and not having a regular doctor?).

Table 6. Multivariate results of the intended use of antibiotics from friends and relatives.

Intended Use of Antibiotics from Friends and Relatives		
Predictors §	OR (95% CI)	p-Value
Social Norms		0.054
How many of your friends or relatives get antibiotics from another country?		
None	1 (reference)	1 (reference)
Some	2.52 (0.92–6.93)	0.072
All/Most/About Half	2.51 (1.07–5.85)	0.034
Don't Know/Don't remember	0.95 (0.34–2.64)	0.918
Sociodemographics		
Education		0.017
Less than High School	1 (reference)	1 (reference)
High school or GED	0.53 (0.24–1.19)	0.126
Some College or Above	0.32 (0.14–0.7)	0.004
Prior Non-prescription Use		
No Prior Use	1 (reference)	1 (reference)
Prior Use	10.59 (5.0–22.43)	<0.001
Barriers To Healthcare Access		
For your medical appointments in the last 12 months, how much of a problem are:		
High cost of doctor visits		
Not a problem	1 (reference)	1 (reference)
A problem	3.16 (1.38–7.21)	0.006

§ The following predictors were not significant in the multivariate model: Acculturation (Language Use Subscale, Media Subscale, and Ethnic Social Relations Subscale); Subjective Norms (How many of your friends or relatives get antibiotics without contacting a doctor?); Sociodemographics (Age, Sex, Insurance, and Country of Birth); and Barriers to Healthcare Access (For your medical appointments in the last 12 months, how much of a problem are transportation, a language barrier, and not having a regular doctor?).

Table 7. Multivariate results of the intended use of antibiotics from leftover antibiotic courses.

Intended Use of Antibiotics from Leftover Courses		
Predictors §	OR (95% CI)	p-Value
Prior Non-prescription Use		
No Prior Use	1 (reference)	1 (reference)
Prior Use	7.51 (4.15–13.26)	<0.001
Barriers To Healthcare Access		
For your medical appointments in the last 12 months, how much of a problem are:		
A language barrier		
Not a problem	1 (reference)	1 (reference)
A problem	3.08 (1.03–9.26)	0.006

§ The following predictors were not significant in the multivariate model: Acculturation (Language Use Subscale, Media Subscale, and Ethnic Social Relations Subscale); Subjective Norms (How many of your friends or relatives get antibiotics without contacting a doctor? How many of your friends or relatives get antibiotics from another country?); Sociodemographics (Healthcare System, Insurance, and Country of Birth); and Barriers to Healthcare Access (For your medical appointments in the last 12 months, how much of a problem are long waiting times or the high cost of doctor visits?).

Table 8. Multivariate results of the intended use of antibiotics from any source (US, abroad, friends and relatives, and leftover courses).

Intended Use of Antibiotics from Any Source (US, Abroad, Friends and Relatives, and Leftover Courses)		
Predictors §	OR (95% CI)	p-Value
Acculturation ¶		
Language Use Subscale	0.61 (0.39–0.96)	0.031
Sociodemographics		
Country of Birth		
Born in US	1 (reference)	1 (reference)
Born in other countries ‖	8.47 (2.56–28.02)	<0.001
Prior Non-prescription Use		
No Prior Use	1 (reference)	1 (reference)
Prior Use	12.32 (6.58–23.09)	<0.001

¶ The Short Acculturation Scale for Hispanics is comprised of three subscales (Language Use, Media, and Ethnic Social Relations). Scores range from 1 (all Latinos/Hispanics) to 5 (all non-Latinos/Hispanics). Higher score indicates higher levels of acculturation [20]. ‖ Includes 1 Columbia, 1 Costa Rica, 6 Cuba, 1 Dominican Republic, 14 El Salvador, 6 Guatemala, 15 Honduras, 131 Mexico, 2 Nicaragua, 1 Panama, 1 Peru, and 3 Venezuela (countries are listed in alphabetical order). § The following predictors were not significant and therefore not included in this model: Acculturation (Media Subscale and Ethnic Social Relations Subscale); Social Norms (How many of your friends or relatives get antibiotics from another country?); Sociodemographics (Education); and Barriers to Healthcare Access (For your medical appointments in the last 12 months, how much of a problem are the high cost of doctor visits and a language barrier).

3.3.1. Intended Use of Antibiotics from Stores or Markets in the United States

The high costs of doctor visits (OR 3.1, 95% CI [1.43–6.69], $p = 0.004$) and prior non-prescription antibiotic use (OR 6.3, 95% CI [3.13–12.51], $p < 0.001$) were significant predictors of the intended use of non-prescribed antibiotics purchased in the US. Neither the acculturation subscales nor subjective norms were significant predictors of the intended use of non-prescription antibiotics from stores or markets in the US (Table 4).

3.3.2. Intended Use of Antibiotics Bought without a Prescription from Another Country

Individuals with lower Ethnic and Social Relations subscale scores indicating higher preferences to socialize and associate with other Hispanic individuals had higher odds of the intention to use non-prescribed antibiotics from another country compared to those with higher Ethnic and Social Relations subscale scores (OR 0.54 95% CI [0.33–0.86], $p = 0.009$). In addition, patients with prior non-prescription antibiotic use had 10.5 times higher intended use from other countries (95% CI [5.13–21.46], $p < 0.001$) (Table 5).

3.3.3. Intended Use of Antibiotics from Friends and Relatives

More educated patients with a high school, college, or above education were 68% less likely to use antibiotics from a friend or relative (OR 0.32, 95% CI [0.14–0.70], $p = 0.004$). The high cost of doctor visits during medical appointments was a significant predictor of intention (OR 3.16, 95% CI [1.38–7.21], $p = 0.006$). Patients who reported at least some of their friends or relatives getting non-prescribed antibiotics from other countries had 2.5 times higher odds of intention to use non-prescription antibiotics from friends and relatives (95% CI [1.07–5.85], $p = 0.034$). Additionally, patients with prior non-prescription antibiotic use had over 10.6 times higher odds of intended use from friends and relatives (95% CI [5.0–22.4], $p < 0.001$) (Table 6).

3.3.4. Intended Use of Antibiotics from Leftover Courses

Patients reporting language barriers as a problem during their medical appointment had over three times higher odds of the intention to use antibiotics from leftover prescription sources than patients who did not (95% CI [1.03–9.26], $p = 0.006$). Prior non-prescription antibiotic use was a strong predictor of the intention from leftover courses (OR 7.5 95% CI [4.15–13.26], $p < 0.001$). Neither acculturation subscales nor social norms were significant predictors of the intended use from leftover antibiotic courses (Table 7).

3.3.5. Intended Use of Antibiotics from Any Source (US, Abroad, Friends and Relatives, and Leftover Courses)

Patients born outside the US had 8.5 times higher intention to use non-prescription antibiotics (95% CI [2.56–28.02], $p < 0.001$). Individuals with a higher preference to socialize in Spanish (lower Language Use subscale scores) expressed a higher intention to use non-prescribed antibiotics from any source (overall) in the future compared to those that had a lower preference to socialize in Spanish (higher Language Use subscale scores) (OR 0.61 95% CI [0.39–0.96], $p = 0.031$). Across all sources, prior non-prescription antibiotic use was a very strong predictor of the intention to use non-prescription antibiotics, with patients who reported previous non-prescription antibiotic use having over 12.3 times more intention to use non-prescription antibiotics in the future than patients who did not report prior non-prescription antibiotic use (95% CI [6.6–23.1], $p < 0.001$) (Table 8).

4. Discussion

This study investigated the effects of acculturation and subjective norms on Hispanic individuals' intentions to use antibiotics without a prescription from the following sources: (1) markets in the United States (illegal), (2) other countries, (3) leftovers from previous prescriptions, and (4) friends/relatives. Our results underscore the alarmingly high proportion of Hispanic patients that have reported non-prescription antibiotic use in the past (47%) or intended to use them in the future (54%). We found that lower acculturation (i.e., language use and ethnic and social relations) and subjective norms favoring non-prescription antibiotic use were associated with higher patient intentions to use non-prescription antibiotics in the future. Simultaneously, healthcare system obstacles (i.e., high doctor visit costs and language barriers at the clinics) were associated with higher intended non-prescription antibiotic use.

Individuals of Hispanic heritage are one of the fastest-growing and largest foreign-born ethnic groups and are estimated to represent 25% of the entire US population by 2050 [22]. Across all sources, Hispanic patients born outside the US had nearly 8.5 times more intention to use non-prescribed antibiotics in our study. Similarly, studies in the US, Australia, and the United Kingdom have shown that immigrants may continue to practice self-medication behaviors that were common in their home countries, including using antibiotics without a prescription, for familiarity, convenience, sociocultural, and financial reasons [23–25]. Thus, it is imperative to understand the sociocultural factors that contribute to non-prescription antibiotic use to prevent this potentially unsafe practice. In addition, our results showed that patients' prior non-prescription antibiotic use in the past year was a strong predictor of the intention to use non-prescription antibiotics in the future across all sources (OR 6.26 to 12.32, $p < 0.001$). These collective results pose an opportunity to develop antibiotic stewardship messaging based on the emerging recognition of the role of acculturation and social norms on non-prescription antibiotic use [26]. Healthcare professionals and health educators can promote safe antibiotic use as a social norm during patient–clinician counseling while also providing information on the individual-level harms and risks associated with antibiotic use, including *Clostridium difficile* infection, adverse effects, or drug interactions [26].

This research complements a growing body of literature on the association(s) between acculturation, subjective norms, and health behavior in Hispanic populations. Most prior research on these associations has focused on other health outcomes, including postpartum depression, nutrition, exercise, obesity, and cardiovascular disease (CVD), rather than inappropriate antibiotic use [11,13,27,28]. In this study, acculturation and subjective norms played an important role in Hispanic patients' decisions to use non-prescription antibiotics. Specifically, we found correlations between lower acculturation (language use and ethnic and social relations subscale scores) and higher patient intentions to use non-prescribed antibiotics in the future, which is a novel finding. Similar to our results, a study in Texas found that less acculturated (by generational scores) Hispanic individuals were more likely to purchase antibiotics across the US–Mexico border, presumably without a prescription [11]. The lack of studies exploring the effects of acculturation on antibiotic use warrants further investigation into other ethnic groups across the US and other countries.

Our findings also highlight some specific healthcare barriers, including the high costs of doctor visits, long clinic waits (e.g., to schedule appointments or during doctor visits), and a lack of health insurance or health coverage, which impact Hispanic patients' decisions to use non-prescription antibiotics [3,12]. Patients who experience the burden of high costs during a doctor's visit also had three times higher intended non-prescription antibiotic use from the US and friends and relatives in comparison to patients that did not report high costs during a doctor's visit as a problem. Another study also found that individuals without health insurance were over three times more likely to purchase antibiotics outside the US, presumably without a prescription [11]. In our previous qualitative study, high copayments (for a doctor's visit and subsequent prescription medications), regardless of patients having healthcare coverage, drove some patients to seek informal medical advice and source non-prescription medications using their social networks [12]. Future research should leverage and promote appropriate antibiotic use as a social norm for Hispanic patients with and without healthcare coverage [13,29]. Specifically, engaging Hispanic communities with individuals whom they trust, such as community pharmacists and community healthcare workers (i.e., "promotoras"), in community stewardship interventions can help patients navigate the complex healthcare system [12,29]. A comprehensive approach that improves access to primary care may reduce non-prescription antibiotic use [12,29]. Moreover, antimicrobial stewardship programs administered by multidisciplinary teams [30] in hospital settings have led to beneficial clinical and economic impacts [31,32]. Therefore, implementing stewardship programs in outpatient settings could lead to similar outcomes, such as reducing inappropriate antibiotic use and limiting antimicrobial resistance.

Our study also identified the language barriers that Hispanic individuals may face during a doctor's visit. Patients reporting language barriers as a problem during their healthcare visit reported three times more intended non-prescription antibiotic use from leftover sources. Hispanic patients' negative healthcare experiences can have detrimental consequences. For instance, a recent Pew research study showed that approximately 50% of Hispanic Americans had negative healthcare experiences and difficulties getting needed healthcare, and 30% of Hispanic adults reported having to "speak up" (voice their concerns) to their doctors to get appropriate care [33]. For patients experiencing language barriers or limited English proficiency, this could be particularly discouraging, promoting alternative medical-seeking behaviors [12]. Similarly, compared to bilingual or English-only speaking

Hispanic individuals surveyed, about 81% of the Spanish-speaking adults preferred seeing Spanish-speaking healthcare providers [33]. Addressing language barriers with language-concordant healthcare initiatives is important to mitigate communication pitfalls in medical care and has been shown to improve health outcomes [34].

Our study has certain limitations. First, our study does not compare Hispanic ethnic subgroups, and these communities encompass diverse cultures, backgrounds, and experiences. However, according to the US census and the Texas Demographics Center, Mexicans are the largest ethnic subgroup, representing 62% of all Hispanic people living in the US and 83% of all Hispanic people in Texas; thus, the Hispanic patients in this survey may represent the largest US Hispanic demographic subgroup [35,36]. Second, we did not account for immigration history or generational status (e.g., we did not ask patients about their parents' or grandparents' ancestry or when people first came to the US). To adjust for this, we calculated the median years lived in the US, but this factor was not a significant predictor of patient intentions to use non-prescription antibiotics. Third, the SASH scale may not account for all aspects of acculturation. Additionally, the SASH scale does not have any measures regarding the cultural context surrounding where study participants received their care (e.g., clinics and pharmacies). Nevertheless, the SASH scale has been found to have both high internal consistency and validity in measuring the language, media, and ethnic and social relations aspects of acculturation in many studies across a wide array of Hispanic subgroups [13,20,28]. Lastly, a social desirability response bias may have occurred despite our best efforts to phrase questions neutrally. Thus, the true prevalence rate of non-prescription antibiotic use may be underestimated, because patients may have had concerns about the legality or otherwise disclosing these behaviors or participating in the survey.

In summary, our results indicate that lower acculturation and subjective norms favoring non-prescription antibiotic use were associated with higher Hispanic patient intentions to use non-prescription antibiotics in the future. In addition, healthcare system obstacles, such as the high costs of doctor visits and language barriers, were associated with a higher intended non-prescription antibiotic use among Hispanic patients.

In conclusion, this study adds value to the scientific literature on the association(s) between acculturation, subjective norms, and health behavior in Hispanic populations. Reducing non-prescription antibiotic use in Hispanic communities in the US will require a multifaceted approach considering the sociocultural and healthcare barriers that influence non-prescription antibiotic use. Future stewardship interventions can leverage social and cultural factors to promote appropriate antibiotic use normative behaviors in Hispanic communities to reduce adverse health effects and antimicrobial resistance.

Author Contributions: Conceptualization, L.A.L., L.G., B.W.T., S.N. and M.K.P.-O.; methodology, L.A.L. and L.G.; software, L.A.L.; validation, L.A.L.; formal analysis, L.A.L.; investigation, L.A.L.; resources, K.O. and J.S.; data curation, K.O., J.S. and O.A.; writing—original draft preparation, L.A.L.; writing—review and editing, L.A.L., L.G., B.W.T., S.N., R.Z., K.O., J.S. and M.K.P.-O.; visualization, L.A.L. and K.O.; supervision, L.G.; project administration, L.G., B.W.T., J.S. and K.O.; and funding acquisition, L.G., R.Z. and B.W.T. All authors have read and agreed to the published version of the manuscript.

Funding: This work was supported by grant number R01HS026901 from the Agency for Healthcare Research and Quality. The content is solely the responsibility of the authors and does not necessarily represent the official views of the Agency for Healthcare Research and Quality. L.L.'s work was supported by the Ruth L. Kirschstein National Research Service Award (NRSA T-32 6T32HC10031). B.W.T.'s work was supported in part by the U.S. Department of Veterans Affairs Health Services Research and Development Service (grant no. CIN 13-413) at the Center for Innovations in Quality, Effectiveness, and Safety. The contents presented herein do not represent the views of the U.S. Department of Veterans Affairs or the U.S. government.

Institutional Review Board Statement: The study was conducted in accordance with the Declaration of Helsinki and approved by the Institutional Review Board (or Ethics Committee) of Baylor College of Medicine and Affiliated Hospitals (protocol H-45709).

Informed Consent Statement: Informed consent was obtained from all subjects involved in the study.

Data Availability Statement: The data presented in this study are available on request from the corresponding author. The data are not publicly available due to privacy and ethical restrictions.

Conflicts of Interest: B.W.T. reports grants or contracts from the VA Health Services Research & Development, Agency for Healthcare Research and Quality R18, Craig H. Neilson Foundation, Genentech, and Peptilogics, Inc.; payment from George Washington ID Board for a Review Course; travel support for meeting attendance from the VA Office of Research & Development and the Infectious Diseases Society of America; and an unpaid role on a DSMB for CSP #2004. L.G. reports grants or contracts from the Agency for Healthcare Research and Quality (AHRQ) R18, Craig H. Neilsen Foundation, and a research education grant (1R25AA028203-01) from the National Institute on Alcohol Abuse and Alcoholism Award. All other authors report no potential conflicts.

Appendix A. Survey Questions

Sociodemographic Questions:

1. How old are you? ____
2. Sex
   - ☐ Male
   - ☐ Female
   - ☐ Other: _____
3. Do you consider yourself to be Hispanic/Latino?
   - ☐ Yes
   - ☐ No
4. Which category best describes your race?
   - ☐ Black or African American
   - ☐ White
   - ☐ Declined
   - ☐ Other, please specify: _____
5. What is the highest level of education you have completed?
   - ☐ Never attended school
   - ☐ Grades 1 through 5 (Elementary)
   - ☐ Grades 6 through 8 (Middle School)
   - ☐ Grades 9 through 11 (Some High School)
   - ☐ Grades 12 or GED (High School graduate)
   - ☐ College 1 year to 3 years (Some college or technical school)
   - ☐ College 4 years or more (College graduate)
6. What was the total annual income in your household in the past year?
   - ☐ Less than $20,000
   - ☐ $20,000 or more but less than $40,000
   - ☐ $40,000 or more but less than $60,000
   - ☐ $60,000 or more but less than $100,000
   - ☐ More than $100,000
   - ☐ Don't know/prefer not to say
7. Which of the following health insurance plans do you have? (Mark all that apply)
   - ☐ Medicaid
   - ☐ Medicare
   - ☐ Harris Health System/Gold card* *County Financial Assistance program*
   - ☐ None
   - ☐ Other: _____
8. Where were you born?
   - ☐ United States

☐ Other, please specify: _____

9. How many years have you lived in the United States? _____

Previous use of antibiotics without a prescription:

1. When was your most recent experience with taking an antibiotic without contacting a doctor/dentist/nurse? (Please include occasions where you took leftover antibiotics)
    ☐ Never
    ☐ Less than 6 months ago
    ☐ Between 6 and 12 months ago
    ☐ More than 12 months but less than 2 years ago
    ☐ At least 2 years ago
    ☐ I don't remember

Intention to use antibiotics without a prescription:

1. If you were feeling sick, would you take antibiotics in the following situations without contacting a doctor/nurse/dentist/clinic?

	Yes	No	Don't Know
You can buy antibiotics without a prescription in the United States.			
You can buy antibiotics without a prescription in another country. If yes, please specify:			
Friends/relatives give you antibiotics.			
You have leftover antibiotics from a previous prescription.			

Social Norms Questions:

1. How many of your friends or relatives use antibiotics without contacting a doctor? For example: Do they use leftover antibiotics from a previous prescription, use antibiotics they bought at a flea market, or use antibiotics they bought on the Internet?
    ☐ All
    ☐ Most
    ☐ About half
    ☐ Some
    ☐ None
    ☐ Don't remember/Don't know

2. How many of your friends or relatives get antibiotics from another country? Please specify the country/countries:
    ☐ Most
    ☐ About half
    ☐ Some
    ☐ None
    ☐ Don't remember/ Don't know

Brief Health Literacy Screen measure:

1. How often do you have problems learning about your medical condition because of difficulty understanding written information?
    ☐ Never
    ☐ Occasionally
    ☐ Sometimes
    ☐ Often
    ☐ Always

2. How confident are you filling out medical forms by yourself?
    ☐ Extremely
    ☐ Quite a bit

☐ Somewhat
☐ A little bit
☐ Not at all

3. How often do you have someone help you read clinic or hospital materials?
☐ Never
☐ Occasionally
☐ Sometimes
☐ Often
☐ Always

Barriers to care questions specific to the patient population of the safety-net healthcare system:

1. For your medical appointments in the last 12 months, how much of a problem is each of the following for you?

	Not a problem	Minor problem	Major problem	Not applicable
1(a) Transportation				
1(b) Long waiting times in the clinic				
1(c) High cost of doctor visit				
1(d) Language barrier				
1(e) Not having a regular doctor				

Acculturation Questions

The following questions have been approved by previous research studies. This set of questions is used to measure the level at which an individual has adopted the traits and characteristics shared by a society. The Short Acculturation Scale for Hispanics is comprised of three subscales (Language Use, Media, and Ethnic Social Relations). Scores range from 1 (all Latinos/Hispanics)–5 (all non-Latinos/Hispanics).

		Only Spanish	Spanish better than English	Both equally	English better than Spanish	Only English
1.	In general, what language(s) do you read and speak?					
2.	What was the language you used as a child?					
3.	What language(s) do you usually speak at home?					
4.	In what language do you usually think?					
5.	What language do you usually speak with your friends?					
6.	In what language(s) are the TV programs you usually watch?					
7.	What language(s) are the radio programs you usually listen to?					
8.	In general, in what language(s) are the movies, TV and radio programs you prefer to watch and listen to?					
9.	Your close friends are:					
10.	You prefer going to social gatherings/parties at which people are:					
11.	The persons you visit or who visit you are:					
12.	If you could choose your children's friends, you would want them to be:					

Appendix B. Short Acculturation Scale for Hispanics Reliability Statistics

Acculturation Scores	Median (IQR‡)	Corrected Cronbach's Alpha †	If item Deleted Cronbach's Alpha †
Short Acculturation Scale for Hispanics * (n = 259)			
Language Use Subscale Score	2.00 (1.20–3.20)	0.939	0.939
Individual Language Subscale Questions			
In general, what language(s) do you read and speak?	2.00 (2.00–3.00)	0.900	0.916
What was the language you used as a child?	1.00 (1.00–2.00)	0.750	0.939
What language(s) do you usually speak at home?	2.00 (1.00–4.00)	0.813	0.929
In what language do you usually think?	2.00 (1.00–4.00)	0.879	0.917
What language do you usually speak with your friends?	2.00 (1.00–4.00)	0.862	0.920
Media Subscale Score	3.00 (1.33–4.00)	0.969	0.969
Individual Media Subscale Questions			
In what language(s) are the TV programs you usually watch?	3.00 (1.00–4.00)	0.953	0.940
What language(s) are the radio programs you usually listen to?	3.00 (1.00–4.00)	0.910	0.971
In general, in what language(s) are the movies, TV and radio programs you prefer to watch and listen to?	3.00 (1.00–4.00)	0.938	0.951
Ethnic Social Relations Subscale Score †	2.33 (2.00–3.00)	0.754	0.754
Individual Ethnic Social Relation Questions			
Your close friends are:	2.00 (2.00–3.00)	0.709	0.598
You prefer going to social gatherings/parties at which people are:	3.00 (2.00–3.00)	0.593	0.673
The persons you visit or who visit you are:	2.00 (2.00–3.00)	0.709	0.598
If you could choose your children's friends, you would want them to be: †	3.00 (3.00–3.00)	0.263	0.817
(n = 254)			
Acculturation Subscale Aggregate Score †	2.44 (1.67–3.29)		0.939

* The Short Acculturation Scale for Hispanics is comprised of three subscales (Language Use, Media, and Ethnic Social Relations). Scores range from 1 (Only Spanish) to 5 (Only English) for the Language and Media Subscales and 1 (all Latinos/Hispanics) to 5 (all non Latinos/Hispanics) for the Ethnic Social Relations subscale. A higher score indicates higher levels of acculturation [20]. ‡ Interquartile Range. † Questions relating to each subscale score were included following the Marin et al. method that uses the principal components analysis (PCA) [20]. The PCA revealed the questions that accurately described each subscore (e.g., language, television and media, and social acculturation subscores). All questions with interitem correlation (IC) scores above 0.5 (except question 12, IC = 0.3) were included in the development of the subscores with the highest reliability (Cronbach's alpha > 0.8).

Appendix C. Patient Reported Barriers to Healthcare Access and Patient-Doctor Communication (n = 262)

	Total No. (%)
Barriers To Healthcare Access In The Last 12 Months (n = 262 *)	
For your medical appointments in the last 12 months, how much of a problem is transportation?	
Not a problem	220 (83.7)
A problem	42 (15.9)
For your medical appointments in the last 12 months, how much of a problem is long waiting times?	
Not a problem	195 (74.1)
A problem	67 (25.5)
For your medical appointments in the last 12 months, how much of a problem is high cost of doctor visits?	
Not a problem	220 (83.7)
A problem	42 (16.0)
For your medical appointments in the last 12 months, how much of a problem is a language barrier.	
Not a problem	242 (92.0)
A problem	20 (7.6)
For your medical appointments in the last 12 months, how much of a problem is not having a regular doctor?	
Not a problem	250 (95.4)
A problem	12 (4.6)

* One patient did not answer these questions.

Appendix D. Univariate Regression Results

	Bought without a Prescription in the US		From Another Country		From Friends/Relatives		From Leftover		Overall Intended Use	
Predictor	OR (95% CI)	p-Value *	OR (95% CI)	p-Value *	OR (95% CI)	p-Value *	OR (95% CI)	p-Value *	OR (95% CI)	p-Value *
Age (y)	0.97 (0.95–0.10)	**0.015**	0.98 (0.96–1.00)	**0.073**	0.98 (0.96–1.00)	**0.056**	0.10 (0.98–1.02)	0.710	0.99 (0.97–1.01)	0.167
Sex										
Female	1 (reference)		1 (reference)		1 (reference)		1 (reference)		1 (reference)	
Male	0.97 (0.51–1.87)	0.931	1.04 (0.56–1.94)	0.908	0.57 (0.31–1.04)	**0.068**	0.82 (0.48–1.43)	0.489	0.76 (0.43–1.32)	0.328
Education										
Less than high school	1 (reference)		1 (reference)		1 (reference)		1 (reference)		1 (reference)	
High school or GED	1.42 (0.68–2.97)	0.352	0.91 (0.46–1.80)	0.783	0.82 (0.40–1.65)	0.569	1.28 (0.72–2.29)	0.398	1.31 (0.74–2.34)	0.358
Some college and above	2.21 (1.04–4.71)	**0.039**	1.80 (0.90–3.58)	**0.094**	1.92 (0.96–3.86)	**0.065**	1.30 (0.69–2.43)	0.414	1.27 (0.68–2.38)	0.450
Healthcare System										
Public	1 (reference)		1 (reference)		1 (reference)		1 (reference)		1 (reference)	
Private	0.32 (0.11–0.94)	**0.038**	0.74 (0.34–1.65)	0.463	0.57 (0.24–1.35)	0.202	0.22 (0.10–0.50)	**<0.001**	0.33 (0.16–0.67)	**0.002**
Insurance										
Private or Medicare	1 (reference)		1 (reference)		1 (reference)		1 (reference)		1 (reference)	
Medicaid or county assistance program §	2.20 (1.07–4.53)	**0.032**	1.33 (0.70–2.50)	0.385	1.85 (0.94–3.68)	**0.077**	1.35 (0.78–2.33)	0.285	1.30 (0.75–2.24)	0.350
Self-pay	0.38 (0.05–3.19)	0.374	1.12 (0.32–3.92)	0.862	1.56 (0.44–5.63)	0.493	0.08 (0.01–0.66)	**0.019**	0.43 (0.14–1.36)	0.151

Predictor	Univariate Analysis								Overall Intended Use	
	Bought without a Prescription in the US		From Another Country		From Friends/Relatives		From Leftover			
	OR (95% CI)	p-Value *	OR (95% CI)	p-Value *	OR (95% CI)	p-Value *	OR (95% CI)	p-Value *	OR (95% CI)	p-Value *
Country of birth										
Born in the US	1 (reference)		1 (reference)		1 (reference)		1 (reference)		1 (reference)	
Born in other countries ‖	1.71 (0.94–3.11)	0.081	1.14 (0.63–2.05)	0.663	1.68 (0.94–3.01)	0.082	2.19 (1.28–3.73)	0.004	2.45 (1.41–4.26)	**0.002**
Years Lived in the USA (n = 182)	1.00 (0.99–1.02)	0.646	0.98 (0.97–1.00)	0.077	1.00 (0.98–1.01)	0.666	1.02 (1.00–1.03)	0.030	1.01 (1.00–1.03)	0.184
Survey language										
English	1 (reference)		1 (reference)		1 (reference)		1 (reference)		1 (reference)	
Spanish	1.75 (0.98–3.13)	0.059	1.02 (0.59–1.18)	0.942	1.27 (0.72–2.23)	0.403	1.78 (1.08–2.92)	0.023	1.81 (1.10–3.00)	**0.020**
Prior Non-Prescription Antibiotic Use										
No Prior Use	1 (reference)		1 (reference)		1 (reference)		1 (reference)		1 (reference)	
Prior Use	0.17 (0.08–0.33)	<0.001	0.11 (0.53–0.21)	<0.001	0.12 (0.06–0.24)	<0.001	0.13 (0.07–0.22)	<0.001	0.09 (0.05–0.15)	**<0.001**
Acculturation Scale ¶										
Language Use Subscale	1.18 (0.94–1.50)	0.161	0.93 (0.74–1.18)	0.561	1.05 (0.83–1.32)	0.686	1.26 (1.02–1.55)	0.029	1.24 (1.00–1.53)	**0.047**
Media Subscale	1.14 (0.93–1.40)	0.209	0.97 (0.80–1.18)	0.767	1.10 (0.91–1.35)	0.328	1.19 (1.00–1.42)	0.052	1.12 (0.94–1.34)	0.189
Ethnic Social Relations Subscale	0.80 (0.53–1.22)	0.295	0.68 (0.45–1.01)	0.057	0.82 (0.54–1.23)	0.336	1.08 (0.75–1.54)	0.682	1.00 (0.70–1.43)	0.996
Total Acculturation	1.16 (0.86–1.57)	0.340	0.88 (0.66–1.18)	0.400	1.07 (0.80–1.43)	0.674	1.30 (1.00–1.68)	0.050	1.21 (0.94–1.57)	0.141
Social Norms Questions										
How many of your friends or relatives use antibiotics without contacting a doctor?										
None	1 (reference)		1 (reference)		1 (reference)		1 (reference)		1 (reference)	
Don't Remember/Don't Know	2.07 (0.69–6.19)	0.193	2.02 (0.77–5.33)	0.155	1.20 (0.48–3.01)	0.693	1.10 (0.49–2.48)	0.817	0.93 (0.42–2.06)	0.853
All/Most/About half	2.01 (0.66–6.12)	0.220	1.75 (0.65–4.73)	0.269	2.27 (0.94–5.43)	0.067	1.53 (0.67–3.50)	0.309	1.20 (0.56–2.86)	0.580
Some	2.26 (0.80–6.42)	0.126	1.52 (0.59–3.87)	0.384	2.00 (0.96–4.19)	0.066	1.66 (0.78–3.56)	0.190	1.11 (0.52–2.34)	0.795
How many of your friends or relatives get antibiotics from another country?										
None	1 (reference)		1 (reference)		1 (reference)		1 (reference)		1 (reference)	
Don't Remember/Don't Know	1.10 (0.44–2.72)	0.838	1.89 (0.82–4.39)	0.138	1.41 (0.49–4.04)	0.523	1.01 (0.49–2.09)	0.974	1.07 (0.52–2.21)	0.853
All / Most / About half	1.66 (0.69–4.02)	0.262	1.86 (0.78–4.45)	0.165	2.29 (0.81–6.42)	0.116	1.19 (0.56–2.52)	0.657	1.32 (0.62–2.81)	0.478
Some	1.4 (0.67–2.96)	0.365	1.74 (0.84–3.61)	0.137	2.13 (0.80–5.66)	0.128	1.22 (0.66–2.23)	0.526	1.19 (0.65–2.18)	0.575
Barriers To Healthcare Access In The Last 12 Months										
For your medical appointments in the last 12 months, how much of a problem is [ ]?										
Transportation										
Not a problem	1 (reference)		1 (reference)		1 (reference)		1 (reference)		1 (reference)	
A problem	0.61 (0.29–1.26)	0.178	0.78 (0.38–1.60)	0.499	0.62 (0.30–1.26)	0.187	0.79 (0.41–1.52)	0.475	0.62 (0.31–1.23)	0.171
Long waiting times										
Not a problem	1 (reference)		1 (reference)		1 (reference)		1 (reference)		1 (reference)	
A problem	0.75 (0.39–1.42)	0.372	0.99 (0.53–1.85)	0.975	0.99 (0.52–1.87)	0.968	1.47 (0.83–2.58)	0.183	1.14 (0.65–1.98)	0.656
High cost of doctor visits										
Not a problem	1 (reference)		1 (reference)		1 (reference)		1 (reference)		1 (reference)	
A problem	0.36 (0.18–0.72)	**0.004**	0.53 (0.26–1.06)	0.072	0.42 (0.21–0.84)	0.015	0.63 (0.32–1.22)	0.167	0.62 (0.31–1.23)	0.171
A language barrier										
Not a problem	1 (reference)		1 (reference)		1 (reference)		1 (reference)		1 (reference)	
A problem	0.73 (0.25–2.13)	0.568	0.41 (0.16–1.04)	0.061	0.51 (0.19–1.34)	0.172	0.33 (0.12–0.90)	0.031	0.35 (0.12–0.99)	**0.049**
Not having a regular doctor										
Not a problem	1 (reference)		1 (reference)		1 (reference)		1 (reference)		1 (reference)	
A problem	2.19 (0.87–5.52)	0.096	1.81 (0.75–4.38)	0.191	3.52 (1.47–8.46)	0.005	0.95 (0.41–2.20)	0.207	1.00 (0.43–2.32)	0.995
Health Literacy										
Adequate health literacy ‡	1 (reference)		1 (reference)		1 (reference)		1 (reference)		1 (reference)	
Inadequate health literacy ‡	1.10 (0.56–2.17)	0.778	0.93 (0.50–1.74)	0.821	0.93 (0.49–1.76)	0.821	1.15 (0.65–2.01)	0.637	1.21 (0.69–2.13)	0.502

* Results shown in boldface type have a p-value of <0.2 in the univariate analyses and were thus included in the multivariate analysis. ¶ The Short Acculturation Scale for Hispanics is comprised of three subscales (Language Use, Media, and Ethnic Social Relations). Scores range from 1 (all non-Latinos/Hispanics) to 5 (all Latinos/Hispanics). Higher score indicates higher levels of acculturation [20]. § County Financial Assistance Program: Includes those who have benefits from the county, allowing access to public clinic providers at either very low cost or no cost. ‖ Includes 1 Columbia, 1 Costa Rica, 6 Cuba, 1 Dominican Republic, 14 El Salvador, 6 Guatemala, 15 Honduras, 131 Mexico, 2 Nicaragua, 1 Panama, 1 Peru, and 3 Venezuela (countries are listed in alphabetical order). ‡ Calculated using the three questions from the Brief Health literacy Screen measure [18,19].

References

1. Morgan, D.J.; Okeke, I.N.; Laxminarayan, R.; Perencevich, E.N.; Weisenberg, S. Non-prescription antimicrobial use worldwide: A systematic review. *Lancet Infect. Dis.* **2011**, *11*, 692–701. [CrossRef] [PubMed]
2. Sun, R.; Yao, T.; Zhou, X.; Harbarth, S.; Lin, L. Non-biomedical factors affecting antibiotic use in the community: A mixed-methods systematic review and meta-analysis. *Clin. Microbiol. Infect.* **2022**, *28*, 345–354. [CrossRef] [PubMed]
3. Grigoryan, L.; Paasche-Orlow, M.K.; Alquicira, O.; Laytner, L.; Schlueter, M.; Street, R.L.; Salinas, J.; Barning, K.; Mahmood, H.; Porter, T.W.; et al. Antibiotic use without a Prescription: A multi-site Survey of Patient, Health System, and Encounter Characteristics. *Clin. Infect. Dis.* **2023**, *77*, 510–517. [CrossRef] [PubMed]
4. Blumenthal, K.G.; Peter, J.G.; Trubiano, J.A.; Phillips, E.J. Antibiotic allergy. *Lancet* **2019**, *393*, 183–198. [CrossRef]
5. Yang, L.; Bajinka, O.; Jarju, P.O.; Tan, Y.; Taal, A.M.; Ozdemir, G. The varying effects of antibiotics on gut microbiota. *AMB Express* **2021**, *11*, 116. [CrossRef]
6. WHO. Antimicrobial Resistance. Available online: https://www.who.int/news-room/fact-sheets/detail/antimicrobial-resistance (accessed on 13 September 2022).
7. Ahmed, I.; King, R.; Akter, S.; Akter, R.; Aggarwal, V.R. Determinants of antibiotic self-medication: A systematic review and meta-analysis. *Res. Social. Adm. Pharm.* **2023**, *19*, 1007–1017. [CrossRef]
8. Anderson, A. Antibiotic Self-Medication and Antibiotic Resistance: Multilevel Regression Analysis of Repeat Cross-Sectional Survey Data in Europe. *REGION* **2021**, *8*, 121–145. [CrossRef]
9. Grigoryan, L.; Germanos, G.; Zoorob, R.; Juneja, S.; Raphael, J.L.; Paasche-Orlow, M.K.; Trautner, B.W. Use of Antibiotics Without a Prescription in the U.S. Population: A Scoping Review. *Ann. Intern. Med.* **2019**, *171*, 257–263. [CrossRef]
10. Watkins, L.K.F.; Sanchez, G.V.; Albert, A.P.; Roberts, R.M.; Hicks, L.A. Knowledge and attitudes regarding antibiotic use among adult consumers, adult Hispanic consumers, and health care providers—United States, 2012–2013. *Morb. Mortal. Wkly. Rep.* **2015**, *64*, 767. [CrossRef]
11. Essigmann, H.T.; Aguilar, D.A.; Perkison, W.B.; Bay, K.G.; Deaton, M.R.; Brown, S.A.; Hanis, C.L.; Brown, E.L. Epidemiology of Antibiotic Use and Drivers of Cross-Border Procurement in a Mexican American Border Community. *Front. Public. Health* **2022**, *10*, 832266. [CrossRef]
12. Laytner, L.; Chen, P.; Nash, S.; Paasche-Orlow, M.K.; Street, R.; Zoorob, R.; Trautner, B.; Grigoryan, L. Perspectives on Non-Prescription Antibiotic Use among Hispanic Patients in the Houston Metroplex. *J. Am. Board. Fam. Med.* **2023**, *36*, 390–404. [CrossRef]
13. Abraído-Lanza, A.F.; Echeverría, S.E.; Flórez, K.R. Latino Immigrants, Acculturation, and Health: Promising New Directions in Research. *Annu. Rev. Public Health* **2016**, *37*, 219–236. [CrossRef] [PubMed]
14. Abraído-Lanza, A.F.; Armbrister, A.N.; Flórez, K.R.; Aguirre, A.N. Toward a theory-driven model of acculturation in public health research. *Am. J. Public. Health* **2006**, *96*, 1342–1346. [CrossRef]
15. Ham, M.; Jeger, M.; Frajman Ivković, A. The role of subjective norms in forming the intention to purchase green food. *Econ. Res.-Ekon. Istraživanja* **2015**, *28*, 738–748. [CrossRef]
16. Zoorob, R.; Grigoryan, L.; Nash, S.; Trautner, B.W. Nonprescription Antimicrobial Use in a Primary Care Population in the United States. *Antimicrob. Agents Chemother.* **2016**, *60*, 5527–5532. [CrossRef]
17. Kilbourne, A.M.; Switzer, G.; Hyman, K.; Crowley-Matoka, M.; Fine, M.J. Advancing health disparities research within the health care system: A conceptual framework. *Am. J. Public. Health* **2006**, *96*, 2113–2121. [CrossRef]
18. Chew, L.D.; Bradley, K.A.; Boyko, E.J. Brief questions to identify patients with inadequate health literacy. *Fam. Med.* **2004**, *36*, 588–594.
19. Chew, L.D.; Griffin, J.M.; Partin, M.R.; Noorbaloochi, S.; Grill, J.P.; Snyder, A.; Bradley, K.A.; Nugent, S.M.; Baines, A.D.; Vanryn, M. Validation of screening questions for limited health literacy in a large VA outpatient population. *J. Gen. Intern. Med.* **2008**, *23*, 561–566. [CrossRef] [PubMed]
20. Marin, G.; Sabogal, F.; Marin, B.V.; Otero-Sabogal, R.; Perez-Stable, E.J. Development of a Short Acculturation Scale for Hispanics. *Hisp. J. Behav. Sci.* **1987**, *9*, 183–205. [CrossRef]
21. IBM Corp. *IBM SPSS Statistics for Windows, Version 28.0*; IBM Corp: Armonk, NY, USA, 2021.
22. Zong, J. A Mosaic, Not a Monolith: A Profile of the U.S. Latino Population, 2000–2020. Available online: https://latino.ucla.edu/research/latino-population-2000-2020/#:~:text=Since%20then%2C%20Latinos%20have%20been,population%20(see%20Figure%201) (accessed on 12 June 2023).
23. Sanchez, J. Self-Medication Practices among a Sample of Latino Migrant Workers in South Florida. *Front. Public Health* **2014**, *2*, 108. [CrossRef]
24. Hu, J.; Wang, Z. Non-prescribed antibiotic use and general practitioner service utilisation among Chinese migrants in Australia. *Aust. J. Prim. Health* **2016**, *22*, 434–439. [CrossRef] [PubMed]
25. Lindenmeyer, A.; Redwood, S.; Griffith, L.; Ahmed, S.; Phillimore, J. Recent migrants' perspectives on antibiotic use and prescribing in primary care: A qualitative study. *Br. J. Gen. Pract.* **2016**, *66*, e802–e809. [CrossRef]
26. Miller, B.J.; Carson, K.A.; Keller, S. Educating Patients on Unnecessary Antibiotics: Personalizing Potential Harm Aids Patient Understanding. *J. Am. Board. Fam. Med.* **2020**, *33*, 969–977. [CrossRef]

27. Liyanage-Don, N.A.; Cornelius, T.; Romero, E.K.; Alcantara, C.; Kronish, I.M. Association of Hispanic ethnicity and linguistic acculturation with cardiovascular medication adherence in patients with suspected acute coronary syndrome. *Prev. Med. Rep.* **2021**, *23*, 101455. [CrossRef] [PubMed]
28. Lara, M.; Gamboa, C.; Kahramanian, M.I.; Morales, L.S.; Bautista, D.E. Acculturation and Latino health in the United States: A review of the literature and its sociopolitical context. *Annu. Rev. Public. Health* **2005**, *26*, 367–397. [CrossRef]
29. Rodriguez-Alcalá, M.E.; Qin, H.; Jeanetta, S. The Role of Acculturation and Social Capital in Access to Health Care: A Meta-study on Hispanics in the US. *J. Community Health* **2019**, *44*, 1224–1252. [CrossRef]
30. MacDougall, C.; Polk, R.E. Antimicrobial stewardship programs in health care systems. *Clin. Microbiol. Rev.* **2005**, *18*, 638–656. [CrossRef]
31. Nathwani, D.; Varghese, D.; Stephens, J.; Ansari, W.; Martin, S.; Charbonneau, C. Value of hospital antimicrobial stewardship programs [ASPs]: A systematic review. *Antimicrob. Resist. Infect. Control* **2019**, *8*, 35. [CrossRef] [PubMed]
32. Albano, G.D.; Midiri, M.; Zerbo, S.; Matteini, E.; Passavanti, G.; Curcio, R.; Curreri, L.; Albano, S.; Argo, A.; Cadelo, M. Implementation of A Year-Long Antimicrobial Stewardship Program in A 227-Bed Community Hospital in Southern Italy. *Int. J. Environ. Res. Public Health* **2023**, *20*, 996. [CrossRef] [PubMed]
33. Cary, F.; Lopez, M.H. *Hispanic Americans' Trust in and Engagement with Science*; PEW Research Center: Washington, DC, USA, 2022.
34. Diamond, L.; Izquierdo, K.; Canfield, D.; Matsoukas, K.; Gany, F. A Systematic Review of the Impact of Patient–Physician Non-English Language Concordance on Quality of Care and Outcomes. *J. Gen. Intern. Med.* **2019**, *34*, 1591–1606. [CrossRef]
35. Office of Minority Health (OMH). Profile: Hispanic/Latino Americans. Available online: https://minorityhealth.hhs.gov/omh/browse.aspx?lvl=3&lvlid=64#:~:text=This%20group%20represents%2018.9%20percent,group%20after%20non%2DHispanic%20whites (accessed on 11 July 2023).
36. Texas Demographics Center (TDC). Hispanic Heritage Month: Hispanic Americans in Texas. Available online: https://demographics.texas.gov/Infographics/2021/HispanicHeritage (accessed on 11 July 2023).

Disclaimer/Publisher's Note: The statements, opinions and data contained in all publications are solely those of the individual author(s) and contributor(s) and not of MDPI and/or the editor(s). MDPI and/or the editor(s) disclaim responsibility for any injury to people or property resulting from any ideas, methods, instructions or products referred to in the content.

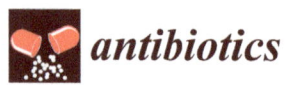

Article

Antibiotic Use in Pregnancy: A Global Survey on Antibiotic Prescription Practices in Antenatal Care

Carlotta Gamberini [1,†], Sabine Donders [1,†], Salwan Al-Nasiry [2], Alena Kamenshchikova [3,†] and Elena Ambrosino [1,*,†]

1. Institute for Public Health Genomics (IPHG), Department of Genetics and Cell Biology, Research School GROW for Oncology and Reproduction, Faculty of Health, Medicine & Life Sciences, Maastricht University, 6229 ER Maastricht, The Netherlands; c.gamberini@maastrichtuniversity.nl (C.G.); spl.donders@alumni.maastrichtuniversity.nl (S.D.)
2. Department of Obstetrics and Gynecology, Research School GROW for Oncology and Reproduction, Maastricht University Medical Centre+, 6229 HX Maastricht, The Netherlands; salwan.alnasiry@mumc.nl
3. Department of Health, Ethics and Society, School of Public Health and Primary Care, Maastricht University, 6229 ER Maastricht, The Netherlands; a.kamenshchikova@maastrichtuniversity.nl
* Correspondence: e.ambrosino@maastrichtuniversity.nl
† These authors contributed equally to this work.

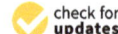

Citation: Gamberini, C.; Donders, S.; Al-Nasiry, S.; Kamenshchikova, A.; Ambrosino, E. Antibiotic Use in Pregnancy: A Global Survey on Antibiotic Prescription Practices in Antenatal Care. *Antibiotics* **2023**, *12*, 831. https://doi.org/10.3390/antibiotics12050831

Academic Editors: Masafumi Seki, Juan Manuel Vázquez-Lago, Ana Estany-Gestal and Angel Salgado-Barreira

Received: 3 April 2023
Revised: 25 April 2023
Accepted: 26 April 2023
Published: 29 April 2023

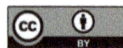

Copyright: © 2023 by the authors. Licensee MDPI, Basel, Switzerland. This article is an open access article distributed under the terms and conditions of the Creative Commons Attribution (CC BY) license (https:// creativecommons.org/licenses/by/ 4.0/).

Abstract: Antibiotic prescription and use practices in the antenatal care setting varies across countries and populations and has the potential to significantly contribute to the global spread of antibiotic resistance. This study aims to explore how healthcare practitioners make decisions about antibiotic prescriptions for pregnant women and what factors play a role in this process. A cross-sectional exploratory survey consisting of 23 questions, including 4 free-text and 19 multiple-choice questions, was distributed online. Quantitative data were collected through multiple-choice questions and was used to identify the most common infections diagnosed and the type of antibiotics prescribed. Qualitative data were gathered through free-text answers to identify gaps, challenges, and suggestions, and the data were analyzed using thematic analysis. A total of 137 complete surveys mostly from gynecologists/obstetricians from 22 different countries were included in the analysis. Overall, national and international clinical guidelines and hospital guidelines/protocols were the most frequently used sources of information. This study highlights the crucial role of laboratory results and guidelines at different levels and emphasizes region-specific challenges and recommendations. These findings underscore the pressing need for tailored interventions to support antibiotic prescribers in their decision-making practice and to address emerging resistance.

Keywords: antibiotic resistance; antenatal care; antibiotic prescription practices

1. Introduction

Antibiotic use in pregnancy has been globally on the rise in the last decade [1], including during pregnancy [2]. According to previous studies, antibiotics account for approximately 80% of drug prescriptions during pregnancy, with an estimated 20–40% of expectant mothers receiving them across different countries in recent years [3]. Antibiotics are powerful drugs used to treat infections; as such, they have contributed to the saving of countless of lives, including those of pregnant women. Indeed, the unique immunologic and physiologic characteristics of pregnancy are associated with high rates of serious and sometimes fatal outcomes from a variety of infectious diseases [3–5]. Untreated infections during pregnancy and delivery are key contributors to maternal and neonatal morbidity and mortality and can largely be prevented by improving the quality of antenatal care (ANC), which aims to be effective, safe, and efficient through judicious use of medications [6,7]. Some of the most common maternal infections are urinary tract infections (UTIs), respiratory tract infections (RTIs), sexually transmitted infections (STIs), bacterial vaginosis (BV), and group B streptococcus infections (GBS) [8,9].

Maternal mortality rates remain high worldwide, with around 300,000 women dying in 2017 according to the World Health Organization (WHO) [10], and global estimates suggest that in 2014, infections were the third leading cause of maternal mortality, or 10.7% of all maternal deaths [11]. In 2019, the WHO reported that around 70 pregnant women per 1000 live births had an infection that required hospitalization. The same report identified that in high-income countries, 11 women per 1000 live births with an infection had adverse maternal outcomes; meanwhile, in low- and middle-income countries, up to 15 women per 1000 births were impacted [10].

Antibiotic treatment is widely accepted as the best way to treat the majority of bacterial infections. Because many antibiotic regimens have similar efficacy, the choice for the type of antibiotic is based on pharmacokinetics, safety, and cost [12]. When considering antibiotic use during pregnancy, antibiotic safety for the mother and fetus is critical because some drugs can be teratogenic or harmful to the developing fetus [13]. Several factors can influence the risk of teratogenicity, including gestational period, dose and duration of therapy, genetic predisposition, environmental factors, and the degree of drug transfer across the placenta [14,15]. Antibiotic prescriptions should therefore be carefully assessed on an individual basis, comparing the advantages and the risks to both the fetus and mother. In certain instances, antibiotic use has been linked to an increased prevalence of neonatal necrotizing enterocolitis, while in others it has been linked to a lower rate of lung problems and serious cerebral abnormalities when compared to non-antibiotic-treated mothers [16].

While antibiotics are essential drugs for the treatment of infectious diseases, data on antibiotic efficacy and safety during pregnancy are extremely limited, including the gestational age they are consumed. In part, this is due to legal and ethical concerns restricting research on pregnant women [17,18]. Typically, clinical and epidemiological studies on drug safety are conducted on non-pregnant women, with results extrapolated to pregnant women [19]. Only 10% of pharmaceuticals sold since 1980 are thought to have collected appropriate data on risks when used in pregnancy, while over 98% of medications lack adequate pharmacokinetic or safety data on dosing in pregnant women [20].

In the context of global maternal and childcare, the selection of optimal antibiotics, their dosages, the duration of therapy, and the balance between costs and benefits are crucial factors to acknowledge. Guidelines play an important role in ensuring that antibiotics are administered correctly. Schuts et al. [21] described the relationship between prescribing antibiotics according to guidelines and a significantly lower risk of mortality in hospitals overall. In addition, compliance with clinical practice and guidelines is an indicator of high-quality treatment in hospitalized patients [22,23]. Although global attention to ANC therapeutic needs is gradually increasing, there are still gaps, primarily in knowledge, that undermine the development or attainment of guidelines to direct physicians' practices.

Adequate antibiotic prescription is crucial to ensure that the right patient receives the right antibiotics at the right time in order to optimize clinical outcomes, while also helping to limit further increases in antibiotic resistance. In fact, as antibiotics reduce the risk of serious morbidity and mortality in a population, they also facilitate the evolution and spread of antibiotic-resistant bacteria, and antibiotic over-prescription hastens this process. Pregnant women and newborns require special consideration. As such, understanding how these issues overlap is urgent, and investigating the role that ANC providers play is empirical. How and when providers prescribe drugs, including antibiotics, is a multifactorial and complex process. Previous research has identified a variety of factors influencing antibiotic prescriptions in hospitals and primary care, including physician-specific and patient-related factors, including the availability of diagnostic tools, local antibiotic resistance data, patient satisfaction, and cultural and organizational factors.

This study investigated how ANC providers in various countries make decisions about antibiotic prescriptions for pregnant women. Improved understandings of antibiotic prescription practices can help healthcare providers better tailor their practices to the specific needs of patients, resulting in improved maternal and neonatal health outcomes. By suggesting evidence-based recommendations for ANC providers, this study can help explore current practices and needs for improvements at the policy and institutional levels to support antibiotic prescribers in their decision-making processes and improve the consistency of care. This, in turn, can lead to more reliable outcomes and a more evidence-based approach to healthcare management and policy development. By having a better understanding of the factors that influence antibiotic prescription decisions, healthcare managers can develop targeted interventions that improve the quality of care and patient outcomes.

2. Results

2.1. Respondents' Characteristics

In total, 161 survey responses were received. However, 24 survey responses were excluded from further analysis as they had missing answers on more than 90 per cent of the questions. In total, 137 healthcare professionals participated in this study, representing 22 different countries from four WHO regions: the European Region (8); the Eastern Mediterranean Region (2); the African Region (7); and the Region of the Americas (5), of which there were several from Central and South America and one respondent from Canada. See Appendix C for a map of the geographical distribution of the survey. Most of the respondents were gynecologists/obstetricians (84.7%). Other professions included gynecologists in training (5.1%), general practitioners (3.6%), public health professionals, and one antimicrobial resistance (AMR) fellow (1.5%) (Table 1).

Table 1. Summary of the main characteristics of healthcare providers who participated in the survey (n = 137).

Characteristic	Total (N = 137), n (%)
Gender	
Male	44 (32.1)
Female	93 (67.9)
Non-binary	0 (0)
Prefer not to say	0 (0)
Age	
20–29	12 (8.8)
30–39	39 (28.5)
40–49	22 (16.1)
50+	60 (43.8)
Other	4 (2.9)
Profession	
Gynecologist/obstetrician	116 (84.7)
General practitioner	5 (3.6)
Midwife	2 (1.5)
Nurse	1 (0.7)
Other	13 (9.5)
Country of practice (WHO region)	
Region of the Americas	16 (11.7)
European Region	101 (73.8)
African Region	8 (5.8)
Eastern Mediterranean Region	12 (8.8)

2.2. Practices of Antibiotic Prescription

The main themes and factors that influenced antibiotic prescribing practice in the study population are summarized in Figure 1.

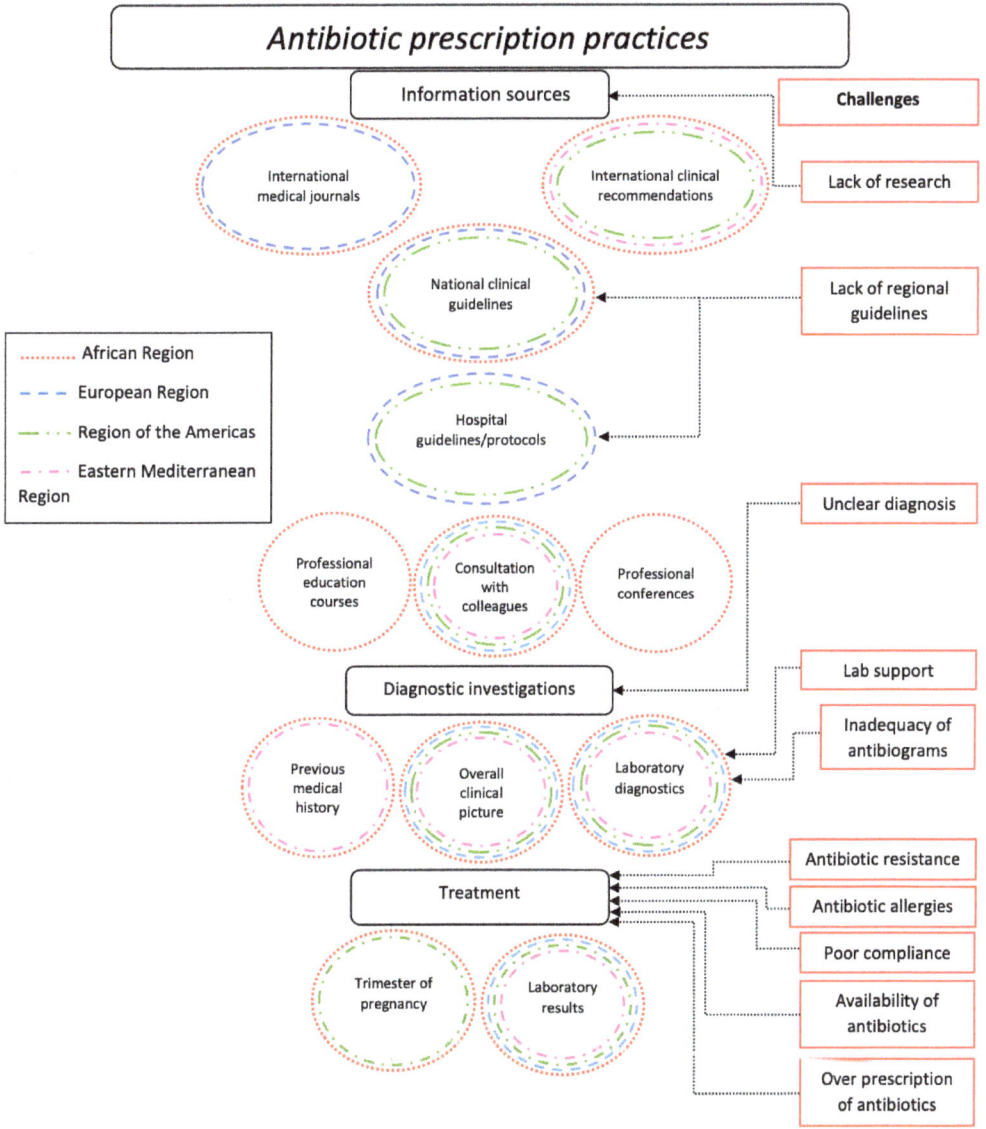

Figure 1. Visual representation of the most common reasons for prescribing antibiotics and the factors that influenced providers' decision making in each case and the challenges described.

2.2.1. Diagnostics

Bacterial infections were the most diagnosed infections (81%) across all WHO regions. Fungal infections were only reported (10.9%) in the European and Eastern Mediterranean regions.

Participants from the European and Eastern Mediterranean Regions reported diagnosing infections more than once per month, those from the African Region at least once a week, and from the Americas both routinely and regularly. Most of the respondents (60.6%) diagnosed infections in pregnant women more than once a month. A little over a third of all respondents (35.8%) diagnosed infections more than once a week. In the African Region, half of the respondents indicated that they diagnosed an infection more than once a week.

In this study, laboratory diagnostics and clinical presentation were the most frequently considered factors for diagnosing suspected infections in pregnant women across all four WHO regions. Regarding laboratory access, the majority of respondents (71.5%) reported having easy and prompt access to laboratory diagnostics. However, regional discrepancies were observed, with 50% (4 out of 8) of the respondents from the African Region indicating partial access and 37.5% (3 out of 8) reporting easy access.

Within the African Region, specific challenges were identified in Zimbabwe, where adequate laboratory support was lacking, as well as in Nigeria, where delays in receiving laboratory investigation results were reported. In Uganda, respondents reported non-adherence to ministry guidelines on antibiotic use for pregnant mothers, lengthy laboratory investigation times, and a reliance on clinical presentations to make diagnostic judgments. It is unclear whether similar challenges exist in other countries, and further investigation is warranted to contextualize these findings.

In the Americas, 56.3% (9 out of 16) of respondents reported easy access to laboratory diagnostics, while the remaining 6 respondents reported partial access. There was no discernible difference between North and South America in this regard. On the other hand, all four respondents who reported difficult access to laboratory diagnostics originated from the European Region, and all were gynecologists/obstetricians from Italy. These findings may have important implications for the development of region-specific interventions to improve laboratory access and facilitate appropriate antibiotic prescribing practices. National clinical guidelines were also frequently taken into consideration (52.6%), as well as previous medical history (38.0%). One respondent from the American Region mentioned lifestyle and diet as additional elements taken into consideration during diagnosis.

2.2.2. Treatment

Across the four WHO regions, the most common infections that required antibiotic treatment were UTIs (67.9%). Other infections requiring antibiotic treatments included BV (5.8%), candidiasis (4.4%), asymptomatic bacteriuria (2.2%), and vaginitis (2.2%). In another 5.8% of cases, the free-text response of *Escherichia coli* infections was provided. It is important to note is that *Escherichia coli* infections are often associated with UTIs and therefore likely contribute to the response chosen most often.

The majority of respondents across all four WHO regions indicated prescribing broad-spectrum antibiotics more often (56.9%) than narrow spectrum (31.4%). Data showed that out of the 34 respondents who indicated partial or difficult access to laboratory diagnostics, 24 (70.6%) indicated prescribing broad-spectrum antibiotics most often, versus 6 respondents who indicated prescribing narrow-spectrum antibiotics more often.

Just over a quarter of the total respondents (28.5%) never referred pregnant women with a suspected infection to a colleague, while over half rarely did. Out of 14 respondents who regularly/routinely referred patients to another specialist, 9 (64.3%) were gynecologists/obstetricians, but only 5 out of 21 (23.8%) of respondents with a different occupation referred patients regularly/routinely. These 5 included a nurse (1), lab technician/AMR fellow (1), midwife (1), gynecologist in training (1), and general practitioner (1)

In case of referral, this was most often carried out by an infectious disease specialist (46%). Other patients were referred to gynecologists (12.4%), female urologists (5.1%), and pathologists (0.7%).

2.2.3. Indicators Considered when Prescribing Antibiotics

Different factors were considered by practitioners when prescribing antibiotics to pregnant women, including laboratory results (73.7%), overall clinical picture (46.7%), trimester of pregnancy (43.1%), national clinical guidelines (40.1%), and international clinical recommendations (35.8%). There were, however, some differences across the four WHO regions. National clinical guidelines were indicated as more important by the

European Region (44.6%) and the Americas (43.8%) compared to the African (25.0%) and the Eastern Mediterranean (8.3%) Regions. Additionally, international clinical guidelines were not mentioned by respondents from the African Region.

2.2.4. Consultations

Respondents were asked more specifically about the frequency of consultations with colleagues. About two thirds of all respondents (61.3%) consulted with colleagues before prescribing antibiotics to a pregnant woman, whereas about one quarter (29.9%) indicated that they never did. This trend was visible across almost all age groups, 20–29 years of age (66.7% vs. 8.3%), 30–39 years of age (76.9% vs. 15.4%), and 40–49 years of age (59.1% vs. 27.3%). Only in the age group of 50+ was the proportion of respondents consulting with colleagues similar to those who did not (48.3% vs. 45.0%).

When consulting with colleagues, respondents mentioned doing so most often with a gynecologist (33.6%) or a microbiologist (32.1%). Other colleagues mentioned were infectious disease specialists and midwives. Most of the respondents who consulted with colleagues did so rarely (38.7%). In the American, European, and African Regions, around twenty per cent of the respondents consulted with colleagues more than once a month, whereas only one of the respondents from the Eastern Mediterranean Region consulted more than two to three times a year with colleagues. Overall, only a small number of respondents (4.4%) consulted weekly with colleagues.

2.2.5. Reasons for Switching between Hospital and National Guidelines

Among the respondents, 22 reported instances of non-adherence to hospital and national guidelines. Reasons for not following guidelines varied across regions. In Europe, reasons included concerns about allergies, antibiotic resistance, and unclear policies. In Switzerland, antibiotics were used cautiously, and alternative strategies were discussed with patients whenever possible. In Italy, antibiotic resistance was a primary concern, while allergies were cited as a reason for non-adherence in Belgium and Lithuania. In the Netherlands, second or third choice antibiotics were used in cases of allergy or resistance based on guidelines or consultation with a microbiologist. However, the guidelines themselves were sometimes unclear or subject to discussion, particularly in cases of preventive antibiotics, such as with preterm rupture of membranes. For instance, a respondent from the Netherlands explained the challenges related to guidelines use in pregnancy in an open question:

"Particularly with preventive antibiotics, there is sometimes discussion in guidelines. For example, in case of preterm ruptured membranes. Previously, the advice was to treat, then not for a while, and now there is a review in which the option is considered again. This is based on the same trials. So, it is not always clear what the best policy is." (The Netherlands; translated from Dutch.)

Respondents from the Americas mentioned natural remedies and non-response to antibiotics from guidelines as reasons for deviation. Based on the experience from the respondent from Canada, clients were supported to make informed choices and if they chose to try natural remedies or aromatherapy first, antibiotics were used only if the first treatment was not successful. In Uruguay, deviation from guidelines occurred sometimes due to non response to the proposed treatment. In the Eastern Mediterranean Region, some respondents reported deviation due to personal experiences and lack of response to antibiotics. In Iraq and Lebanon, treatment decisions were made based on culture results. In the African Region, respondents mentioned resistance and drug availability as reasons for deviation. In Zimbabwe, overuse of Ceftriaxone led to resistance. An example of a respondent from Nigeria has provided insight into the difficulties surrounding medication and drug availability by responding to an open-ended question.

"Working in rural areas within LMICs (low and middle-income countries) often requires prescriptions based on available medications amongst other considerations." (Nigeria.)

It is important to note that the reasons for deviation may differ based on the healthcare setting and not just because of overuse or misuse of antibiotics. Therefore, guidelines should be contextualized according to the specific setting to ensure appropriate and effective use of antibiotics.

2.3. Challenges of Diagnostics/Antibiotic Treatment

Twenty-eight respondents (22.4%) reported encountering challenges related to the diagnosis and/or prescription of antibiotics for pregnant women in their daily practice, with variations across different WHO regions. Many respondents from the African Region (71.4%) reported facing such challenges, whereas in the European Region and Eastern Mediterranean Region, a relatively smaller proportion of respondents (11.5% and 20.0%, respectively) reported facing similar challenges. In the Region of the Americas, nearly half of the respondents (42.9%) reported encountering such challenges. In Europe, challenges related to the diagnosis of infections and/or antibiotic prescription for pregnant women included inadequacy of antibiograms, allergies, and resistance. Specifically, respondents from Switzerland identified challenges related to atypical pneumonia, preterm labor, preterm rupture of membranes, appendicitis, and asymptomatic UTIs. In Italy, inadequate use antibiograms were reported.

"Antibiograms often investigate antibiotics that cannot be prescribed during pregnancy" (Italy; translated from Italian.)

In the Netherlands, challenges included unknown allergies to antibiotics and the need to switch medications due to lack of clinical improvement, as well as a lack of studies on proper dosage for pregnant women and the degree of transmission to the child.

"- Not unequivocal best policy—There is a lack of studies on proper dosing for pregnant women and on the extent of transmission to the child. During delivery, leucocytes and CRP are routinely elevated, which makes differentiation between infection and inflammation due to delivery not always possible." (The Netherlands; translated from Dutch)

In the Eastern Mediterranean Region, poor compliance and disagreement pose challenges. In Iraq, poor compliance and limited investigations available, or the unavailability of certain medications, were identified as issues. In Lebanon, resistance patterns present in patients and conflicting laboratory test results that do not fit with symptoms pose challenges that require collaboration and resolution.

In the African Region, challenges included lack of lab support, delays in lab results, resistance, and recurrent UTI. Respondents from Uganda reported not adhering to ministry guidelines on antibiotic use for pregnant women due to long delays in lab investigations. Zimbabwe faces a lack of adequate laboratory support, while respondents from Nigeria experience delays in laboratory investigations. In Ethiopia, selecting antibiotics that are not associated with congenital malformations in case of resistance development poses a challenge in the first trimester of pregnancy. In Liberia, pregnant women presenting with recurrent UTI were identified as a challenge that requires urine culture and sensitivity tests. It is important to note that these findings are based on the experiences reported by our respondents in Ethiopia and Liberia and may not be representative of the entire countries.

In the Americas, challenges included resistance, sensitivity, lack of consideration for diet, and lifestyle factors. Specifically, respondents from the Dominican Republic reported challenges when faced with sensitivity to antibiotics not recommended for the appropriate trimester of pregnancy in urine or vaginal culture reports. In Uruguay, challenges include uncertainty around whether patients are immunized or experiencing toxoplasmosis reinfection, as well as multi-resistant germs that require treatment with antibiotics not ideal in pregnancy.

"When I have a report of a urine or vaginal culture that gives me sensitivity to antibiotics not recommended for the corresponding trimester of pregnancy." (Dominican Republic; translated from Spanish.)

"There are multi-resistant germs that make it necessary to treat with antibiotics that are not ideal in pregnancy." (Uruguay; translated from Spanish.)

2.4. Sources of Information

The results indicate that national clinical guidelines (67.1%), international clinical guidelines (63.5%), and hospital guidelines/protocols (56.2%) were the most frequently used sources of information among healthcare professionals. Professional education courses were also identified as a commonly used source of information (42.3%). However, there were differences in the sources of information used between the four WHO regions. In Europe, national clinical guidelines (71.3%), international clinical recommendations (61.4%), and hospital guidelines (60.4%) were the top three sources of information. In the Eastern Mediterranean Region, international clinical recommendations (58.3%), professional conferences (41.7%), and hospital guidelines (41.7%) were the most used sources. In Africa, where there is limited resource availability, healthcare professionals heavily rely on professional education courses (87.5%), followed by international clinical recommendations (75.0%) and national clinical guidelines (62.5%). In the Americas, both national clinical guidelines and international clinical recommendations were equally used (75.0%), while hospital guidelines were used by 50.0% of healthcare professionals.

2.5. Recommendations

The respondents' recommendations indicate an urgent need for support in the form of guidelines, access to resources, and training manuals to aid in decision making regarding the diagnosis and treatment of infections in pregnant women. The reduction in antibiotic use was suggested in Canada and Belgium, while considerations for resistance when prescribing were recommended in Uruguay and Italy. Italy also called for more specific guidelines for resistant bacteria. More uniform and better guidelines for prescription during pregnancy, increased education for healthcare professionals and patients, and improved lab accessibility were also recommended.

"Taking into account antibiotic resistance. Taking into account the unavailability in Italy of amoxicillin for prevention of Streptococcus agalactia infection in labor." (Italy; translated from Italian.)

"Publish updated national/regional pocket guidelines based on local epidemiology. Establish a national registry on (severe) pregnancy infections treated in inpatient settings." (Italy; translated from Italian.)

Several specific recommendations were provided by different countries, such as non-antibiotic therapy in pregnant women in Switzerland, utilizing culture and sensitivity testing by clinicians in Uganda and Belgium, limiting the use of antibiotics and prioritizing the results of the antibiogram in the Netherlands, and refraining from prescribing first-line antibiotics, which are the standard antibiotics that are typically prescribed as a first course of treatment for a particular infection, without a proper diagnosis, in Mozambique.

"Hospital develop antibiograms for mothers and should be adhered to. Culture and sensitivity testing should be fully utilized by the clinicians." (Uganda.)

Respondents from Uruguay suggested better treatment of UTIs during pregnancy, along with following national and international clinical guidelines and avoiding prophylactic antibiotic use.

Respondents from Italy recommended teratology courses, establishing a national registry of hospitalized infections in pregnancy. Considering the risk of AMR and the limited availability of antibiotics, it may not be advisable to rely solely on antibiotic treatment to prevent GBS infection. More specificity of therapy and options in case of resistance, as well as easily accessible guidelines, were also recommended in Italy. In Lebanon, teaching patients and teamwork were suggested, while upgrading laboratory services, especially culture and sensitivity, was recommended in Liberia.

Respondents from the Dominican Republic emphasized the importance of following guidelines, using logical judgment, and continually updating medical practices. Finally, respondents from Canada recommended considering treatment with natural remedies before antibiotics, if appropriate and suitable for the patient.

3. Discussion

The primary objective of this study was to present a comprehensive overview of diverse antibiotic prescription practices for pregnant women among healthcare professionals from different regions of the globe.

In the context of diagnosing and treating infections in pregnant women, most healthcare professionals reported engaging in such practices as part of their routine clinical activities. Despite considerable similarity in responses across respondents from various WHO regions, there were notable differences observed, specifically with respect to the accessibility of laboratory diagnostic testing. Respondents from the Regions of the Americas, Europe, and Eastern Mediterranean commonly reported easy and rapid access to laboratory diagnostic testing, whereas others reported limited access. However, caution is needed when generalizing the findings, as the percentage of those reporting limited access was low in all regions. The challenges faced by respondents from the African Region in accessing laboratory diagnostic testing were also reflected in issues related to prescribing antibiotics. These disparities in laboratory diagnostic accessibility align with the concept of the global diagnostic gap, which describes the unequal distribution of diagnostic resources worldwide [24]. Individuals residing in larger urban areas or with higher socioeconomic status generally enjoy better access to laboratory diagnostic testing, whereas those from rural areas or with lower socioeconomic status are disproportionately affected [25]. Insufficient access to high-quality laboratory diagnostic testing can have significant implications for pregnant women's care, potentially leading to inaccurate diagnoses and inappropriate treatment regimens [26]. Such circumstances may also contribute to the emergence of antimicrobial resistance.

Notably, UTIs were the most treated infections across all four WHO regions, which is consistent with previous research that identifies UTIs as the most prevalent infections among pregnant women [27]. The majority of respondents reported prescribing broad-spectrum antibiotics most frequently, which aligns with empirical treatment practices observed in the general population. However, research has also shown that once laboratory diagnostic results are obtained, clinicians often shift to prescribing narrow-spectrum antibiotics [28]. This pattern was not reported in the present study. Additionally, some respondents discussed the applicability of guidelines and the potential adverse clinical outcomes of prescribing certain antibiotics during pregnancy, particularly in specific trimesters.

A few respondents In our study also mentioned the inadequacy of antibiograms for infections during pregnancy. According to them, antibiograms often fail to evaluate antibiotics that are safe to use during pregnancy, while some of the evaluated antibiotics are contraindicated during pregnancy due to their teratogenic effects [29]. Moreover, resistance to commonly used antibiotics among prevalent bacterial strains is widespread, limiting the choice of antibiotics during pregnancy. Although β-lactam antibiotics are generally considered safe during pregnancy, resistance rates to these antibiotics are rapidly increasing [30]. Furthermore, little is known about the effects of many antibiotics on maternal and fetal health. A study reported that the vast majority of antibiotics approved by the Food and Drug Administration (FDA) had an 'undetermined' potential to cause fetal abnormalities [31]. This lack of evidence-based information on the safety and efficacy of most drugs during pregnancy has resulted in insufficient support for decision-making processes concerning antibiotic prescriptions for pregnant women, as described by other studies [32,33]

In terms of sources of information, variations were observed among the four WHO regions in our study. National clinical guidelines, international clinical guidelines, and hospital guidelines/protocols were the most frequently consulted sources of information overall. However, in the African Region, professional education courses were the most used source, while professional conferences and education courses were among the top three sources in the Eastern Mediterranean Region. The lower utilization of national and institutional clinical guidelines in the African Region may be attributed to the limited availability of standardized treatment guidelines in many African Union member states [34]. Similarly, the lack of clear guidelines regarding dosage and duration of antibiotic treatment in Lebanon has been identified as a potential reason for the low reliance on national and institutional guidelines in the Eastern Mediterranean Region. These findings suggest that healthcare professionals follow established guidelines and training procedures that prioritize diagnostic accuracy in identifying infections [35]. However, it is important to note that the specific guidelines or training protocols followed by healthcare professionals may vary depending on their location, setting, or specialty. Therefore, it may be beneficial to further explore the underlying factors that contribute to these diagnostic practices and to consider potential improvements or modifications to existing guidelines or training programs to ensure optimal diagnosis and treatment of infections in pregnant women.

The survey also revealed that approximately one third of the respondents consulted colleagues before prescribing antibiotics to pregnant women, with gynecologists and microbiologists being the most frequently consulted. Previous research identified four key characteristics of consultation with colleagues, including the influence of colleagues, social team dynamics, hierarchy, and reputational risk [36]. However, our study did not explore the specific motivations for consulting with colleagues among the respondents. The process of referral and consultation can vary significantly across different countries and healthcare systems. Referral and consultation mechanisms may differ based on factors such as the organization of healthcare systems, the availability of specialists, and the criteria for referral [37]. For instance, in some countries, patients may require a referral from a primary care physician before seeing a specialist, while in others, patients may be able to directly access specialists without a referral. Additionally, the process of consultation may involve various methods of communication, such as telephone, electronic messaging, or face-to-face meetings. These differences in referral and consultation processes may have implications for the quality and timeliness of care that patients receive, and healthcare professionals may need to adapt their practices based on the specific systems in which they work. One possible explanation for the trend in higher proportions of respondents consulting with colleagues among younger age groups compared to older age groups could be the difference in experience and confidence levels in their respective fields. Younger individuals who are newer to their professions may be more likely to seek guidance from colleagues to gain knowledge and build their confidence, while older individuals with more experience may have already developed a more independent decision-making process. However, further research would be needed to confirm this hypothesis.

The prescription practices of antibiotics can vary greatly between countries due to differences in regulatory frameworks, healthcare systems, and cultural norms. For instance, some countries have more stringent regulations regarding antibiotic use, which may result in lower rates of prescription and a greater emphasis on non-antibiotic treatments. Several countries have implemented strategies to promote appropriate antibiotic use, resulting in lower rates of antibiotic use and a greater emphasis on non-antibiotic treatments. For example, in the Netherlands, there is a strong emphasis on responsible antibiotic use, which has led to lower rates of antibiotic use in the general population [38,39]. In Canada, initiatives focused on education and awareness have been implemented to promote appropriate antibiotic use, resulting in more conservative prescribing practices compared to the United States [40]. Contrary to the conventional assumption that behavioral factors, such as education, are the main drivers of antibiotic practices, recent research suggests that these practices should be examined from the perspective of infrastructural constraints. In other words, systemic factors, including the availability of healthcare facilities, drug supply chains, and laboratory diagnostic capacity, are important determinants of antibiotic use, in addition to individual-level factors [41,42]. While some countries may have more relaxed regulations that encourage the use of antibiotics, leading to higher rates of prescription, there are also systemic factors that contribute to inappropriate antibiotic use. For instance, in Nigeria, there may be infrastructural challenges, such as limited access to healthcare facilities and qualified medical personnel, which further exacerbates the overuse and misuse of antibiotics [43]. Similarly, in Uganda, infrastructure challenges, such as inadequate drug supply chains, limited laboratory diagnostic capacity, and insufficient staffing also contribute to inappropriate antibiotic use [44]. In Italy, systemic factors such as inadequate prescribing guidelines and a lack of antimicrobial stewardship programs may also play a significant role in driving inappropriate antibiotic use [45,46].

The differences in prescription practices may have significant implications for the emergence and spread of antibiotic resistance, as well as for patient outcomes. Currently available guidelines and support were evaluated by the majority of the respondents in our study, who appeared either completely or somewhat satisfied. However, some respondents expressed some dissatisfaction, and provided recommendations for improving the diagnostics and treatment of pregnant women with bacterial infections. The findings are consistent with previous research, which has shown an improvement in AMR awareness among healthcare professionals over time [36,47]. Despite this, our respondents highlighted a need for better guidance and support for the treatment of resistant bacteria in pregnant women. To address this need, it is recommended that local guidelines are developed specifically for the most frequently occurring (resistant) bacterial strains.

Moreover, the respondents in this study exhibited an awareness of the importance of careful use of antibiotics, particularly in cases of prophylaxis, as a means of curbing the emergence of antibiotic resistance. Research conducted previously has indicated that antibiotics are often administered routinely to women in labor in low- and middle-income countries, regardless of the complexity of delivery [48]. This practice of prophylactic antibiotic use could have a detrimental effect on the emergence of antibiotic resistance. Therefore, raising awareness about safe and effective antibiotic use could help prevent antibiotic resistance. Additionally, a few respondents identified the need for high-quality and easily accessible laboratory tests to ensure appropriate antibiotic prescribing. As Kollef [28] suggested, initial broad-spectrum antibiotic treatment should be narrowed or adjusted based on the results of culture and sensitivity tests to minimize the risk of death due to ineffective initial treatment, as well as the risk of antibiotic resistance resulting from prolonged use of broad-spectrum antibiotics.

An online survey was utilized to collect data for this study due to its global scope. However, this method may have introduced sampling bias. The decision to participate in the survey could have been affected by access to the internet and technological proficiency, potentially dissuading certain medical professionals from contributing to the study, particularly those in areas with limited internet connectivity. This could have led to distorted survey results, particularly in relation to information sources used for diagnostics and antibiotic treatment. One potential limitation is the relatively low number of responses received despite our international recruitment efforts. We recognize that a larger sample size would have provided a more representative and diverse range of perspectives on the determinants of antimicrobial use and resistance; the limited number of responses should be considered when interpreting the findings of our study. Another limitation of our study is that we did not collect specific information on the names or families of the antimicrobials used in our sample. As a result, we were unable to classify the antimicrobials according to the WHO AWaRe classification (WHO access, watch, reserve, classification of antibiotics for evaluation and monitoring of use), which could provide valuable information on their appropriateness and potential impact on antimicrobial resistance.

Furthermore, this study is limited by significant variations in the number of respondents across the different WHO regions. Many of the respondents were from the European

Region, with many of those respondents originating from Italy. Some of the researchers' Italian background may have resulted in more responses from Italy to the post they shared on social media, and snowball sampling may have compounded this effect. As a result, the study's findings may not be representative of the global population. Finally, while acknowledging the diversity of gender identities among patients, the present study employs the term 'pregnant women' to refer to this population. This choice is justified on several grounds. The term 'pregnant women' is widely used in ANC facilities worldwide. Therefore, it was deemed appropriate to adopt this terminology consistently in the survey and subsequent paper. Notably, this terminology does not preclude individuals identifying as a different gender to be included.

4. Materials and Methods

A cross-sectional online survey was carried out among healthcare providers working in ANC from different countries around the globe between 1 June 2022 and 1 January 2023.

4.1. Online Survey

The online survey consisted of 23 questions, including 4 free-text answers and 19 multiple-choice questions. It focused on three aspects: practices of antibiotic prescription, sources of information, and recommendations for future practices. The survey was first developed in English, after which it was shared with a multidisciplinary group of healthcare professionals for feedback and to ensure the quality of the questions. The finalized survey was translated with the support of native speakers into six more languages: Dutch, German, French, Spanish, Portuguese, and Italian. A further quality check was performed to ensure the content was consistent across translations and to ensure the absence of grammatical or spelling errors. The survey was generated online using Qualtrics XM (Qualtrics, Provo, UT, USA, 2022). See Appendix A for the survey.

4.2. Study Population

The study population consisted of healthcare practitioners working in ANC with no geographical limitation. To reach a broad number of participants, a combination of purposive sampling and snowball sampling was used. Participants were recruited on a voluntary basis and were invited to participate via email, by contacting professional organizations/networks, or by sharing the information on social media platforms (LinkedIn, Twitter, and Facebook). Email addresses of practitioners or networks were gathered from the main researchers' personal networks, as well as the International Federation of Gynaecology and Obstetrics (FIGO) website, which was utilized to compile an email list of member countries. The Gynécologie Suisse SSGO (Swiss association of gynecology) shared the project information on their monthly newsletter. The email and an information leaflet (in each of the seven languages) included a link to the online survey, a brief explanation of the project, its major goals, and the researchers' names and contact information. Participants were also invited to share the email and information flyer with their professional networks to recruit more participants.

4.3. Data Analysis

Quantitative and qualitative data on prescription practices and decision-making tools were obtained using closed and open-ended questions. Data were utilized to identify the key ideas that influence antibiotic prescribing behavior. Quantitative data were gathered and analyzed using descriptive statistics (frequencies and percentages) in IBM SPSS Statistics 27 (Armonk, NY, USA: IBM Corp). Because of the heterogeneous number of responses across countries, data were reported per WHO region.

To generate common themes from qualitative data, descriptive thematic analysis of free-text responses was used. DeepL Translator (DeepL Translate, n.d.) was used to translate free-text responses to English, and the translations were reviewed by native speakers. Initially, a deductive approach was utilized to develop general themes based on survey question topics. Following that, an inductive approach was used to discover additional (sub)themes based on responses. A coding technique was established after reading the answers several times. An overview of the main themes and factors was developed (Figure 1).

In the context of antibiotic prescribing practices, the term "rarely" was used to indicate a frequency of 2 to 3 diagnoses per year, while "regularly" denoted a frequency of more than 1 diagnosis per month, and "routinely" signified a frequency of more than once a week. These terms were used to describe the frequency with which healthcare providers diagnose infections and subsequently prescribe antibiotics.

4.4. Ethical Considerations

The study received ethical approval from Maastricht University Medical Ethics Review Committee (FHML- REC/2022/001). Informed consent was obtained from each respondent prior to participation in the survey (Appendix B). The participants had to agree online before going forward with the survey, and they were informed that they could stop at any time by closing the browser. Participants were also informed about the purpose of the study, that participation was voluntary, and that all data collected would be confidential.

5. Conclusions

This study sheds light on the decision-making process underlying antibiotic prescription among healthcare practitioners in ANC globally. Data suggest that consultation of laboratory test results and adherence to guidelines were among the most important factors in this process. The study also identified differences in practices and challenges across four WHO regions, indicating the need for region-specific guidance. Furthermore, this study highlights the need for continued efforts to prevent the emergence of AMR within ANC through the implementation of effective and safe antibiotic use practices. This exploratory work provides important insights that can be used to inform the development of targeted interventions and policies to improve the care of pregnant women worldwide. This study can stimulate further research on this topic, including studies on the effectiveness of current guidelines and the development of better guidelines for antibiotic prescription to pregnant women. Research should also investigate the significance of patient expectations in the decision-making process of healthcare practitioners regarding antibiotic prescriptions as this can have implications for the emergence and spread of AMR. Lastly, this study can be beneficial to researchers working on global health issues as it highlights the importance of identifying challenges and regional differences in the implementation of guidelines for antibiotic prescription in ANC.

Author Contributions: Conceptualization, E.A. and A.K.; methodology, E.A. and A.K.; investigation, C.G. and S.D.; resources, C.G. and S.D.; data curation, C.G. and S.D.; writing—original draft preparation, C.G. and S.D.; writing—review and editing, C.G., S.A.-N., A.K., and E.A.; supervision, E.A. and A.K. All authors have read and agreed to the published version of the manuscript.

Funding: This research received no external funding.

Institutional Review Board Statement: The study was conducted in accordance with the Declaration of Helsinki and approved by the Institutional Review Board (Maastricht University Medical Ethics Review Committee) of Maastricht University (FHML- REC/2022/001 and date of approval).

Informed Consent Statement: Informed consent was obtained from all subjects involved in the study.

Data Availability Statement: Data are contained within the article.

Acknowledgments: We would like to thank all participants for taking the time to participate in this study.

Conflicts of Interest: The authors declare no conflict of interest.

Appendix A. Survey

I. Demographics

1. Age (years):
20–29
30–39
40–49
50+
Other

2. Gender
Female
Male
Non-binary
Do not want to say.

3. Occupation
General practitioner
Gynecologist/Obstetrician
Nurse
Midwife
Other (please indicate) _____

4. Country of practice
Please indicate _____

II. Practices of Antibiotic Prescription

5. In your practice, do you have to diagnose infections in pregnant women?
1. Yes
2. No, we transfer to (please indicate) (if this answer is chosen, you can skip to question 15)
3. Other (please indicate) ___

6. How often do you diagnose infections in pregnant women?
1. Rarely (2–3 times a year)
2. Regularly (>1x a month)
3. Routinely (>1x a week)

7. In your practice, do you have to treat infections in pregnant women?
1. Yes
2. No
3. Other (please indicate) _____

8. What are the most common infections (Urinary Tract Infection (UTI), Reproductive Tract Infections (RTI), vaginal) that you managed in pregnant women?
1. Bacterial infections (e.g., bacterial vaginosis, chlamydia trachomatis, urinary tract infections, etc.)
2. Viral infections (e.g., Herpes Simplex, genital warts, etc.)
3. Parasitic infections (e.g., malaria, helminth infections, etc.)
4. Fungal infections (e.g., vulvovaginal candidiasis)
5. Difficult to say
6. Other (please indicate) _____

9. Which of the following elements do you usually consider when diagnosing a suspected infection in pregnant women? (Multiple answers possible)
1. Overall clinical picture
2. Previous medical history
3. National clinical guidelines
4. International clinical recommendations
5. Previous work experience with similar cases
6. Laboratory diagnostics
7. Other (please indicate) _____

10. Do you have easy access to laboratory diagnostics?
1. Yes, I have easy access to quick laboratory diagnostics
2. Partial access, not always quick
3. No, difficult to get access to laboratory diagnostics and it takes a long time
4. No, lack of finances
5. Other (please indicate) _____

11. Which of the following indicators do you usually consider when prescribing antibiotics to a pregnant woman? (Maximum 3 main indicators)
1. Overall clinical picture
2. The trimester of pregnancy
3. Previous history of infectious diseases
4. Laboratory results
5. National clinical guidelines
6. International clinical recommendations
7. Previous work experiences with similar cases
8. Other (please indicate) _____

12. What is the most common disease that you cure via antibiotics in your practice?
_____

13. What type of antibiotics do you prescribe most often to pregnant women?
1. Broad spectrum
2. Narrow spectrum
3. Difficult to say

14. Did you ever switched from the treatment advice given through the hospital/national guideline? Why?
1. No
2. Yes, please explain

15. Have you experienced any specific challenges related to diagnostic of infections and/or antibiotic prescription for pregnant women?
1. Yes, please explain
_____

2. No

16. To which specialist do you usually refer pregnant women with suspected infections?
1. Gynaecologist
2. Female urologist
3. Infectious diseases specialist
3. Other (please indicate) _____

17. How often do you refer pregnant women with suspected infections to a specialist?
1. Rarely (2–3 times a year)
2. Regularly (>1x a month)
3. Routinely (>1x a week)

III. Sources of Information

18. What sources of information do you usually use to inform yourself on diagnostic and treatment options for infectious diseases in pregnant women? (Multiple answers possible)
1. National clinical guidelines
2. International clinical recommendations
3. Pharmaceutical representatives
4. National medical journals
5. International medical journals
6. Professional conferences
7. Conversations with colleagues
8. Professional education courses
9. Hospital guidelines/protocols
10. Other (please indicate) _____

19. Do you (sometimes) consult with colleagues before prescribing antibiotics to a pregnant woman?
1. Yes
2. No (if this answer is chosen, you can skip to question 20)

20. If you answered yes to question number 17, how often do you consult your collogues before prescribing antibiotics?
1. Rarely
2. Regularly
3. Routinely

21. What colleagues you may consult with about antibiotic prescription for pregnant women? (Multiple answers possible)
1. Microbiologists
2. Pharmacist
3. Urologist
4. Gynecologist
5. None
6. Other (please indicate) _____

IV. Recommendations

22. Are you satisfied with the current support and guidelines that you use in your practice for diagnostic and treatment of infections in pregnant women?
1. Completely satisfied
2. Somewhat satisfied
3. Somewhat unsatisfied
4. Completely unsatisfied
5. Neutral

23. Are there any recommendations/suggestions that you would like to propose to improve practices of diagnostics and treatment in pregnant women?
1. Yes, please elaborate _____
2. No

Thank you for sharing your experience!

Appendix B. Informed Consent/Information Form

Thank you for showing your interest in the project MIcrobes in MOthers (MIMO)-Global aiming to understand practices of antibiotic prescription in antenatal care in different countries. The knowledge acquired through this project will be used to formulate recommendations for the improvement of clinical guidelines on antibiotic prescriptions. Before agreeing to take part, please read the information below.

The survey will take at most 15/20 min. Your participation is optional, and you can decide the pace and time to fill in the survey. At any time in the process, you can stop the survey, simply by closing the browser. You can also skip any question you do not wish to answer.

All data collected in this project will be handled in confidence by the project team, following the EU General Data Protection Regulation (GDPR) and no identifiable information is collected.

This project is coordinated by Elena Ambrosino (e.ambrosino@maastrichtuniversity.nl) and Alena Kamenshchikova (a.kamenshchikova@maastrichtuniversity.nl) from Maastricht University, the Netherlands. You can reach out to them if you have any questions.

By pressing 'Start the survey' you are giving your consent for processing your answers within the scope of MIMO project

Appendix C. Geographical Distribution of Survey Responses

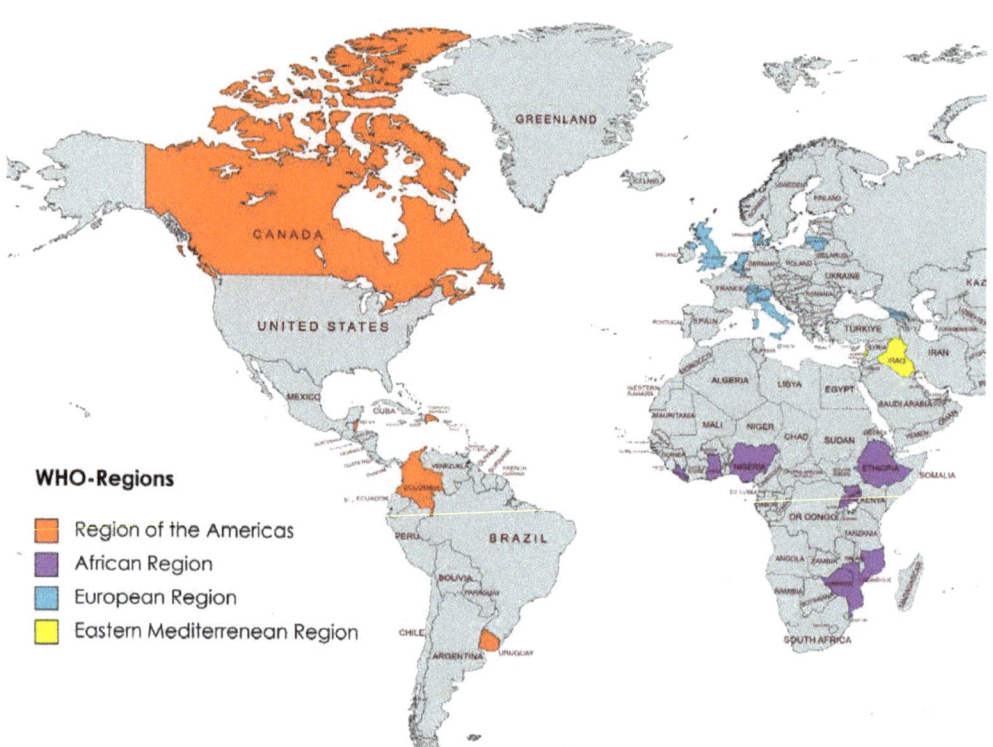

Figure A1. TitleAdapted from https://www.mapchart.net/world.html (*World Map - Simple*, 2023). Countries of practice: Canada (1), Dominican Republic (1), Colombia (1), Uruguay (12), Italy (65), Switzerland (12), The Netherlands (13), Belgium (2), United Kingdom (3), Georgia (1), Denmark (1), Lithuania (4), Uganda (1), Ghana (1), Mozambique (1), Ethiopia (1), Nigeria (2), Zimbabwe (1), Liberia (1), Lebanon (10), Iraq (2).

References

1. Broe, A.; Pottegård, A.; Lamont, R.F.; Jørgensen, J.S.; Damkier, P. Increasing Use antibiotics in pregnancy during the period 2000-2010: Prevalence, timing, category, and demographics. *Bjog* **2014**, *121*, 988–996. [CrossRef] [PubMed]
2. Kuperman, A.A.; Koren, O. Antibiotic use during pregnancy: How bad is it? *BMC Med.* **2016**, *14*, 91. [CrossRef] [PubMed]
3. Yu, P.A.; Tran, E.L.; Parker, C.M.; Kim, H.-J.; Yee, E.L.; Smith, P.W.; Russell, Z.; A Nelson, C.; Broussard, C.S.; Yu, Y.C.; et al. Safety of antimicrobials during pregnancy: A systematic review of antimicrobials considered for treatment and postexposure prophylaxis of plague. *Clin. Infect. Dis.* **2020**, *70* (Suppl. S1), S37–S50. [CrossRef] [PubMed]
4. Furfaro, L.L.; Chang, B.J.; Payne, M.S. Applications for bacteriophage therapy during pregnancy and the perinatal period. *Front. Microbiol.* **2018**, *8*, 2660. [CrossRef] [PubMed]
5. Cantarutti, A.; Rea, F.; Franchi, M.; Beccalli, B.; Locatelli, A.; Corrao, G. Use of antibiotic treatment in pregnancy and the risk of several neonatal outcomes: A population-based study. *Int. J. Environ. Res. Public. Health* **2021**, *18*, 12621. [CrossRef]
6. Harbison, A.F.; Polly, D.M.; Musselman, M.E. Antiinfective therapy for pregnant or lactating patients in the emergency department. *Am. J. Health-Syst. Pharm.* **2015**, *72*, 189–197. [CrossRef]
7. Lamont, H.F.; Blogg, H.J.; Lamont, R.F. Safety of antimicrobial treatment during pregnancy: A current review of resistance, immunomodulation and teratogenicity. *Expert. Opin. Drug. Saf.* **2014**, *13*, 1569–1581. [CrossRef]
8. Lee, A.C.; Mullany, L.C.; Koffi, A.K.; Rafiqullah, I.; Khanam, R.; Folger, L.V.; Rahman, M.; Mitra, D.K.; Labrique, A.; Christian, P. Urinary tract infections in pregnancy in a rural population of Bangladesh: Population-based prevalence, risk factors, etiology, and antibiotic resistance. *BMC Pregnancy Childbirth* **2019**, *20*, 1. [CrossRef]
9. Heikkilä, A.M. Antibiotics in pregnanc—A prospective cohort study on the policy of antibiotic prescription. *Ann. Med.* **1993**, *25*, 467–471. [CrossRef]

10. WHO. *Trends in Maternal Mortality 2000 to 2017: Estimates by WHO, UNICEF, UNFPA*; Executive Summary; World Bank Group and the United Nations Population Division: Geneva, Switzerland, 2019.
11. Say, L.; Chou, D.; Getmmill, A.; Tunçalp, Ö.; Moller, A.-B.; Daniels, J.; Gülmezoglu, A.M.; Temmerman, M.; Alkema, L. Global causes of maternal death: A WHO systematic analysis. *Lancet Glob. Health* **2014**, *2*, e323–e333. [CrossRef]
12. Vidal, A.C.; Murphy, S.K.; Murtha, A.P.; Schildkraut, J.M.; Soubry, A.; Huang, Z.; Neelon, S.E.B.; Fuemmeler, B.; Iversen, E.; Wang, F.; et al. Associations between antibiotic exposure during pregnancy, birth weight and aberrant methylation at imprinted genes among offspring. *Int. J. Obes.* **2013**, *37*, 907–913. [CrossRef]
13. Holderness, M.; Straughan, J.L. *South African Medicines Formulary*; Medical Association of South Africa, Publications Division: Pretoria, South Africa, 1991.
14. Amann, U.; Egen-Lappe, V.; Strunz-Lehner, C.; Hasford, J. Antibiotics in pregnancy: Analysis of potential risks and determinants in a large German statutory sickness fund population. *Pharmacoepidemiol. Drug. Saf.* **2006**, *15*, 327–337. [CrossRef]
15. Ledger, W.J.; Blaser, M.J. Are we using too many antibiotics during pregnancy? *Bjog* **2013**, *120*, 1450–1452. [CrossRef] [PubMed]
16. Esmaeilizand, R.; Shah, P.S.; Seshia, M.; Yee, W.; Yoon, E.W.; Dow, K. Antibiotic exposure and development of necrotizing enterocolitis in very preterm neonates. *Paediatr. Child. Health* **2018**, *23*, e56–e61. [CrossRef] [PubMed]
17. Bookstaver, P.B.; Bland, C.M.; Griffin, B.; Stover, K.R.; Eiland, L.S.; McLaughlin, M. A Review of Antibiotic Use in Pregnancy. *Pharmacotherapy* **2015**, *35*, 1052–1062. [CrossRef]
18. Crider, K.S.; Cleves, M.A.; Reefhuis, J.; Berry, R.J.; Hobbs, C.A.; Hu, D.J. Antibacterial medication use during pregnancy and risk of birth defects: National Birth Defects Prevention Study. *Arch. Pediatr. Adolesc. Med.* **2009**, *163*, 978–985. [CrossRef]
19. Ayad, M.; Costantine, M.M. Epidemiology of medications use in pregnancy. *Semin. Perinatol.* **2015**, *39*, 508–511. [CrossRef] [PubMed]
20. Sheffield, J.S.; Sietgel, D.; Mirochnick, M.; Heine, R.P.; Nguyen, C.; Bergman, K.L.; Savic, R.M.; Long, J.; Dooley, K.E.; Nesin, M. Designing drug trials: Considerations for pregnant women. *Clin. Infect. Dis.* **2014**, *59* (Suppl. S7), S437–S444. [CrossRef] [PubMed]
21. Schuts, E.C.; Hulscher, M.E.J.L.; Mouton, J.W.; Verduin, C.M.; Stuart, J.W.T.C.; Overdiek, H.W.P.M.; van der Linden, P.D.; Natsch, S.; Hertogh, C.M.P.M.; Wolfs, T.F.W.; et al. Current evidence on hospital antimicrobial stewardship objectives: A systematic review and meta-analysis. *Lancet Infect. Dis* **2016**, *16*, 847–856. [CrossRef]
22. Hermanides, H.S.; Hulscher, M.E.; Schouten, J.A.; Prins, J.M.; Geerlings, S.E. Development of quality indicators for the antibiotic treatment of complicated urinary tract infections: A first step to measure and improve care. *Clin. Infect. Dis.* **2008**, *46*, 703–711. [CrossRef]
23. Mensah, K.B.; Opoku-Agyeman, K.; Ansah, C. Antibiotic use during pregnancy: A retrospective study of prescription patterns and birth outcomes at an antenatal clinic in rural Ghana. *J. Pharm. Policy Pract.* **2017**, *10*, 24. [CrossRef] [PubMed]
24. The Lancet Health Global. Essential diagnostics: Mind the gap. *Lancet Glob. Health* **2021**, *9*, e1474. [CrossRef] [PubMed]
25. Fleming, K.A.; Horton, S.; Wilson, M.L.; Atun, R.; DeStigter, K.; Flanigan, J.; Sayed, N.; Adam, P.; Aguilar, B.; Andronikou, S.; et al. The Lancet Commission on diagnostics: Transforming access to diagnostics. *Lancet* **2021**, *398*, 1997–2050. [CrossRef] [PubMed]
26. Menéndez, C.; Quintó, L.; Castillo, P.; Fernandes, F.; Carrilho, C.; Ismail, M.R.; Lorenzoni, C.; Hurtado, J.C.; Rakislova, N.; Munguambe, K.; et al. Quality of care and maternal mortality in a tertiary-level hospital in Mozambique: A retrospective study of clinicopathological discrepancies. *Lancet Global Health* **2020**, *8*, e965–e972. [CrossRef] [PubMed]
27. Habak, P.J.; Griggs, R.P., Jr. *Urinary Tract. Infection In Pregnancy, StatPearls ed.*; StatPearls Publishing: Treasure Island, FL, USA, 2022. Available online: https://www.ncbi.nlm.nih.gov/books/NBK537047/ (accessed on 13 February 2023).
28. Kollef, M.H. Broad-Spectrum Antimicrobials and the Treatment of Serious Bacterial Infections: Getting It Right Up Front. *Clin. Infect. Dis.* **2008**, *47* (Suppl. S1), S3–S13. [CrossRef]
29. Dashe, J.S.; Gilstrap, L.C. Antibiotic Use in Pregnancy. *Obstet. Gynecol. Clin. North. Am.* **1997**, *24*, 617–629. [CrossRef] [PubMed]
30. Rizvi, M.; Khan, F.; Shukla, I.; Malik, A.; Shaheen. Rising prevalence of antimicrobial resistance in urinary tract infections during pregnancy: Necessity for exploring newer treatment options. *J. Lab. Physicians* **2011**, *3*, 98–103. [CrossRef]
31. Lo, W.Y.; Friedman, J.M. Teratogenicity of recently introduced medications in human pregnancy. *Obstet. Gynecol.* **2002**, *100*, 465–473. [CrossRef]
32. Dathe, K.; Schaefer, C. The Use of Medication in Pregnancy. *Dtsch. Arztebl. Int.* **2019**, *116*, 783–790. [CrossRef]
33. Lynch, M.M.; Squiers, L.B.; Kosa, K.M.; Dolina, S.; Read, J.G.; Broussard, C.S.; Frey, M.T.; Polen, K.N.; Lind, J.N.; Gilboa, S.M.; et al. Making Decisions About Medication Use During Pregnancy: Implications for Communication Strategies. *Matern. Child. Health J.* **2018**, *22*, 92–100. [CrossRef]
34. Craig, J.; Hiban, K.; Frost, I.; Kapoor, G.; Alimi, Y.; Varma, J.K. Comparison of national antimicrobial treatment guidelines, African Union. *Bull. World Health Organ.* **2022**, *100*, 50–59. [CrossRef]
35. Saleh, N.; Awada, S.; Awwad, R.; Jibai, S.; Arfoul, C.; Zaiter, L.; Dib, W.; Salameh, P. Evaluation of antibiotic prescription in the Lebanese community: A pilot study. *Infect. Ecol. Epidemiol.* **2015**, *5*, 27094. [CrossRef]
36. Warremana, E.; Lambregtsa, M.; Wouters, R.; Visser, L.; Staats, H.; van Dijk, E.; de Boer, M. Determinants of in-hospital antibiotic prescription behaviour: A systematic review and formation of a comprehensive framework. *Clin. Microbiol. Infect.* **2019**, *25*, 538–545. [CrossRef]
37. Seyed-Nezhad, M.; Ahmadi, B.; Akbari-Sari, A. Factors affecting the successful implementation of the referral system: A scoping review. *J. Fam. Med. Prim. Care* **2021**, *10*, 4364–4375. (In English) [CrossRef]

38. Van den Broek d'Obrenan, J.; Verheij, T.J.M.; Numans, M.E.; van der Velden, A.W. Antibiotic use in Dutch primary care: Relation between diagnosis, consultation and treatment. *J. Antimicrob. Chemother.* **2014**, *69*, 1701–1707. [CrossRef] [PubMed]
39. Van Rijn, M.; Haverkate, M.; Achterberg, P.; Timen, A. The public uptake of information about antibiotic resistance in the Netherlands. *Public. Underst. Sci.* **2019**, *28*, 486–503. [CrossRef] [PubMed]
40. Federal Action Plan On Antimicrobial Resistance And Use In Canada. 2015. Available online: https://www.canada.ca/en/health-canada/services/publications/drugs-health-products/federal-action-plan-antimicrobial-resistance-canada.html (accessed on 21 February 2023).
41. Chandler, C.I.R. Current accounts of antimicrobial resistance: Stabilisation, individualisation and antibiotics as infrastructure. *Palgrave Commun.* **2019**, *5*, 53. [CrossRef] [PubMed]
42. Willis, L.D.; Chandler, C. Quick fix for care, productivity, hygiene and inequality: Reframing the entrenched problem of antibiotic overuse. *BMJ Glob. Health* **2019**, *4*, e001590. [CrossRef]
43. Ajibola, O.; Omisakin, O.A.; Eze, A.A.; Omoleke, S.A. Self-Medication with Antibiotics, Attitude and Knowledge of Antibiotic Resistance among Community Residents and Undergraduate Students in Northwest Nigeria. *Diseases* **2018**, *6*, 32. Available online: https://www.mdpi.com/2079-9721/6/2/32 (accessed on 21 February 2023). [CrossRef] [PubMed]
44. Obakiro, S.B.; Napyo, A.; Wilberforce, M.J.; Adongo, P.; Kiyimba, K.; Anthierens, S.; Kostyanev, T.; Waako, P.; Van Royen, P. Are antibiotic prescription practices in Eastern Uganda concordant with the national standard treatment guidelines? A cross-sectional retrospective study. *J. Glob. Antimicrob. Resist.* **2022**, *29*, 513–519. [CrossRef]
45. Barchitta, M.; Sabbatucci, M.; Furiozzi, F.; Iannazzo, S.; Maugeri, A.; Maraglino, F.; Prato, R.; Agodi, A.; Pantosti, A. Knowledge, attitudes and behaviors on antibiotic use and resistance among healthcare workers in Italy, 2019: Investigation by a clustering method. *Antimicrob. Resist. Infect. Control.* **2021**, *10*, 134. [CrossRef] [PubMed]
46. Menichetti, F.; Falcone, M.; Lopalco, P.; Tascini, C.; Pan, A.; Busani, L.; Viaggi, B.; Rossolini, G.M.; Arena, F.; Novelli, A.; et al. The GISA call to action for the appropriate use of antimicrobials and the control of antimicrobial resistance in Italy. *Int. J. Antimicrob. Agents* **2018**, *52*, 127–134. [CrossRef] [PubMed]
47. Pouwels, K.; Hopkins, S.; Llewelyn, M.; Walker, A.; McNulty, C.; Robotham, J. Duration of antibiotic treatment for common infections in English primary care: Cross sectional analysis and comparison with guidelines. *BMJ* **2019**, *364*, 1440. [CrossRef] [PubMed]
48. Graham, W.J.; Morrison, E.; Dancer, S.; Afsana, K.; Aulakh, A.; Campbell, O.M.R.; Cross, S.; Ellis, R.; Enkubahiri, S.; Fekad, B.; et al. What are the threats from antimicrobial resistance for maternity units in low- and middle- income countries? *Glob. Health Action.* **2016**, *9*, 33381. [CrossRef]

Disclaimer/Publisher's Note: The statements, opinions and data contained in all publications are solely those of the individual author(s) and contributor(s) and not of MDPI and/or the editor(s). MDPI and/or the editor(s) disclaim responsibility for any injury to people or property resulting from any ideas, methods, instructions or products referred to in the content.

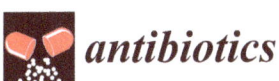

Article

Associations between Polycystic Ovary Syndrome (PCOS) and Antibiotic Use: Results from the UAEHFS

Nirmin F. Juber [1,*], Abdishakur Abdulle [1], Amar Ahmad [1], Fatme AlAnouti [2], Tom Loney [3], Youssef Idaghdour [1], Yvonne Valles [1] and Raghib Ali [1,4]

[1] Public Health Research Center, New York University Abu Dhabi, Abu Dhabi P.O. Box 129188, United Arab Emirates; aa192@nyu.edu (A.A.); asa12@nyu.edu (A.A.); yi3@nyu.edu (Y.I.); yv8@nyu.edu (Y.V.); ra107@nyu.edu (R.A.)
[2] College of Natural and Health Sciences, Zayed University, Abu Dhabi P.O. Box 19282, United Arab Emirates; fatme.alanouti@zu.ac.ae
[3] College of Medicine, Mohammed Bin Rashid University of Medicine and Health Sciences, Dubai Health, Dubai P.O. Box 505055, United Arab Emirates; tom.loney@mbru.ac.ae
[4] MRC Epidemiology Unit, University of Cambridge, Cambridge CB2 0SL, UK
* Correspondence: nirmin.juber@nyu.edu; Tel.: +971-2-6287631

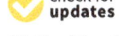

Citation: Juber, N.F.; Abdulle, A.; Ahmad, A.; AlAnouti, F.; Loney, T.; Idaghdour, Y.; Valles, Y.; Ali, R. Associations between Polycystic Ovary Syndrome (PCOS) and Antibiotic Use: Results from the UAEHFS. *Antibiotics* 2024, *13*, 397. https://doi.org/10.3390/antibiotics13050397

Academic Editors: Juan Manuel Vázquez-Lago, Ana Estany-Gestal and Angel Salgado-Barreira

Received: 30 March 2024
Revised: 21 April 2024
Accepted: 22 April 2024
Published: 26 April 2024

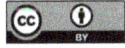

Copyright: © 2024 by the authors. Licensee MDPI, Basel, Switzerland. This article is an open access article distributed under the terms and conditions of the Creative Commons Attribution (CC BY) license (https://creativecommons.org/licenses/by/4.0/).

Abstract: Women with polycystic ovary syndrome (PCOS) have a higher susceptibility to infections compared to those without PCOS. Studies evaluating antibiotic use based on PCOS status are scarce. Therefore, we aimed to (i) assess the associations between self-reported PCOS and antibiotic use, and (ii) whether PCOS treatment and the age at PCOS diagnosis modified the associations above. This cross-sectional analysis used the United Arab Emirates Healthy Future Study (UAEHFS) conducted from February 2016 to March 2023 involving 2063 Emirati women aged 18–62 years. We performed ordinal logistic regressions under unadjusted and demographic-health-characteristic-adjusted models to obtain the odds ratios (ORs) and 95% confidence intervals (CIs) to analyze PCOS and antibiotic use. Subgroup analyses were performed by treatment status and age at diagnosis. We found that women with PCOS were 55% more likely to frequently take a course of antibiotics in the past year (aOR 1.55; 95% CI 1.26–1.90). Similar likelihoods were also found among those being treated for PCOS and those without treatment but with a PCOS diagnosis at ≤25 years. Our study suggests that PCOS was associated with an increased use of antibiotics among Emirati women. Understanding the frequent antibiotic use susceptibility among those with PCOS may improve antibiotic use surveillance and promote antibiotic stewardship in these at-risk individuals.

Keywords: antibiotic use; polycystic ovary syndrome; PCOS; global health; epidemiology

1. Introduction

Polycystic ovary syndrome (PCOS) is a common endocrine disorder affecting 4–20% of women of reproductive age worldwide, depending on the diagnostic criteria used [1,2]. The etiology of PCOS is not exactly known; however, adiposity, ovarian follicle development, insulin sensitivity, and chronic systemic inflammation have been proposed as a few possible mechanisms [3]. The common features of PCOS include irregular menstrual cycles, elevated testosterone levels leading to a hormonal imbalance or hyperandrogenism, and metabolic disorders [4–6]. PCOS is a multifactorial disorder with known risk factors including genetic predisposition, dietary factors or nutritional status, and obesity [6–9]. PCOS has been recognized as a chronic metabolic disorder, not just an endocrine disorder, due to the metabolic disturbances that accompany PCOS [10]. The consequences of this metabolic disturbance are that women with PCOS are often burdened with multiple chronic morbidities and multiple medications to treat their conditions [11,12]. The treatment of PCOS usually involves multimodal or combination approaches due to the complex etiology of PCOS, depending on the prevailing PCOS symptoms [9]. Several factors in PCOS treatment need to be considered in treating PCOS effectively, including the gut microbiota composition, as gut dysbiosis is known to be one of the risk factors for PCOS [9,13,14].

Antibiotic use is a major public health concern as the inappropriate use of antibiotics leads to antibiotic resistance, which significantly threatens human health [15]. In 2019, the World Health Organization considered antibiotic resistance as one of the top ten threats to global health [16]. Several factors have been known to be associated with the increase in antibiotic resistance, including excessive antibiotic prescriptions by medical professionals as well as self-prescription or self-medication [17–19]. Frequent antibiotic use has been associated with increased disease risks, such as colorectal cancer risk and second breast cancer events [20,21]. Antibiotics are essential in treating life-threatening conditions caused by bacteria. With the appropriate and effective use of antibiotics, the successful treatment of bacterial infections can be achieved and will improve human health [22]. Therefore, the close surveillance or monitoring of at-risk individuals for increased antibiotic use may improve the effectiveness of antibiotics in the population.

PCOS is a pro-inflammatory state and the endocrine–immune features of this disorder may explain the link between PCOS and infections, hence the antibiotic use [23]. Previous studies reported that women with PCOS had a higher susceptibility to various infections than those without PCOS [11,24,25]. Furthermore, women with PCOS may exhibit obesity [4], and the frequent co-occurrence of obesity with PCOS has been observed [26]. This may lead to increased antibiotic consumption among women diagnosed with PCOS, particularly obese women with PCOS. Studies have shown that a compromised immune response and leptin deficiency in obese individuals were found to be associated with an increased susceptibility to infections [27,28].

To date, there are limited population studies aimed at revealing the link between PCOS status and antibiotic use. To our knowledge, there is no study evaluating the association between PCOS and antibiotic use considering PCOS treatment and PCOS phenotypes, such as PCOS in adolescents and adults. In addition, the roles of comorbidity and obesity in the associations between PCOS and antibiotic use have not been widely discussed. Therefore, we aimed to investigate the associations between PCOS status and antibiotic use with further stratifications by PCOS treatment status and the age at PCOS diagnosis. Further, we performed sensitivity analyses to better reveal the roles of comorbidity and obesity in the associations between PCOS-related status and antibiotic use.

2. Material and Methods

We investigated the associations of PCOS-related status—namely women with PCOS versus those without PCOS, women being treated with PCOS versus those without treatment, and women diagnosed with PCOS earlier in life (at the age of 25 years or younger) versus those diagnosed with PCOS later in life (after the age of 25)—with antibiotic use in the past year.

2.1. Study Design, Participants, and Setting

This was a cross-sectional analysis of the United Arab Emirates Healthy Future Study (UAEHFS) conducted from February 2016 to March 2023. From a complete cohort of 14,376 individuals based on numeration IDs in the UAEHFS, we included 2063 Emirati women aged 18–62 years who provided complete information on PCOS status and antibiotic use in the past year; a complete case method (Figure 1). We excluded women with uncertain responses on PCOS status and antibiotic use in the past year (do not know, prefer not to answer, and missing). The study design and methodology of the UAEHFS are described elsewhere [29]. In brief, the UAEHFS is a population-based multirecruitment center study that recruited Emirati adults aged 18 years or above across the UAE. Participants were asked to fill out the online questionnaire and had some physical measurements assessed in the participating centers. Women who participated in this study were asked whether they were pregnant at the survey time, and only non-pregnant women were recruited into the cohort. Due to the COVID-19 pandemic, the recruitment shifted to being online-based starting in April 2020.

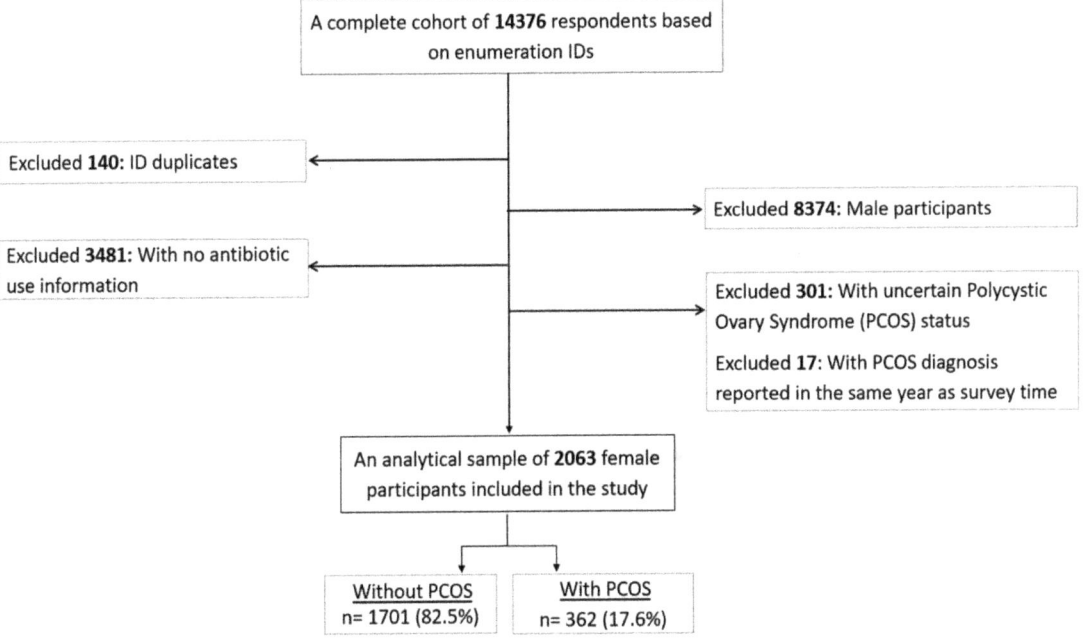

Figure 1. Flowchart of the final analytical sample included in the study.

2.2. *Measurements*

2.2.1. Antibiotic Use as an Outcome Variable

We analyzed self-reported antibiotic use in the past year based on the questionnaire response to "How often have you taken a course of antibiotics in the last year?" (never, once, twice, or three times or more) [30]. We treated antibiotic use as an ordinal outcome due to the ordered categories of the questionnaire responses.

2.2.2. PCOS-Related Status as Exposure Variables

We analyzed self-reported diagnosis of PCOS based on the questionnaire response to: "Has a doctor ever told you that you have polycystic ovarian syndrome or disease?" (yes or no). The self-reported age at PCOS diagnosis was extracted from the questionnaire response to "How old were you when the doctor first told you that you had polycystic ovarian syndrome or disease?". We then used the age of 25 years as a cut-off for PCOS diagnosis categorization, similar to previous epidemiological studies [12,31,32]. Lastly, PCOS treatment status was extracted from the questionnaire item "Are you being treated for polycystic ovarian syndrome or disease?" (yes or no).

2.2.3. Demographic Characteristics and Health Profiles as Third Variables

The questionnaire responses determined age (years in continuous form). Urbanicity was determined based on the questionnaire response to "Where do you and your family live now?" (urban or rural/non-urban areas). Education levels were constructed based on the questionnaire response to "What is the highest level of education that you have completed?". We then categorized education levels into two categories: ≤12 years and >12 years of schooling [33]. Body mass index (BMI) was calculated using the Tanita MC 780 by nurses at the recruitment centers, and we categorized the BMI levels into normal or low BMI (<25 kg/m^2), overweight (25 to <30 kg/m^2), and obese (≥30 kg/m^2) [34]. Overall health was determined based on the questionnaire response to "In general how would you rate your overall health now?" (poor, fair, good, or excellent). We then categorized overall health status into poor/fair or good/excellent categories based on the responses [35]. The smoking variable was determined based on the questionnaire response to "Have you ever smoked cigarettes, even one time?" (yes or no). Next, regular medication use was determined based on the questionnaire responses to the item "Do you regularly take any of the following high blood sugar medication/high cholesterol medication/high blood pressure medication/aspirin/paracetamol/regular prescription medication/vitamins/other supplementations?". We then categorized regular medication use into yes (if at least one previously stated medication was being reported) or no (if no medication was being reported). Lastly, the comorbidity in this study was determined based on the questionnaire response to "Has a doctor ever told you that you had [disease name]?" (yes or no). We included three pro-inflammatory chronic conditions, namely diabetes, high cholesterol, and high blood pressure. Those with comorbidity were defined as individuals who reported at least one of the above-mentioned chronic conditions at the survey time.

2.3. Statistical Analysis

Demographic characteristics and health profiles of study participants based on their PCOS status were evaluated using medians with interquartile ranges (median, IQR) for continuous variables and frequencies with percentages (n, %) for categorical variables. Distributions of antibiotic use in the past year based on PCOS status, as well as by PCOS treatment status and the age at PCOS diagnosis, were evaluated using frequencies with percentages (n, %). We further tested the distribution of our data for the parallel lines assumption for an ordered logistic regression. Since the assumption was met for our data, we then performed ordinal logistic regressions to estimate the odds ratios (ORs) and 95% confidence interval (CI), respectively, for the associations between PCOS status and antibiotic use in the past year among the total participants (main analysis), as well as by PCOS treatment and the age at PCOS diagnosis (stratification analysis). Women without PCOS history were used as a reference group in any analyses. We examined the ORs under two models: unadjusted and adjusted models. The complete case method was used to handle missing values in the regression analyses. We adjusted for current demographic characteristics and health profiles based on the literature and those found in the dataset, namely age [36], urbanicity [37,38], education level [39,40], BMI [12,41], overall health [36], smoking [35,42], and regular medication use [36], as these variables are known to be associated with PCOS and antibiotic use based on the literature. All analyses were performed using STATA 17.0 (StataCorp, College Station, TX, USA). p-values of <0.05 were considered statistically significant.

2.4. Ethical Approval

The study and its procedures have been reviewed and approved by the Institutional Review Board at New York University Abu Dhabi, Dubai Health Authority, Ministry of Health and Prevention in the UAE, and Abu Dhabi Health Research and Technology Committee, with the reference number of DOH/HQD/2020/516. Written consent was obtained from participants at the participating recruitment centers or by filling out an online consent form before data collection started.

3. Results

The demographic characteristics and health profiles of the study participants based on PCOS status are shown in Table 1. Compared to women without PCOS, those with PCOS were older (28.5 ± 8.1 vs. 22.0 ± 8.1 years) and a greater proportion resided in urban areas (90.1% vs. 85.9%), had higher education levels or >12 years of schooling (65.7% vs. 53.9%), had a higher BMI (26.6 ± 6.6 vs. 23.9 ± 6.6 kg/m^2), were in poor or fair health

(27.9% vs. 25.0%), reported having ever smoked (13.3% vs. 8.7%), and reported regular medication use (68.2% vs. 58.7%).

Table 1. Demographic characteristics and health profiles of study participants based on PCOS status.

Demographic Characteristics and Health Profiles	Without PCOS (n = 1701, 82.5%)	With PCOS (n = 362, 17.6%)
Demographic characteristics		
Age, median (IQR range), year	22.0 (20–31)	28.5 (23–36)
Urbanicity		
Rural or non-urban areas	240 (14.1)	36 (9.9)
Urban areas	1461 (85.9)	326 (90.1)
Education		
12 years of schooling or below	785 (46.2)	121 (33.4)
Above 12 years of schooling	916 (53.9)	241 (66.6)
Health profiles		
BMI, median (IQR range), kg/m^2	23.9 (20.4–28.9)	26.6 (23.0–30.9)
BMI categories, without missing category, reported		
Normal BMI or below (<25 kg/m^2)	835 (49.1)	125 (34.5)
Overweight (25 kg/m^2 to <30 kg/m^2)	335 (19.7)	85 (23.5)
Obese (30 kg/m^2 or above)	313 (18.4)	99 (27.4)
Overall health status		
Poor or fair	426 (25.0)	101 (27.9)
Excellent or good	1275 (75.0)	261 (72.1)
Smoking, without missing category reported		
Never	1410 (82.9)	280 (77.4)
Ever	148 (8.7)	48 (13.3)
Regular medication use *		
No	702 (41.3)	115 (31.8)
Yes	999 (58.7)	247 (68.2)

* Consumed at least one of the following medications: high blood sugar medication, high cholesterol medication, high blood pressure medication, aspirin, paracetamol, regular prescription medication, vitamins, or other supplementations.

In addition, the proportion of antibiotics used in the past year among study participants based on PCOS status, PCOS treatment status, and the age at PCOS diagnosis are shown in Figure 2. A third of participants reported never having a course of antibiotics in the past year. Meanwhile, 17% reported having two or more antibiotic courses in the past year (frequent users). In PCOS status stratification, more women with PCOS were reported as frequent antibiotic users compared to women without PCOS (20.2% vs. 16.3%). Women being treated for PCOS as well as those with PCOS diagnosed at ≥25 years were more likely to report being frequent antibiotic users compared to their respective counterparts (25.8% versus 21.9% in the PCOS treatment group and 26.9% versus 20.9% in the age at PCOS diagnosis group).

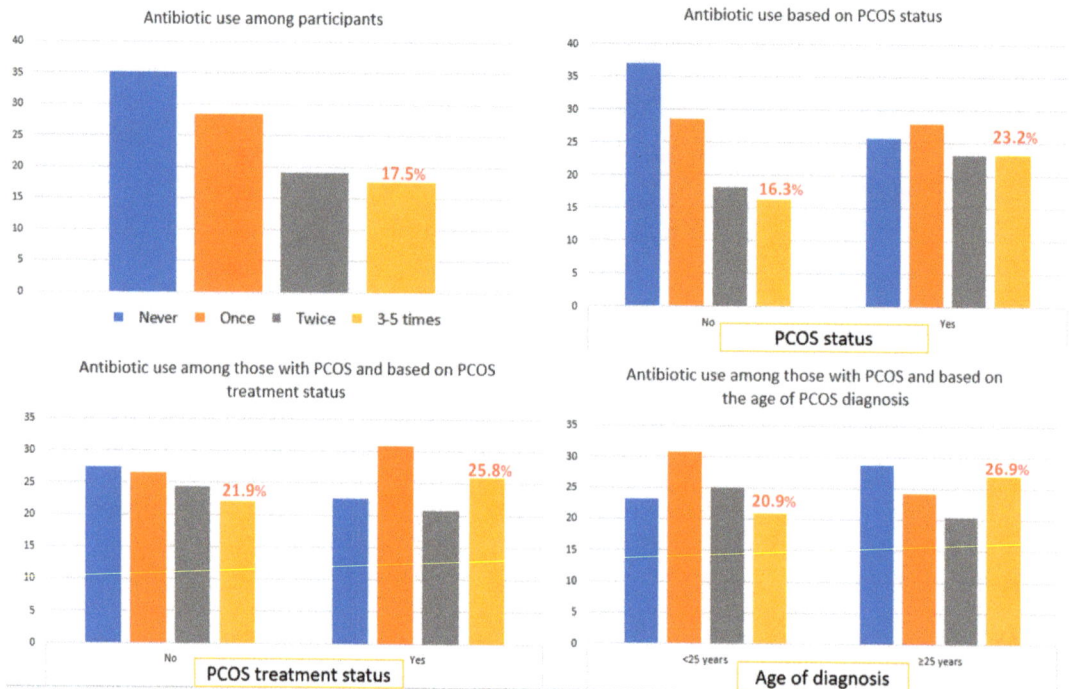

Figure 2. Antibiotic use in the past year among study participants, based on PCOS-related status.

The associations between PCOS status and antibiotic use in the past year among participants (main analysis), as well as PCOS treatment status and the age at PCOS diagnosis (stratified analyses), are presented in Table 2. Women with PCOS were 55% more likely to frequently take a course of antibiotics in the past year compared to women without PCOS. Similar likelihoods were also observed in all stratified analyses, except in the ≥25 years at PCOS diagnosis group. The strongest association between PCOS and antibiotic use was observed among women being treated for PCOS, compared to those without PCOS, history after adjusting for confounding factors (aOR = 1.70; 95% CI: 1.22–2.38).

Table 2. Crude and adjusted ordinal logistic regression analysis of the associations between antibiotic use in the past year and PCOS status among total participants (main analysis), as well as PCOS treatment status and the age at PCOS diagnosis (stratified analysis). Reference group in all analyses: women without PCOS history.

	Antibiotic Use in the Past Year			
	Crude Model OR (95% CI)	*p*-Value	**Adjusted Model *** OR (95% CI)	*p*-Value
Main analysis				
Without PCOS (*n* = 1701)	(Reference)		(Reference)	
With PCOS (*n* = 362)	1.65 [1.34–2.02]	<0.001	1.55 [1.26–1.90]	<0.001
PCOS-treatment-stratified models				
No				
Without PCOS (*n* = 1701)	(Reference)		(Reference)	
Without PCOS treatment (*n* = 242)	1.57 [1.23–1.99]	<0.001	1.46 [1.14–1.87]	0.003

Table 2. Cont.

	Antibiotic Use in the Past Year			
	Crude Model	p-Value	Adjusted Model *	p-Value
	OR (95% CI)		OR (95% CI)	
Yes				
Without PCOS (n = 1701)	(Reference)		(Reference)	
Being treated for PCOS (n = 120)	1.81 [1.30–2.52]	<0.001	1.70 [1.22–2.38]	0.002
Age-of-PCOS-diagnosis-stratified models				
<25 years of age				
Without PCOS (n = 1701)	(Reference)		(Reference)	
PCOS diagnosed at <25 years (n = 211)	1.65 [1.28–2.13]	<0.001	1.60 [1.24–2.07]	<0.001
>25 years of age				
Without PCOS (n = 1701)	(Reference)		(Reference)	
PCOS diagnosed at ≥25 years (n = 108)	1.66 [1.17–2.37]	0.005	1.44 [0.99–2.10]	0.055

* Adjusted for age (continuous), urbanicity (rural/urban), education level (≤12 years/>12 years), BMI category (normal or below; overweight/obese), overall health status (excellent, good/fair, or poor), smoking (no/yes), and regular medication use (no/yes). Statistical significance at the 0.05 level is marked in **bold**.

Similar regression analysis strategies restricted only among those reported comorbidities are highlighted in Table 3. In all adjusted models, the previously observed significant association between PCOS and antibiotic use in the past year persisted, even after considering the comorbid conditions. In this comorbidity-stratified analysis and referring to the main regression analysis, the greatest increase in the magnitude of the associations between PCOS and antibiotic use was observed among women with PCOS diagnosed at ≤25 years of age compared to those without PCOS history (aOR = 2.09; 95% CI: 1.30–3.36).

Table 3. Crude and adjusted ordinal logistic regression analysis of the associations between antibiotic use in the past year and PCOS status, restricted only among participants with a history of diabetes, high cholesterol, and high blood pressure). Reference group: women with at least one of comorbidity of diabetes, high cholesterol, or high blood pressure and with no PCOS history, n = 470.

	Antibiotic Use in the Past Year			
	Crude Model	p-Value	Adjusted Model *	p-Value
	OR (95% CI)		OR (95% CI)	
Main analysis				
Without PCOS (n = 338)	(Reference)		(Reference)	
With PCOS (n = 132)	1.78 [1.24–2.55]	0.002	1.69 [1.17–2.46]	0.006
PCOS-treatment-stratified models				
No				
Without PCOS (n = 338)	(Reference)		(Reference)	
Without PCOS treatment (n = 88)	1.68 [1.10–2.57]	0.017	1.59 [1.03–2.46]	0.038
Yes				
Without PCOS (n = 338)	(Reference)		(Reference)	
Being treated for PCOS (n = 44)	1.95 [1.12–3.39]	0.018	1.87 [1.06–3.30]	0.031

Table 3. Cont.

	Antibiotic Use in the Past Year			
	Crude Model	p-Value	Adjusted Model *	p-Value
	OR (95% CI)		OR (95% CI)	
Age-at-PCOS-diagnosis-stratified models				
<25 years of age				
Without PCOS (*n* = 338)	(Reference)		(Reference)	
PCOS diagnosed at <25 years (*n* = 68)	**2.08 [1.32–3.28]**	**0.002**	**2.09 [1.30–3.36]**	**0.002**
>25 years of age				
Without PCOS (*n* = 338)	(Reference)		(Reference)	
PCOS diagnosed at ≥25 year (*n* = 47)	1.51 [0.86–2.64]	0.154	1.31 [0.73–2.36]	0.363

* Adjusted for age (continuous), urbanicity (rural/urban), education levels (≤12 years/>12 years), BMI category (normal or below/overweight/obese), overall health status (excellent or good/fair or poor), smoking (no/yes), regular medication use (no/yes). Statistically significance at the 0.05 is marked in **bold**.

Lastly, a restricted analysis to assess the possibility of whether obesity mediates the associations between PCOS-related status and antibiotic use are presented in Table 4. This table shows the ORs for the associations between PCOS status and antibiotic use in the past year, restricted only among obese participants, in the main analysis and stratified analyses by PCOS treatment status and the age at PCOS diagnosis. All statistically significant associations found in the previous analyses disappeared if the analysis was restricted to only obese women with PCOS versus obese participants without PCOS. In this obesity-stratified analysis and referring to the main regression analysis, interestingly, the greatest decrease in the magnitude of the associations between PCOS and antibiotic use was observed among women being treated for PCOS, compared to those without PCOS history (aOR = 1.19; 95% CI: 0.57–2.46).

Table 4. Crude and adjusted ordinal logistic regression analysis of the associations between antibiotic use in the past year and PCOS status, restricted only among obese participants, in the main analysis and stratified by PCOS treatment status and age at PCOS diagnosis (reference group: obese women without PCOS history); *n* = 412.

	Antibiotic Use in the Past Year			
	Crude Model	p-Value	Adjusted Model *	p-Value
	OR (95% CI)		OR (95% CI)	
Main analysis				
Without PCOS (*n* = 313)	(Reference)		(Reference)	
With PCOS (*n* = 99)	1.50 [0.99–2.27]	0.054	1.42 [0.93–2.17]	0.109
PCOS-treatment-stratified models				
No				
Without PCOS (*n* = 313)	(Reference)		(Reference)	
Without PCOS treatment (*n* = 71)	**1.61 [1.01–2.58]**	**0.050**	1.50 [0.92–2.44]	0.103
Yes				
Without PCOS (*n* = 313)	(Reference)		(Reference)	
Being treated for PCOS (*n* = 28)	1.28 [0.63–2.63]	0.494	1.19 [0.57–2.46]	0.641

Table 4. Cont.

	Antibiotic Use in the Past Year			
	Crude Model	p-Value	Adjusted Model *	p-Value
	OR (95% CI)		OR (95% CI)	
Age-at-PCOS-diagnosis-stratified models				
<25 years of age				
Without PCOS (n = 313)	(Reference)		(Reference)	
PCOS diagnosed at <25 years (n =48)	1.28 [0.74–2.21]	0.375	1.24 [0.71–2.17]	0.446
>25 years of age				
Without PCOS (n = 313)	(Reference)		(Reference)	
PCOS diagnosed at ≥25 years (n = 39)	1.76 [0.94–3.29]	0.076	1.70 [0.87–3.32]	0.119

* Adjusted for age (continuous), urbanicity (rural/urban), education level (≤12 years/>12 years), BMI level (continuous), overall health status (excellent or good/fair or poor), smoking (no/yes), and regular medication use (no/yes). Statistical significance at the 0.05 level is marked in **bold**.

4. Discussion

The crude prevalence of self-reported PCOS in this cross-sectional study was 17.6% (Table 1). The prevalence in this study is similar to a UAE study involving Emiratis and non-Emirati nationals aged ≥18 years, which reported 18.6% physician-diagnosed PCOS prevalence [43]. In contrast, other UAE studies among university students aged 15–25 years and adults aged ≥25 years reported 13.0% to 27.6% PCOS prevalence [12,44,45]. The differences in diagnostic criteria, sample characteristics or age inclusion criteria, and sampling designs may contribute to the wide range of PCOS prevalence observed in the UAE. Middle Easterners are known to have a higher PCOS prevalence compared to other ethnicities [46], ranging from 6.1% to 16.0% depending on the diagnostic criteria of PCOS [47]. A previous study found certain factors promoting PCOS pathogenesis pertinent to the UAE population, including vitamin D deficiency and obesity [4,46]. Our study also showed that women with PCOS had a higher percentage of being obese, compared to those without PCOS (Table 1). Obesity is known to be a risk factor and a manifestation of PCOS [46]. A current study found that 39.6% of Emirati women are classified as obese [48]. This phenomenon contributes to an increasing rate of PCOS in this country since obesity increases PCOS susceptibility [46].

We found that women with PCOS were 55% more likely to frequently take a course of antibiotics in the past year compared to those without PCOS. In addition, we observed more women with PCOS reported as "frequent users" of antibiotics (those who had taken antibiotics at least three times in the past year), compared to those without PCOS (Figure 2). A previous study reported that women with PCOS had a higher susceptibility to infections than those without PCOS [11,24,25]. PCOS is a pro-inflammatory endocrine disorder and the altered immune features in those affected by PCOS may explain their susceptibility to infections [23], hence more frequent users of antibiotics among women with PCOS than in the control group. On the one hand, we noted that women with PCOS had a higher percentage of reported regular medication use (Table 1), compared to those without PCOS. Our results are in agreement with previous studies that also found similar findings and highlighted that women with PCOS are burdened with medication use and comorbidity [11]. This study reported that women with PCOS are known to take more dermatological and hormonal medications compared to those without PCOS [11]. On the other hand, we also found that more women with PCOS reported being in poorer health, compared to those without PCOS. A previous cohort study in the UK revealed that any comorbidity increased antibiotic prescriptions by 62% among women in primary care settings [49]. Hence, there is a possibility that the increased antibiotic use among those with PCOS in our study was related to their comorbidities. However, we addressed this possibility by performing a sensitivity analysis evaluating only those who reported diabetes, cholesterol, or high blood pressure (Table 3), and we found similar results to that of the main regression analysis (Table 2). With higher magnitudes of associations observed in all strata, this may suggest the possibility of comorbidities modifying the associations between PCOS-related status and antibiotic use. Addressing inappropriate antibiotic use in individuals with PCOS could contribute to broader efforts to combat antibiotic resistance. Future antibiotic resistome studies to identify existing mechanisms of the resistance [50], especially linking them to certain conditions such as PCOS, are needed to address existing antibiotic threats more effectively.

In the PCOS treatment stratification, we found that women being treated for PCOS and those without treatment had a significantly increased likelihood of more frequently taking a course of antibiotics in the past year compared to women without PCOS. We found that those without PCOS treatment had a 46% increased likelihood of more frequently taking a course of antibiotics in the past years compared to those without PCOS. In our study, two-thirds of those with PCOS reported not being treated for PCOS. We have a similar finding to a Korean study that revealed two-thirds of women with PCOS were untreated, including without regular exercise as the basic form of PCOS management [51]. However, a higher magnitude of association was observed in the treated PCOS group with a 70% increased likelihood of more frequently taking a course of antibiotics in the past year (Table 2). To provide further evidence to confirm this observation, we also found a higher proportion of frequent antibiotic users among women being treated for PCOS, compared to those without treatment (Figure 2). This finding raised an important question of whether antibiotic prescription is an integral part of PCOS treatment. PCOS treatment is rarely mono-therapeutic, depending on PCOS signs and symptoms; therefore, PCOS treatment must be personalized to meet each patient's needs [9]. Existing treatment modalities for PCOS include surgery, contraceptives, as well as pharmacological and non-pharmacological interventions through improved nutritional or diet and physical activity (lifestyle changes to lose weight) [9,32,45]. The possible links between PCOS and antibiotic use can be explained as follows. The intestinal flora in individuals with PCOS differ from those without PCOS, with a higher abundance of certain gut microbiota that promote PCOS [13,14]. A previous study on human subjects and animal models revealed that removing these microbiota through antibiotics improved PCOS symptoms due to decreased serum testosterone levels [14]. Women with PCOS are known to have elevated testosterone levels [5]; therefore, decreasing testosterone levels has been shown to have positive effects on women with PCOS [4]. Future studies investigating the pattern of antibiotic prescriptions specifically used for PCOS management are recommended to better reveal the efficacy of antibiotics in treating PCOS symptoms.

We stratified the analysis by the age at PCOS diagnosis to better understand two distinct PCOS phenotypes (diagnosed earlier versus later in life) and their associations with antibiotic use. We found that those diagnosed with PCOS before 25 years of age were 60% more likely to frequently take a course of antibiotics in the past year compared to those without PCOS (Table 2). Meanwhile, a marginal association was observed between those diagnosed with PCOS at ≥ 25 years of age, compared to their healthier counterparts. We had 11% missing values for the age at PCOS and lower counts of those with older adults PCOS, and this may contribute to the observed marginal association of PCOS diagnosed at ≥ 25 years of age with antibiotic use. Nevertheless, the magnitude and direction of the association in this category were consistent with the findings in the younger PCOS category (diagnosed with PCOS at <25 years of age). Those with PCOS diagnosed at ≥ 25 years of age had a higher proportion of reporting being frequent antibiotic users, compared to those diagnosed before 25 years (Figure 2). Our findings highlighted two distinct PCOS phenotypes, as previous studies have suggested [52–54]. The expression of PCOS diagnosed in earlier adulthood differs in clinical and endocrinological features from that of PCOS diagnosed in later adulthood [52]. These differences in clinical and biochemical presentations of PCOS with age lead to the age-related diagnostic criteria of PCOS [54]. Previous studies have documented higher androgen levels in younger PCOS compared to older PCOS [55,56], implying elevated testosterone levels in the younger PCOS group. This may, to some extent, explain our findings, as we observed the strongest magnitude of the association between PCOS and antibiotic use among those with PCOS diagnosed in earlier life. Further, in the UAE context, it has been reported that the most prevalent PCOS symptom among women aged 18–25 years is acne [45]. Oral antibiotics have been used to treat acne vulgaris, a type of acne affecting adolescents and young adults [57], and may partially explain our finding of a stronger and more significant association between those with PCOS diagnosed before the age of 25 years and antibiotic use. In this study, we did not have any information on certain types of antibiotics and whether their prescription was indicated to treat PCOS symptoms among women affected by this hormonal disorder. Therefore, the findings in this study should be interpreted carefully. Better studies to confirm our findings, with complete information on the types of antibiotics and the purpose of antibiotic prescriptions among those affected with PCOS are highly recommended.

Lastly, we performed the same regression analysis among only obese participants to address the possibility of obesity mediating the associations between PCOS-related status and antibiotic use in the past year. We found that all significances in the previously observed associations in the PCOS status, PCOS treatment, and the age at PCOS diagnosis groups disappeared if the analyses were restricted only to those with obesity (Table 4). These findings suggested the possibility of obesity mediates the associations between PCOS-related status and antibiotic use. With the greatest decrease in the magnitude of association was found in the PCOS treatment group, suggesting the stronger role of obesity in mediating the association between PCOS treatment and antibiotic use. Obesity is linked to PCOS in many ways, including low-grade inflammation that leads to insulin resistance and metabolic disorders [58]. The exact link between the pro-inflammatory state of obesity and infections leading to antibiotic use is still unclear. However, a compromised immune response and leptin deficiency in obese individuals were suggested as possible mechanisms of the link between frequent antibiotic use among those living with obesity [27,28]. In addition, the pharmacodynamic parameters, such as volume of distribution and clearance in many commonly used antimicrobials, and the rate of metabolism in individuals with obesity differ from those in the normal weight category [59]. Therefore, it is possible that being obese may lead to inadequate antibiotic dosing [27]. With the frequent co-occurence of obesity with PCOS [26], the appropriateness of antibiotic dosing among those with PCOS merits special attention and further investigation.

Strengths and Limitations

To our knowledge, this is the first population-based study to investigate the associations between PCOS status and antibiotic use with further stratification by PCOS treatment and the age at PCOS diagnosis among the Emirati population. We were able to examine the associations between PCOS-related status and antibiotic use in the past year with clear temporality. We only included PCOS diagnosis at least one year before the survey time to the recall of antibiotic use in the past year, to avoid the overlapping timeline. However, our large sample size made it possible to perform multiple stratification analyses. We were also able to control for important confounding factors based on the literature. Our study has several limitations. Our findings are specific to Emirati females aged 18–62 years and may not be generalizable to other populations. We conducted a cross-sectional sectional study; therefore, we could establish associations but not causation. Next, the diagnosis of PCOS in our study was based on self-reports, raising the concern of accuracy and diagnosis bias. However, a meta-analysis study found that self-reported PCOS was consistent with diagnosis using the Rotterdam or other criteria [60]. To better address the recall error and cohort effect, we adjusted for age in the adjusted model. In addition, this study might also be prone to possible selection bias due to the convenience sampling design that we used. However, we increased the representativeness of our sample through recruitment in multiple centers across the UAE. Next, there was also a possibility that those with severe PCOS or comorbidity and acute infections might not be able to participate in this study due to their limiting conditions. Further, we do not have any information on the types of antibiotics, the duration of use, or the quantity or total dosage for each course. Lastly, residual confounding factors are possible due to the observational nature of our study, including PCOS severity as it has been found to be associated with PCOS-related microbial pathways [61].

5. Conclusions

Our study suggests that PCOS was associated with increased use of antibiotics among Emirati women, especially among women treated for PCOS or without treatment and those diagnosed before the age of 25 years. Understanding the frequent antibiotic use susceptibility among those with PCOS may improve antibiotic use surveillance and promote antibiotic stewardship in these at-risk individuals. Future studies to evaluate the appropriateness of antibiotic prescriptions among those with PCOS merits further investigations, particularly within the context of the global problem of inappropriate antibiotic use (misuse or overuse) that may lead to antibiotic resistance. Lastly, further longitudinal or experimental studies would be needed to establish a causal relationship to better address the link between PCOS and antibiotic use.

Author Contributions: Conceptualization, N.F.J.; data acquisition, A.A. (Abdishakur Abdulle), A.A. (Amar Ahmad), Y.I., Y.V. and R.A.; data curation, N.F.J.; data interpretation, A.A. (Abdishakur Abdulle), A.A. (Amar Ahmad), F.A., T.L., Y.I., Y.V. and R.A.; formal analysis, N.F.J.; investigation, N.F.J., F.A. and T.L.; methodology, N.F.J. and A.A. (Amar Ahmad); project administration, A.A. (Abdishakur Abdulle), Y.I. and R.A.; writing—original draft preparation, N.F.J., writing—review and editing, A.A. (Abdishakur Abdulle), A.A. (Amar Ahmad), F.A., T.L., Y.I., Y.V. and R.A.; funding acquisition, R.A. All authors have read and agreed to the published version of the manuscript.

Funding: This publication is based upon works supported by Tamkeen under Research Institute Grant No. G1206.

Institutional Review Board Statement: The study and its procedures have been reviewed and approved by the Institutional Review Board at New York University Abu Dhabi, Dubai Health Authority, Ministry of Health and Prevention in the UAE, and Abu Dhabi Health Research and Technology Committee, with the reference number of DOH/HQD/2020/516.

Informed Consent Statement: Written consent was obtained from participants at the participating recruitment centers or by filling out an online consent form before data collection started.

Data Availability Statement: The datasets used and/or analyzed during the current study are available from the principle investigators of the UAE Healthy Future Study on reasonable request.

Acknowledgments: The authors would like to thank all members of the Public Health Research Center at New York University Abu Dhabi and those who are actively involved in the UAE Healthy Future Study (UAEHFS). This study would not have been possible without their collective effort.

Conflicts of Interest: The authors declare no conflict of interest. The funders had no role in the design of the study; in the collection, analyses, or interpretation of data; in the writing of the manuscript; or in the decision to publish the results.

References

1. Bozdag, G.; Mumusoglu, S.; Zengin, D.; Karabulut, E.; Yildiz, B.O. The prevalence and phenotypic features of polycystic ovary syndrome: A systematic review and meta-analysis. *Hum. Reprod.* **2016**, *31*, 2841–2855. [CrossRef]
2. Deswal, R.; Narwal, V.; Dang, A.; Pundir, C.S. The prevalence of polycystic ovary syndrome: A brief systematic review. *J. Hum. Reprod. Sci.* **2020**, *13*, 261–271. [CrossRef] [PubMed]
3. Ibáñez, L.; Oberfield, S.E.; Witchel, S.; Auchus, R.J.; Chang, R.J.; Codner, E.; Dabadghao, P.; Darendeliler, F.; Elbarbary, N.S.; Gambineri, A.; et al. An international consortium update: Pathophysiology, diagnosis, and treatment of polycystic ovarian syndrome in adolescence. *Horm. Res. Paediatr.* **2017**, *88*, 371–395. [CrossRef]
4. Mohan, A.; Haider, R.; Fakhor, H.; Hina, F.; Kumar, V.; Jawed, A.; Majumder, K.M.; Ayaz, A.M.; Lal, P.M.M.; Tejwaney, U.P.D.; et al. Vitamin D and polycystic ovary syndrome (PCOS): A review. *Ann. Med. Surg.* **2023**, *85*, 3506–3511. [CrossRef] [PubMed]
5. Baptiste, C.G.; Battista, M.-C.; Trottier, A.; Baillargeon, J.-P. Insulin and hyperandrogenism in women with polycystic ovary syndrome. *J. Steroid Biochem. Mol. Biol.* **2010**, *122*, 42–52. [CrossRef]

6. Yang, J.; Chen, C. Hormonal changes in PCOS. *J. Endocrinol.* **2024**, *261*, e230342. [CrossRef]
7. Sahin, S.B.; Nalkiran, I.; Ayaz, T.; Guzel, A.I.; Eldes, T.; Calapoglu, T.; Nalkiran, H.S. Genetic variations in OLR1 gene associated with PCOS and atherosclerotic risk factors. *J. Investig. Med.* **2023**, *71*, 113–123. [CrossRef] [PubMed]
8. Sanchez-Garrido, M.A.; Tena-Sempere, M. Metabolic dysfunction in polycystic ovary syndrome: Pathogenic role of androgen excess and potential therapeutic strategies. *Mol. Metab.* **2020**, *35*, 100937. [CrossRef]
9. Singh, S.; Pal, N.; Shubham, S.; Sarma, D.K.; Verma, V.; Marotta, F.; Kumar, M. Polycystic ovary syndrome: Etiology, current management, and future therapeutics. *J. Clin. Med.* **2023**, *12*, 1454. [CrossRef]
10. El-Hayek, S.; Bitar, L.; Hamdar, L.H.; Mirza, F.G.; Daoud, G. Poly Cystic Ovarian Syndrome: An Updated Overview. *Front. Physiol.* **2016**, *7*, 124. [CrossRef]
11. Kujanpää, L.; Arffman, R.K.; Pesonen, P.; Korhonen, E.; Karjula, S.; Järvelin, M.R.; Franks, S.; Tapanainen, J.S.; Morin-Papunen, L.; Piltonen, T.T. Women with polycystic ovary syndrome are burdened with multimorbidity and medication use independent of body mass index at late fertile age: A population-based cohort study. *Acta Obstet. Gynecol. Scand.* **2022**, *101*, 728–736. [CrossRef] [PubMed]
12. Juber, N.F.; Abdulle, A.; AlJunaibi, A.; AlNaeemi, A.; Ahmad, A.; Leinberger-Jabari, A.; Al Dhaheri, A.S.; AlZaabi, E.; Al-Maskari, F.; AlAnouti, F.; et al. Association between self-reported polycystic ovary syndrome with chronic diseases among emiratis: A cross-sectional analysis from the UAE healthy future study. *Int. J. Womens Health* **2023**, *15*, 289–298. [CrossRef] [PubMed]
13. Qi, X.; Yun, C.; Sun, L.; Xia, J.; Wu, Q.; Wang, Y.; Wang, L.; Zhang, Y.; Liang, X.; Wang, L.; et al. Gut microbiota–bile acid–interleukin-22 axis orchestrates polycystic ovary syndrome. *Nat. Med.* **2019**, *25*, 1225–1233. [CrossRef] [PubMed]
14. Yang, Y.-L.; Zhou, W.-W.; Wu, S.; Tang, W.-L.; Wang, Z.-W.; Zhou, Z.-Y.; Li, Z.-W.; Huang, Q.-F.; He, Y.; Zhou, H.-W.; et al. Intestinal flora is a key factor in insulin resistance and contributes to the development of polycystic ovary syndrome. *Endocrinology* **2021**, *162*, bqab118. [CrossRef] [PubMed]
15. Tayler, E.; Gregory, R.; Bloom, G.; Salama, P.; Balkhy, H. Universal health coverage: An opportunity to address antimicrobial resistance? *Lancet Glob. Health* **2019**, *7*, e1480–e1481. [CrossRef] [PubMed]
16. World Health Organization. *Ten Threats to Global Health in 2019*; World Health Organization: Geneva, Switzerland, 2019. Available online: https://www.who.int/news-room/spotlight/ten-threats-to-global-health-in-2019 (accessed on 3 March 2024).
17. Iskakova, N.; Khismetova, Z.; Suleymenova, D.; Kozhekenova, Z.; Khamidullina, Z.; Samarova, U.; Glushkova, N.; Semenova, Y. Factors Influencing Antibiotic Consumption in Adult Population of Kazakhstan. *Antibiotics* **2023**, *12*, 560. [CrossRef]
18. Hussain, M.A.; Mohamed, A.O.; Abdelkarim, O.A.; Yousef, B.A.; Babikir, A.A.; Mirghani, M.M.; Mohamed, E.A.; Osman, W.; Mothana, R.A.; Elhag, R. Prevalence and Predictors of Antibiotic Self-Medication in Sudan: A Descriptive Cross-Sectional Study. *Antibiotics* **2023**, *12*, 612. [CrossRef]
19. Abduelkarem, A.R.; Othman, A.M.; Abuelkhair, Z.M.; Ghazal, M.M.; Alzouobi, S.B.; El-Zowalaty, M.E. Prevalence of self-medication with antibiotics among residents in United Arab Emirates. *Infect. Drug Resist.* **2019**, *12*, 3445–3453. [CrossRef] [PubMed]
20. Dik, V.K.; van Oijen, M.G.; Smeets, H.M.; Siersema, P.D. Frequent use of antibiotics is associated with colorectal cancer risk: Results of a nested case–control study. *Dig. Dis. Sci.* **2016**, *61*, 255–264. [CrossRef]
21. Wirtz, H.S.; Buist, D.S.; Gralow, J.R.; Barlow, W.E.; Gray, S.; Chubak, J.; Yu, O.; Bowles, E.J.; Fujii, M.; Boudreau, D.M. Frequent Antibiotic Use and Second Breast Cancer EventsAntibiotics and Second Breast Cancer Events. *Cancer Epidemiol. Biomarkers Prev.* **2013**, *22*, 1588–1599. [CrossRef]
22. Radlinski, L.; Conlon, B. Antibiotic efficacy in the complex infection environment. *Curr. Opin. Microbiol.* **2018**, *42*, 19–24. [CrossRef] [PubMed]
23. Liu, M.; Gao, J.; Zhang, Y.; Li, P.; Wang, H.; Ren, X.; Li, C. Serum levels of TSP-1, NF-κB and TGF-β1 in polycystic ovarian syndrome (PCOS) patients in northern China suggest PCOS is associated with chronic inflammation. *Clin. Endocrinol.* **2015**, *83*, 913–922. [CrossRef] [PubMed]
24. Alahmadi, A. The common pathological factors between polycystic ovary syndrome and COVID-19 infection: A review. *Biosc Biotech. Res. Comm.* **2020**, *13*, 1708–1716. [CrossRef]
25. Subramanian, A.; Anand, A.; Adderley, N.J.; Okoth, K.; Toulis, K.A.; Gokhale, K.; Sainsbury, C.; O'reilly, M.W.; Arlt, W.; Nirantharakumar, K. Increased COVID-19 infections in women with polycystic ovary syndrome: A population-based study. *Eur. J. Endocrinol.* **2021**, *184*, 637–645. [CrossRef] [PubMed]
26. Barber, T.M.; Hanson, P.; Weickert, M.O.; Franks, S. Obesity and Polycystic Ovary Syndrome: Implications for Pathogenesis and Novel Management Strategies. *Clin. Med. Insights Reprod. Health* **2019**, *13*, 1179558119874042. [CrossRef] [PubMed]
27. Falagas, M.E.; Kompoti, M. Obesity and infection. *Lancet Infect. Dis.* **2006**, *6*, 438–446. [CrossRef] [PubMed]
28. Marti, A.; Marcos, A.; Martinez, J.A. Obesity and immune function relationships. *Obes. Rev.* **2001**, *2*, 131–140. [CrossRef]
29. Abdulle, A.; Alnaeemi, A.; Aljunaibi, A.; Al Ali, A.; Al-Saedi, K.; Al-Zaabi, E.; Oumeziane, N.; Al Bastaki, M.; Al-Houqani, M.; Al Maskari, F.; et al. The UAE healthy future study: A pilot for a prospective cohort study of 20,000 United Arab Emirates nationals. *BMC Public. Health* **2018**, *18*, 101. [CrossRef]
30. Hoskin-Parr, L.; Teyhan, A.; Blocker, A.; Henderson, A. Antibiotic exposure in the first two years of life and development of asthma and other allergic diseases by 7.5 yr: A dose-dependent relationship. *Pediatr. Allergy Immunol.* **2013**, *24*, 762–771. [CrossRef]
31. Ahmad, A.K.; Quinn, M.; Kao, C.-N.; Greenwood, E.; Cedars, M.I.; Huddleston, H.G. Improved diagnostic performance for the diagnosis of polycystic ovary syndrome using age-stratified criteria. *Fertil. Steril.* **2019**, *111*, 787–793. [CrossRef]

32. Jena, S.K.; Mishra, L.; Naik, S.S.; Khan, S. Awareness and opinion about polycystic ovarian syndrome (PCOS) among young women: A developing country perspective. *Int. J. Adolesc. Med. Health* **2020**, *33*, 123–126. [CrossRef] [PubMed]
33. Higuita-Gutiérrez, L.F.; Roncancio Villamil, G.E.; Jiménez Quiceno, J.N. Knowledge, attitude, and practice regarding antibiotic use and resistance among medical students in Colombia: A cross-sectional descriptive study. *BMC Public. Health* **2020**, *20*, 1861. [CrossRef] [PubMed]
34. World Health Organization. Obesity: Preventing and Managing the Global Epidemic. Report of a WHO Consultation. *World Health Organ. Tech. Rep. Ser.* **2000**, *1–12*, 1–253. Available online: https://pubmed.ncbi.nlm.nih.gov/11234459/ (accessed on 19 February 2024).
35. Juber, N.F.; Abdulle, A.; Ahmad, A.; Leinberger-Jabari, A.; Dhaheri, A.S.A.; Al-Maskari, F.; AlAnouti, F.; Al-Houqani, M.; Ali, M.H.; El-Shahawy, O.; et al. Associations between Birth Weight and Adult Sleep Characteristics: A Cross-Sectional Analysis from the UAEHFS. *J. Clin. Med.* **2023**, *12*, 5618. [CrossRef]
36. Glintborg, D.; Hass Rubin, K.; Nybo, M.; Abrahamsen, B.; Andersen, M. Morbidity and medicine prescriptions in a nationwide Danish population of patients diagnosed with polycystic ovary syndrome. *Eur. J. Endocrinol.* **2015**, *172*, 627–638. [CrossRef] [PubMed]
37. Clark, A.W.; Durkin, M.J.; Olsen, M.A.; Keller, M.; Ma, Y.; O'Neil, C.A.; Butler, A.M. Rural–urban differences in antibiotic prescribing for uncomplicated urinary tract infection. *Infect. Control. Hosp. Epidemiol.* **2021**, *42*, 1437–1444. [CrossRef]
38. Radha, P.; Devi, R.S.; Madhavi, J. Comparative Study of Prevalence of Polycystic Ovarian Syndrome in Rural and Urban Population. *J. Adv. Med. Dent. Scie. Res.* **2016**, *4*, 90. Available online: https://jamdsr.com/uploadfiles/19.PREVALENCEOFPOLYCYSTICOVARIANSYNDROME.20160310054301.pdf (accessed on 13 March 2024).
39. Chow, S.K.Y.; Tao, X.; Zhu, X.; Niyomyart, A.; Choi, E. How socioeconomic, health seeking behaviours, and educational factors are affecting the knowledge and use of antibiotics in four different cities in Asia. *Antibiotics* **2021**, *10*, 1522. [CrossRef]
40. Bell, G.A.; Sundaram, R.; Mumford, S.L.; Park, H.; Mills, J.; Bell, E.M.; Broadney, M.; Yeung, E.H. Maternal polycystic ovarian syndrome and early offspring development. *Hum. Reprod.* **2018**, *33*, 1307–1315. [CrossRef]
41. Leong, K.S.; Derraik, J.G.; Hofman, P.L.; Cutfield, W.S. Antibiotics, gut microbiome and obesity. *Clin. Endocrinol.* **2018**, *88*, 185–200. [CrossRef]
42. Steinberg, M.B.; Akincigil, A.; Kim, E.J.; Shallis, R.; Delnevo, C.D. Tobacco smoking as a risk factor for increased antibiotic prescription. *Am. J. Prev. Med.* **2016**, *50*, 692–698. [CrossRef]
43. Zaitoun, B.; Al Kubaisi, A.; AlQattan, N.; Alassouli, Y.; Mohammad, A.; Alameeri, H.; Mohammad, G. Polycystic ovarian syndrome awareness among females in the UAE: A cross-sectional study. *BMC Womens Health* **2023**, *23*, 181. [CrossRef]
44. Begum, G.S.; Shariff, A.; Ayman, G.; Mohammad, B.; Housam, R.; Khaled, N. Assessment of Risk Factors for Development of Polycystic Ovarian Syndrome. *Int. J. Contemp. Med. Res.* **2017**, *4*, 164–167. Available online: https://www.ijcmr.com/uploads/7/7/4/6/77464738/ijcmr_1209_feb_6.pdf (accessed on 21 February 2024).
45. Pramodh, S. Exploration of Lifestyle Choices, Reproductive Health Knowledge, and Polycystic Ovary Syndrome (PCOS) Awareness Among Female Emirati University Students. *Int. J. Womens Health* **2020**, *12*, 927–938. [CrossRef] [PubMed]
46. Dalibalta, S.; Abukhaled, Y.; Samara, F. Factors influencing the prevalence of polycystic ovary syndrome (PCOS) in the United Arab Emirates. *Rev. Environ. Health* **2022**, *37*, 311–319. [CrossRef]
47. Ding, T.; Hardiman, P.J.; Petersen, I.; Wang, F.-F.; Qu, F.; Baio, G. The prevalence of polycystic ovary syndrome in reproductive-aged women of different ethnicity: A systematic review and meta-analysis. *Oncotarget* **2017**, *8*, 96351. [CrossRef] [PubMed]
48. Mamdouh, H.; Hussain, H.Y.; Ibrahim, G.M.; Alawadi, F.; Hassanein, M.; Zarooni, A.A.; Al Suwaidi, H.; Hassan, A.; Alsheikh-Ali, A.; Alnakhi, W.K. Prevalence and associated risk factors of overweight and obesity among adult population in Dubai: A population-based cross-sectional survey in Dubai, the United Arab Emirates. *BMJ Open* **2023**, *13*, e062053. [CrossRef] [PubMed]
49. Shallcross, L.; Beckley, N.; Rait, G.; Hayward, A.; Petersen, I. Antibiotic prescribing frequency amongst patients in primary care: A cohort study using electronic health records. *J. Antimicrob. Chemother.* **2017**, *72*, 1818–1824. [CrossRef] [PubMed]
50. Crofts, T.S.; Gasparrini, A.J.; Dantas, G. Next-generation approaches to understand and combat the antibiotic resistome. *Nat. Rev. Microbiol.* **2017**, *15*, 422–434. [CrossRef]
51. Kim, J.J.; Hwang, K.R.; Choi, Y.M.; Moon, S.Y.; Chae, S.J.; Park, C.W.; Kim, H.O.; Choi, D.S.; Kwon, H.C.; Kang, B.M.; et al. Complete phenotypic and metabolic profiles of a large consecutive cohort of untreated Korean women with polycystic ovary syndrome. *Fertil. Steril.* **2014**, *101*, 1424–1430. [CrossRef]
52. Michelmore, K.F. Polycystic ovary syndrome in adolescence and early adulthood. *Hum. Fertil.* **2000**, *3*, 96–100. [CrossRef] [PubMed]
53. Davison, S.L.; Bell, R.; Donath, S.; Montalto, J.; Davis, S.R. Androgen levels in adult females: Changes with age, menopause, and oophorectomy. *J. Clin. Endocrinol. Metab.* **2005**, *90*, 3847–3853. [CrossRef] [PubMed]
54. Hsu, M.-I. Changes in the PCOS phenotype with age. *Steroids* **2013**, *78*, 761–766. [CrossRef] [PubMed]
55. Liang, S.-J.; Hsu, C.-S.; Tzeng, C.-R.; Chen, C.-H.; Hsu, M.-I. Clinical and biochemical presentation of polycystic ovary syndrome in women between the ages of 20 and 40. *Hum. Reprod.* **2011**, *26*, 3443–3449. [CrossRef] [PubMed]
56. Panidis, D.; Tziomalos, K.; Macut, D.; Delkos, D.; Betsas, G.; Misichronis, G.; Katsikis, I. Cross-sectional analysis of the effects of age on the hormonal, metabolic, and ultrasonographic features and the prevalence of the different phenotypes of polycystic ovary syndrome. *Fertil. Steril.* **2012**, *97*, 494–500. [CrossRef] [PubMed]
57. Baldwin, H. Oral antibiotic treatment options for acne vulgaris. *J. Clin. Aesthet. Dermatol.* **2020**, *13*, 26. Available online: https://www.ncbi.nlm.nih.gov/pmc/articles/PMC7577330/ (accessed on 30 March 2024). [PubMed]

58. Hardy, O.T.; Czech, M.P.; Corvera, S. What causes the insulin resistance underlying obesity? *Curr. Opin. Endocrinol. Diabetes Obes.* **2012**, *19*, 81–87. [CrossRef]
59. Pai, M.P.; Bearden, D.T. Antimicrobial dosing considerations in obese adult patients: Insights from the Society of Infectious Diseases Pharmacists. *Pharmacotherapy* **2007**, *27*, 1081–1091. [CrossRef]
60. Chang, S.; Dunaif, A. Diagnosis of Polycystic Ovary Syndrome: Which Criteria to Use and When? *Endocrinol. Metab. Clin. North. Am.* **2021**, *50*, 11–23. [CrossRef]
61. Liyanage, G.S.; Inoue, R.; Fujitani, M.; Ishijima, T.; Shibutani, T.; Abe, K.; Kishida, T.; Okada, S. Effects of soy isoflavones, resistant starch and antibiotics on polycystic ovary syndrome (PCOS)-like features in letrozole-treated rats. *Nutrients* **2021**, *13*, 3759. [CrossRef]

Disclaimer/Publisher's Note: The statements, opinions and data contained in all publications are solely those of the individual author(s) and contributor(s) and not of MDPI and/or the editor(s). MDPI and/or the editor(s) disclaim responsibility for any injury to people or property resulting from any ideas, methods, instructions or products referred to in the content.

MDPI AG
Grosspeteranlage 5
4052 Basel
Switzerland
Tel.: +41 61 683 77 34

Antibiotics Editorial Office
E-mail: antibiotics@mdpi.com
www.mdpi.com/journal/antibiotics

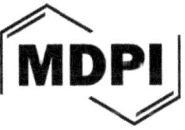

Disclaimer/Publisher's Note: The statements, opinions and data contained in all publications are solely those of the individual author(s) and contributor(s) and not of MDPI and/or the editor(s). MDPI and/or the editor(s) disclaim responsibility for any injury to people or property resulting from any ideas, methods, instructions or products referred to in the content.